Handbook of PLASTIC SURGERY

Peter McKinney, M.D., F.A.C.S.
Associate Professor of Clinical Surgery
Division of Plastic and Reconstructive Surgery
Department of Surgery
Northwestern University Medical School

Bruce Langdon Cunningham, M.D.
Instructor in Surgery
Division of Plastic and Reconstructive Surgery
Department of Surgery
University of Minnesota Medical School

WILLIAMS & WILKINS
Baltimore/London

Made in the United States of America

Library of Congress Cataloging in Publication Data

McKinney, Peter.

Handbook of plastic surgery.

Bibliography: p.
Includes index.
1. Surgery, Plastic. I. Cunningham, Bruce Langdon. II. Title.
RD118.M44 617'.95 81-3383
ISBN 0-683-05865-7 AACR2

Composed and printed at the
Waverly Press, Inc.
Mt. Royal and Guilford Aves.
Baltimore, MD 21202, U.S.A.

DEDICATION

To our students and colleagues

Foreword

The origins of plastic surgery are lost in antiquity. But at least some of the techniques that are employed today, and certainly some of the basic principles, were known and used hundreds and perhaps even thousands of years ago. Our understanding and application of them have expanded over the years, and our success with them has increased with refinements in technique and advances in our general medical knowledge.

The development of plastic surgery as a distinct specialty within the framework of general surgery, came about during World War I, a mere 65 years ago. Its maturation since then has been a wonder to behold. Likewise, the literature of plastic surgery has grown exponentially from occasional scattered articles and books now and then, to a vast library of reference works, sets of principles, scientific reports, recitations of clinical experiences and technical manuals. All of these have value and utility, but their volume, diversity and, at times inaccessibility can be distressing to the student or practitioner who wants an easily understood introduction to the field and a handy guide to everyday clinical problems. The *Handbook of Plastic Surgery* will serve this function.

It is especially pleasant for me to see this book come from the thought and hands of my esteemed associate of many years, who has earned for himself a respected place in plastic surgery, and one of our former residents whose future in our specialty we view with great expectations. Their sound understanding of this subject and the clarity of its presentation make this a volume with great practical value for students and practitioners in many fields of surgery.

B. Herold Griffith, M.D., Professor of Surgery
Chief, Division of Plastic, Reconstructive
and Maxillofacial Surgery
Northwestern University Medical School

Chicago 1981

Preface

Few clinical fields have expanded as rapidly as plastic and reconstructive surgery. Advances in technology and increased sophistication in the application of the basic sciences to clinical work have so broadened the specialty that the body of available information has become immense. The authors believe that a fundamental guide which presents and analyzes the basic principles of plastic and reconstructive surgery can help to catalogue this information. It is a mastery of the underlying concepts, rather than a rote memorization of facts, that will assist younger surgeons in developing their clinical skills.

Many excellent textbooks on plastic surgery exist, but most of them are designed for surgeons already working in the field. These publications contain more technical detail than is appropriate for medical students or for members of the surgical house staff rotating on the Plastic Surgery Service. This book is designed for those groups, as well as for physicians in other fields who want a working knowledge of plastic and reconstructive surgery in order to assist them in the management of emergencies or elective incisions, or in counseling patients concerning a plastic surgical procedure.

The concepts underlying the book were developed in a large teaching hospital where input from medical students, surgical house staff and academic plastic surgeons was readily available. Many of the concepts were first presented in a series of lectures given by the senior author to medical students at Northwestern University. It is through questions and responses of these students that many of the explanations have been simplified and refined.

The illustrations, all original drawings commissioned for this work, are designed to clarify and extend many oт the principles developed in the text.

Peter McKinney, M.D., F.A.C.S.
Bruce L. Cunningham, M.D.

Spring 1981

Introduction

To obtain maximum benefit from this book, the reader should take the time to thoroughly digest, in a leisurely manner, Section I, Basic Concepts (Chapters 1 through 7) before proceeding to Section II, Clinical Entities (Chapters 8 through 16). In Section I the authors have spared the reader the burden of having to memorize endless detailed data by presenting instead a core of information embodying the basic concepts applicable to all forms of plastic and reconstructive surgery. In spite of our lifting that burden, understanding the concepts presented here will require a certain amount of time and effort, but the rewards will far outweigh the initial investment.

In plastic surgery the technical details vary for each surgical procedure, yet every operation adheres to the same basic principles. The careful reader will come to appreciate that fact when he approaches the second section of the book and comes to see that each specific procedure follows, in its own way, the basic concepts outlined in Section I.

The second section provides basic information that physicians in other fields can apply to their own specialties. For example, the portion of Chapter 9 outlining current concepts and techniques in breast reconstruction contains information of value to the surgeon who performs mastectomies, as do the paragraphs on the current controversy over subcutaneous mastectomy. For emergency room physicians, Section II provides information which will assist in the management of fractures and lacerations.

Chapter 1, History and Scope, was included to give the reader a historical perspective on modern techniques. This is especially important in the field of plastic surgery because many of the original ideas have been lost and later rediscovered.

Chapter 2, Legal Aspects, could go anywhere (preferably to congressional reform). It is included because it is important that the reader have some working knowledge of the present system as it affects the surgeon.

Logically, the part of Chapter 8 on the psychological aspects of patient selection should be included under Basic Concepts rather than under Clinical Entities. It was placed in the chapter on aesthetic surgery because most pertinent psychological studies have been limited to the psychology of patients seeking such surgery. However, the authors cannot emphasize too strongly that the personality types described in that chapter apply to all plastic surgery patients, and an understanding of the personality differences involved and how to handle them will make for a happier physician/patient relationship.

The illustrations are designed to augment the text and are placed as close as possible to the corresponding references.

A bibliography has not been included because isolated ideas, or ideas supported by only one or two authors, have been generally avoided. The authors have attempted instead to present facts on which there is a consensus. A reading list has been provided for those seeking more detailed information in specific areas.

Acknowledgments

From the time this book was in the planning stage, the authors believed that quality artwork would be crucial to the clarity of the text. We are indebted to Sandra Koperski, A.M.I., who spent many hours in research and execution of the illustrations.

Thanks also to Paula Hamilton and Associates, especially Elizabeth Aulenbach, editor, and Sharon Bierman, word processing specialist, for preparation of the manuscript.

Contents

I. Basic Concepts

CHAPTER 1

History and Scope

The word "plastic" is derived from the Greek word "plastikos" which means "fit for molding." Although von Graefe wrote *Rhinoplastik* in 1818, application of the term to medicine has been attributed to Zeis who published *Handbuch der Plastischen Chirurgia* in 1838. He used the term to signify the ability of the surgeon to mold and refashion parts misshapen by disease or injury.

Early Beginnings

Although the term "plastic surgery" is relatively recent, the concept is not. Modern techniques of plastic surgery are rooted in thousands of years of medicine. The earliest known surgery dates from 10,000 B.C. when the Peruvians performed the first craniotomy by creating burn holes. While the reason for this practice is unclear, the technique resembles methods used today to treat subdural hematoma. New bone formation found in these ancient skulls gives evidence of some of those patients surviving. Reconstructive surgery dates from 1,000 B.C. in ancient India where members of the tilemaker caste reconstructed noses and ear lobes lost in battle. This method was described by Hindu surgeon Susruta around 400 B.C. He employed cheek tissue to replace nasal tips and ear lobes. Repair of cleft lips was described by the Chinese of the Chin dynasty (229-317 A.D.). The famous Persian physician Rhazes described the use of animal gut for ligatures in 900 A.D., although the use of ligatures was suggested by Celsus (circa 25 B.C.-50 A.D.), a Roman, many years earlier.

The practice of medicine spread from India to China and westward through Arabia and Egypt to Europe. Celsus (who, incidentally, was not a physician) discussed reconstructive surgery of the face in his eight-book work entitled *De Re Medicina*. The hemostats used today are not unlike those invented by the Romans of Celsus' time, who had a variety of sophisticated instruments.

In 15th Century Europe, there were reports of nasal reconstructions using arm flaps. This method came to be known as the Italian method because it was popularized by Tagliacozzi of Bologna. He published the first textbook of plastic surgery in 1597 with his *De Curtorum Chirurgia* (Fig. 1-1).

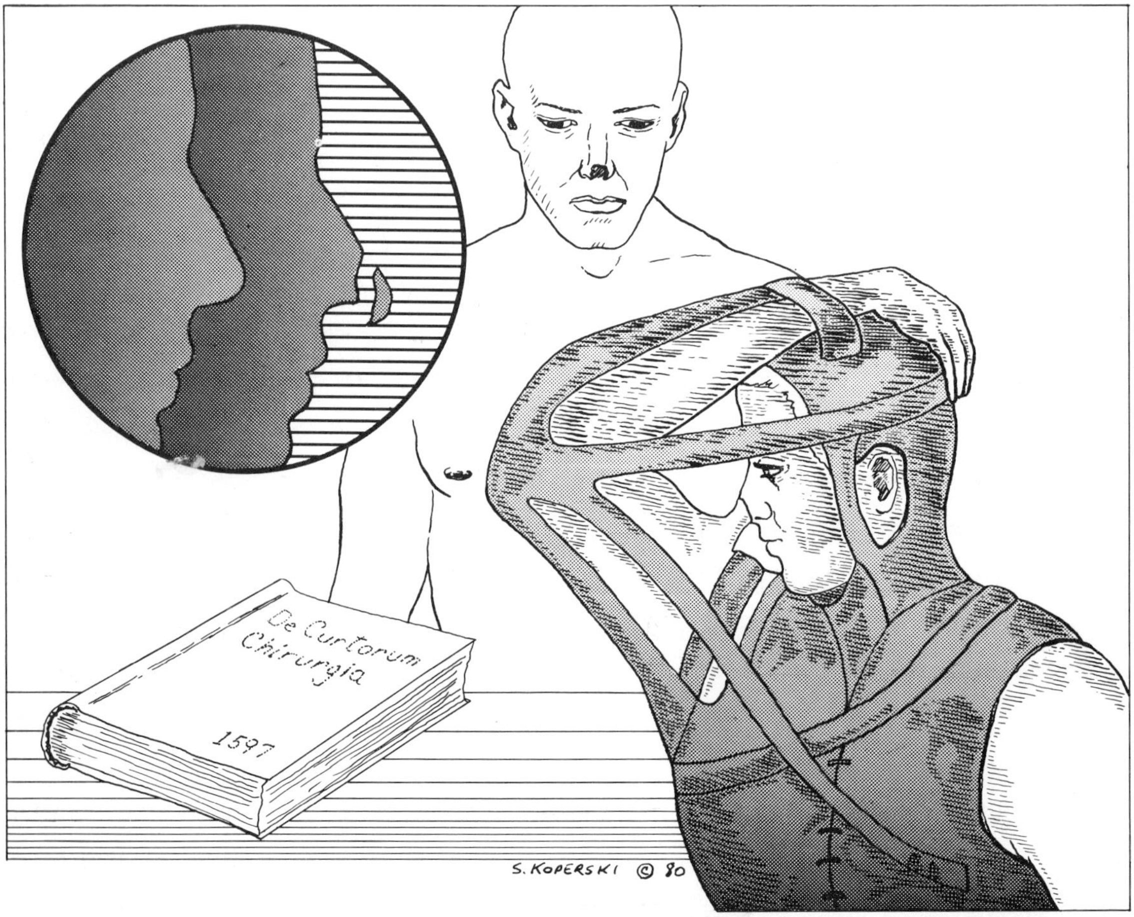

Figure 1-1. **Tagliacozzi's technique of nasal reconstruction.** This method utilized arm tissue and incorporated an ingenious device for immobilizing the arm.

Plastic and reconstructive surgery have not always been eagerly accepted. Although Tagliacozzi's work was in response to a common need (nasal tips were frequently injured in sword fights), it did meet fierce resistance from the powerful church. Tagliacozzi's remains were said to have been exhumed and moved to unconsecrated ground because his work "meddled with the will of God."

The church was not alone in its opposition to reconstructive surgery. The French satirist Voltaire ridiculed Tagliacozzi in a poem, and even Paré, who introduced modern wound care, criticized the surgeon from Bologna.

This same resistance to progress prompted reversal of the first known bone graft for skull reconstruction. In 1668, Van Meekren reconstructed a soldier's defective skull with a bone from a dog's skull. The resultant outcry from the church forced removal of the bone and, ironically, prevented the inevitable failure of this xenograft reconstruction.

Some of these feelings still abound today, especially regarding aesthetic surgery. Actually, Tagliacozzi probably performed the first aesthetic rhinoplasty, albeit for functional purposes. A famous duke had a prominent nasal hump which obscured his vision on that side. Tagliacozzi removed the hump, restoring peripheral vision.

A common punishment for adultery in 18th Century India was the amputation of the nose. Accidental injury to the nose, therefore, was associated with considerable social stigma. In 1794, the *Gentleman's Magazine* published a report of a nasal reconstruction using the skin of the forehead. This technique is still considered one of the best for nasal reconstruction.

In the late 18th and early 19th Centuries surgical activity increased, prompted by the need generated by the military campaigns of the day. Jones introduced techniques of plastic surgery to the American colonies with the publication of his *Plain, Concise Practical Remarks on the Treatments of Wounds and Fractures* in 1775. This was timely information as the Revolutionary War erupted one year later and the book became the military surgeon's bible.

Progress in solving many problems of plastic surgery progressed rapidly. Von Graefe of Berlin performed the first blepharoplasty in 1809. Mettauer of Virginia was the first to repair the soft palate in 1827; and Warren of Boston performed the first hard palate repair in 1843.

Basic plastic surgical research began with Baronio in 1804. He had heard scattered reports of the clinical application of skin grafts in India. He used sheep as a model to experiment with such grafts, discovering that only autografts survived. It is possible that this information was put to use by Bunger in 1823 when he did the first modern skin graft (Fig. 1-2).

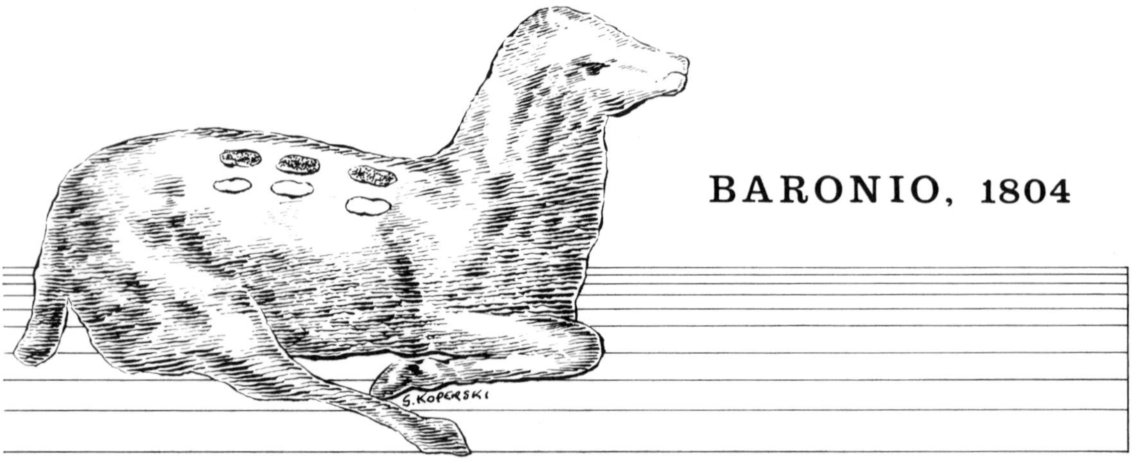

Figure 1-2. **Baronio, in 1804, utilized sheep for the first experiments with skin grafts.** The white grafts from the sheep shown here did survive, a tribute to the principle of autogenous skin grafting. The black grafts are allografts from another sheep and did not survive.

Further advances were made in 1869 when an intern in Paris applied thin sheets of skin to a granulating wound, with subsequent closure of the lesion. This became known as the Reverdin graft in honor of the man who first performed it. Later, thicker, larger grafts were used by Ollier and Thiersch. Wolfe of Glasgow performed the first known full thickness skin graft in 1876, although the ancient surgeons of India had probably used these methods.

Earlier in the 19th Century, Dupuytren (1784-1840) created a classification of burns that we still use today. He also described a contracture of the palm of a hand which bears his name. Hamilton of Buffalo, New York, described a cross leg flap to cover an open fracture of the leg in the mid-19th Century (Fig. 1-3).

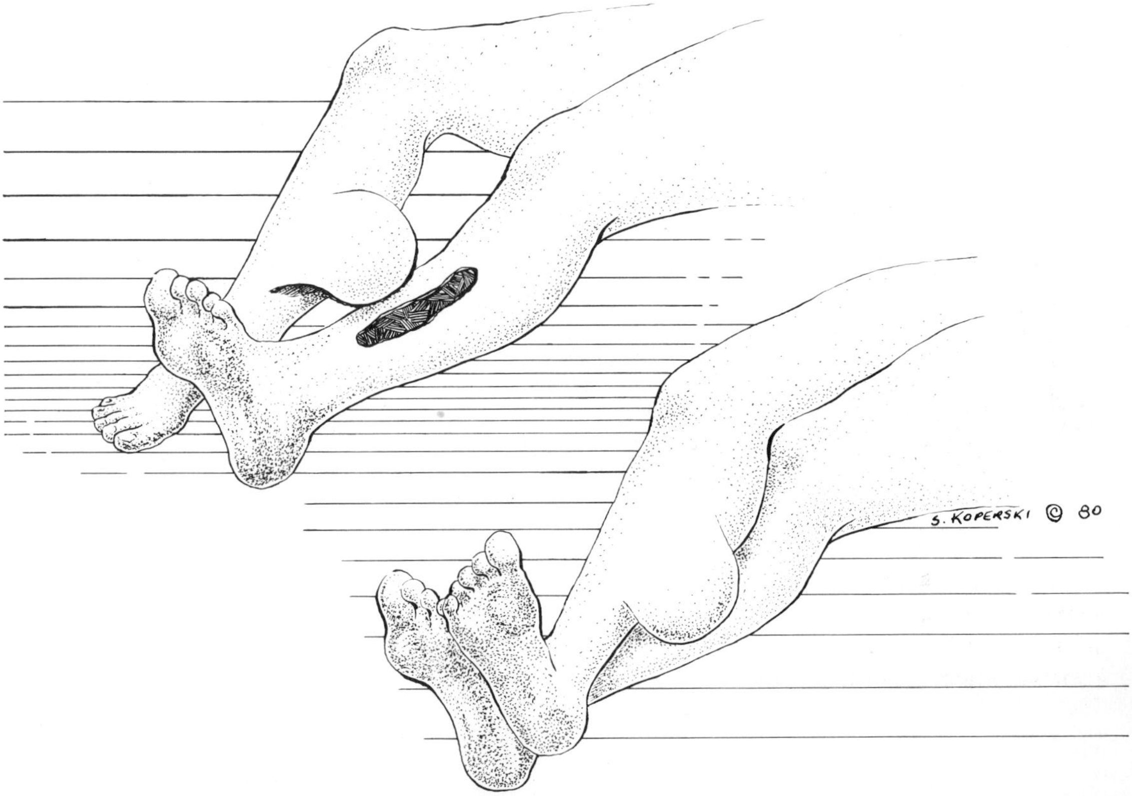

Figure 1-3. **Hamilton's cross leg flap for closing an open fracture.** This landmark procedure was utilized for such wounds for well over a century. Musculocutaneous flaps have only recently superseded this technique in some instances.

Advances of the Last Century

Following these early discoveries, clinical plastic surgical practice began to be incorporated into medical texts. Based on Civil War experiences, Buck of New York published his book *Contributions to Reparative Surgery* in 1876; and in 1887 Roe of Rochester, New York, introduced aesthetic surgery to the United States with his internasal approach to aesthetic rhinoplasty. This method was later adopted by Joseph of Berlin who became known as the father of modern rhinoplasty. Joseph's book on plastic surgery remains a classic.

As usual, war initiated a new era of medical progress. World War I stimulated a burst of reparative work, particularly of the head and neck. Because most of the fighting was conducted in the trenches, the number of facial injuries was staggering. To treat these head injuries, Gillies established the first hospital in England devoted to reconstructive surgery. His dedicated and innovative work, published in *Plastic Surgery of the Face* in 1920, made meaningful life possible for hundreds of maimed soldiers. For this accomplishment he is justly considered the father of modern plastic surgery, and many of his discoveries continue to form the basis of reconstructive surgery today.

During World War I such specialized centers as Gillies' required full-time reconstructive surgeons. Davis became the first full-time academic plastic surgeon and published many of his observations in *Plastic Surgery: Its Principles and Practice* in 1919. Much of our modern understanding of the practical applications of the Z-plasty is based on his papers on the topic.

The widespread use of antibiotics following World War II made the development of more elaborate reconstructive procedures possible. The success of workers like Gillies, who did not have antibiotics, is a tribute to these pioneers in proper wound care and careful surgical techniques.

Recent Developments

While all branches of medicine have benefited from the applications of modern technology, none has done so to the degree of plastic surgery. New inert alloplastic materials have made the reconstruction of bones and the augmentation of soft tissue defects possible. The development of the operating microscope and improvements in suturing material have opened a new era of reconstructive surgery. Amputated fingers can be replaced and large amounts of tissue transplanted using fine sutures and surgical microscopes. It is certain that as new technological advances become available plastic and reconstructive surgeons will be among the first to investigate and implement them.

The scope of plastic surgery is extremely broad, and there is considerable overlap with other subspecialty fields. Plastic surgeons deal with head and neck cancer, congenital malformations, cleft lip and palate, aesthetic surgery, hand surgery, reconstructive surgery, and microsurgery. Plastic surgeons frequently work with pediatric surgeons, urologists, otolaryngologists, ophthalmologists, and orthopedists. The rapidly expanding specialty of plastic surgery requires an awareness of developments in many other fields.

To improve communication between plastic surgeons and other surgeons, specialized medical societies came into being. In 1921, the American Association of Plastic Surgeons, the first group to be devoted exclusively to plastic surgery, was founded. The Plastic Surgery Research Foundation was established in 1955 to provide a forum for ongoing basic research. The American Society of Plastic and Reconstructive Surgeons, founded in 1931, is the largest and most broadly based plastic surgical society in the world. *Plastic and Reconstructive Surgery* began publication in 1946 and was the first American journal devoted entirely to the field of plastic surgery.

The American Board of Plastic Surgery was founded in 1937 for the purpose of evaluating and certifying specialists in plastic surgery. There are now over 2,000 persons board certified in plastic surgery in the United States. To become board certified, a candidate, in addition to completing medical school, must complete three years of a surgical residency plus an approved plastic surgical residency of two to three years, and then pass both written and oral examinations.

While the plastic surgeon of today has more tools at his disposal, including many synthetic materials, the goals remain the same as stated by the famous Renaissance surgeon Tagliacozzi who wrote: "We reconstruct and complete parts which nature hath given but which were destroyed by fate, and we do so not so much for the enjoyment of the eye as for psychic comfort to the afflicted."

This introduction has emphasized two principles of scientific progress as they relate to plastic surgery. First, the techniques employed today have evolved over many centuries and reflect the imagination and hard work of many dedicated individuals. Second, the forging of channels of information exchange has been vital to the development of these new techniques.

One fact remains to be emphasized. It is this: a common thread runs through the entire history of plastic surgery. It takes the form of three standards which translate into three basic principles: meticulous wound management, intelligent scar placement, and careful and precise wound closure. These three principles are expanded in the subsequent chapters. Together they form the foundation of plastic surgery.

CHAPTER 2

Legal Aspects

Until a decade ago medical malpractice was a minor problem. This is reflected in the small number of cases tried before the late 1960s and the relatively low premiums for malpractice insurance up to that time. Five years ago the term "malpractice" suddenly leapt into national focus. Because of the adverse publicity generated, insurance premiums increased from 10 to 30 times and, in some cases, even became unavailable. What had happened to precipitate this state of affairs in the country generally recognized as the world leader in medicine?

Two events unhappily collided. First, the explosive growth in medical knowledge required such an extraordinary number of new technical and scientific abilities that bedside manner and physician/patient rapport sank to low priority items in the medical school curriculum. Second, attorneys discovered this weak link in the chain of medical care. This left the medical profession vulnerable to a legal system that operates essentially as a one-way street.

Our legal system is the only one in the world that allows a "contingency fee," meaning that a percentage of the award is given to the successful attorney. Hence, the plaintiff risks no out-of-pocket expenses, and the defendant finances the entire system. He must pay his attorney to defend him, yet he has virtually no recourse to financial restitution when he wins.

The plaintiffs' attorneys defend this system by pointing to it as being "the poor man's key to the court house." However, statistics compiled by the Illinois Medical Insurance Exchange show that over 70 percent of malpractice suits are lost, dropped or dismissed before trial. Yet, the defendant physicians have no effective way of recovering their legal costs in these situations.

Canada, with virtually the same high standard of medical care and the same population mix as the United States, has not shared in this malpractice crisis. There a plaintiff can be held responsible for defense costs and contingency fees are considered unethical.

Malpractice has been defined as "the failure of one rendering professional services to exercise that degree of skill and learning commonly applied under similar circumstances in the community by the average prudent, reputable member of that profession, with the result of injury, loss or damage." The definition of community is a national one and, if one practices as a specialist, one is judged by national standards of the specialty. Complications and unsatisfactory results are not in themselves considered malpractice.

How can one protect oneself from unfair malpractice suits? As a rule of thumb, if one cannot establish a healthy rapport with the patient, one should not perform surgery. In emergency situations, it is a professional and legal obligation to render care, but in elective situations it is always possible to suggest another opinion. Unfortunately, a higher number of malpractice suits arise from emergency situations than from elective operations.

Written notes and records should be as detailed as possible. X-rays, blood tests, CAT scans, biopsies and anything else that might be used for a defense, although medically of no value in many proven instances, should be obtained until the system changes. Photographic records are particularly important to a plastic surgeon.

It is necessary for every patient to give "informed consent." An absurd term on the face of it, legally this means that the patient has been informed of: (1) the likelihood and seriousness of possible complications, (2) alternative methods of treatment, and (3) the degree to which the proposed treatment meets the standards of medical practice.

It is not necessary to give the same information to all patients. The information given should be geared to the patient's ability to absorb it. In practice, if the patient is told the two most likely complications and the two worst and agrees to the procedure, it would seem reasonable to assume that the patient has given his informed consent. However, the informed consent procedure must always be put in writing.

In one sense, the very existence of malpractice insurance clearly adds to the problem since the money is already sitting there, labelled and, hence, inviting a raid. Yet physicians should carry such insurance for the protection of themselves and their patients. If a problem arises, the carrier should be notified immediately, while medical records and staff recollections are fresh.

Some years ago, plaintiffs' attorneys proclaimed that they would change medical practice. They certainly have. A tragic example is the case of the pediatrician who had to consult seven specialists before a child on public aid could receive emergency treatment. The reason for the pediatrician's problem becomes clear when one realizes that the majority of suits in Cook County, Illinois, are filed by public aid patients or patients in an emergency situation, and also that a child may bring suit many years following the event. The hapless child in the example given represented a triple threat -- he was a public aid recipient, he was in an emergency situation, and he was a minor.

Until the system changes, research and development are seriously hampered in this country because of the threat of suits and, hence, are being done abroad more and more. It is unfortunate that this topic occupies as much space as it does in the context of our specialty, but to be forewarned is to be forearmed.

Changing the rules so that the plaintiff, upon losing the suit, at least pays the defense costs of the winner would help make the process a two-way street, which would help restore order and balance to the system, and would permit the patient to concentrate on getting well rather than on potential quarrels. This rule change was recently enacted in Florida where the loser in a medical malpractice suit now must pay all costs. It is the first instance in this country of a plaintiff being made to assume financial responsibility when he sues.

CHAPTER 3

Fundamental Techniques

Each surgical subspecialty has its own goals and objectives which dictate the techniques employed. Plastic surgery is concerned with optimizing wound healing, whether the ultimate objective is to achieve a functional result or to improve aesthetic appearance. The techniques employed are designed to minimize damage to healthy tissue and to facilitate the healing of injured tissue.

Instruments and Equipment

Because cells are sensitive to mechanical forces, surgical instruments can inadvertently cause cellular necrosis. Excessive injury can be prevented by gentle handling of tissue. The instruments commonly utilized by plastic surgeons for small wounds are: fine double-prong hooks, small forceps for retracting tissue, hemostats small enough to clamp only the severed vessels, small scissors to accurately dissect tissue and cut sutures, needle holders of small scale, and No. 15 and No. 11 knife blades.

A change in scale is indicated for larger wounds such as a breast reconstruction. Here longer instruments of similar design are utilized. These may include No. 10 knife blades and larger needle holders, and scissors and forceps which accommodate the larger dissection and larger needles.

Instruments of appropriate scale and design will facilitate accurate dissection and focus attention on the anatomical details at hand. This is not meant to imply that one must be painfully slow in dissecting, but only to point out that accuracy and gentle retraction preserve the tissue and promote wound healing (Fig. 3-1).

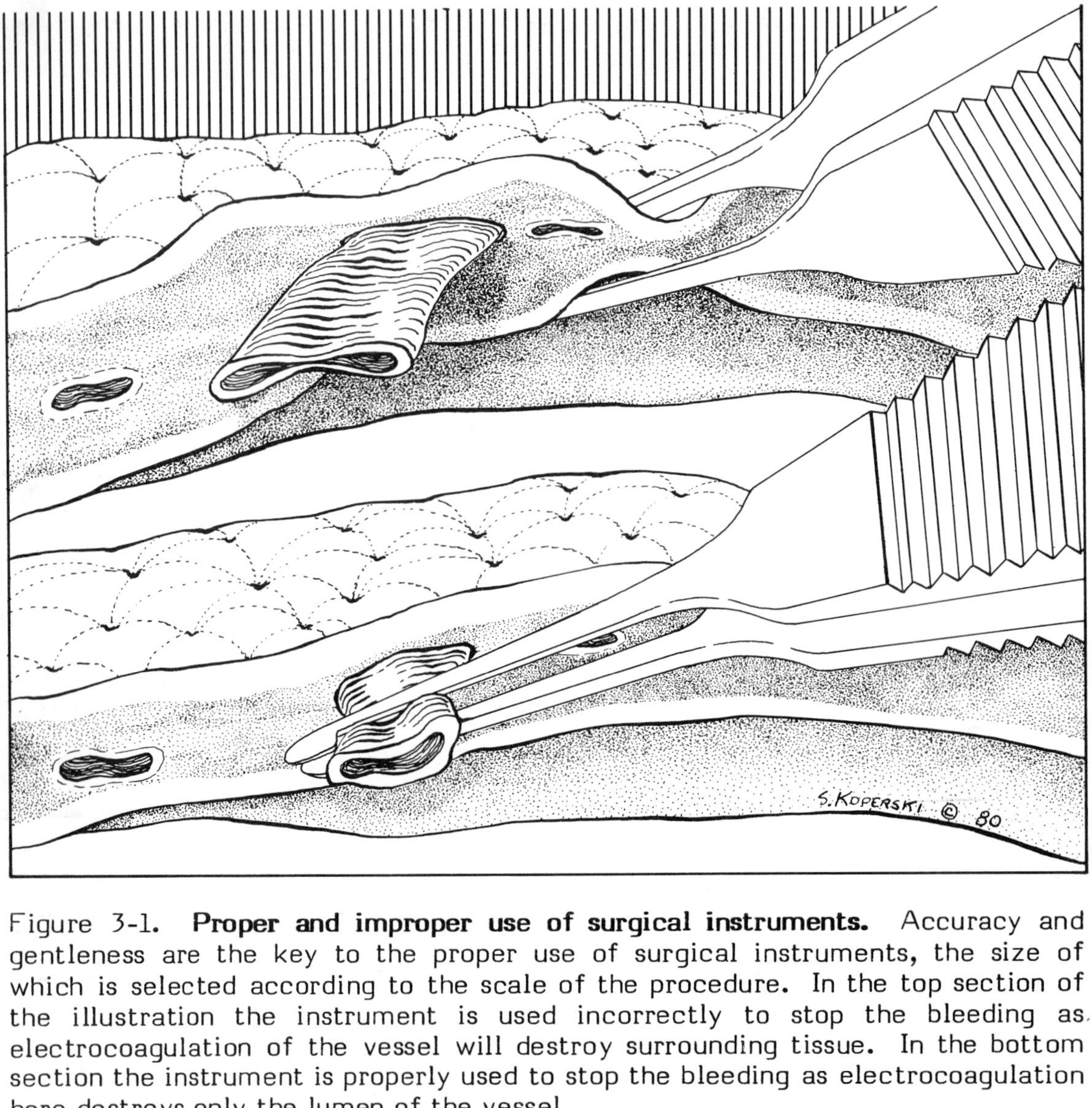

Figure 3-1. **Proper and improper use of surgical instruments.** Accuracy and gentleness are the key to the proper use of surgical instruments, the size of which is selected according to the scale of the procedure. In the top section of the illustration the instrument is used incorrectly to stop the bleeding as electrocoagulation of the vessel will destroy surrounding tissue. In the bottom section the instrument is properly used to stop the bleeding as electrocoagulation here destroys only the lumen of the vessel.

For accurate work on small structures, glasses which provide 1.5X to 4X power magnification are most helpful. These are adequate for most general purposes. Glasses at this magnification combine a comfortable working distance with a good depth and adequate field circumference. For smaller structures, the operating microscope is necessary. This allows magnification up to 40X. Zoom lenses with magnification of 10X to 26X are used for anastomosing small vessels or approximating small nerves.

A comfortable position, both for the patient and for the surgeon, is extremely important for successful surgery. This is especially true of emergency situations where makeshift arrangements often lead to fatigue which, in turn, compromises the result. The most important adjunct to comfort is a good light source. This can be either ceiling mounted, attached to the surgical retractors, or attached to a headband worn by the surgeon.

The operating room table should be placed in a recumbent position and should be adequately padded so that the patient can rest comfortably. If the room is particularly cold, especially under conditions requiring general anesthesia with its attendant vasodilatation, the patient should lie on a heating pad. The table height should be adjustable so that the surgeon can work at elbow height and not be forced into an unnatural, cramped position. An adjustable padded stool with wheels is often useful to both the surgeon and his assistants. It is sometimes helpful if the surgeon is able to alternate between a standing and a sitting position during a long procedure.

Finally, the surgeon should make sure he has adequate help to assist with retraction and instrument handling as well as for consultation when required. Most of the time an intravenous line, electrocardiogram, and blood pressure monitoring equipment will control much of the procedure so that the surgeon can concentrate fully on the work at hand.

Anesthetics

Local anesthesia is most commonly used for plastic surgery. Face lifts, breast reconstructions, staged reconstructions of the face, and hand surgery are examples of the wide range of procedures that can be performed under local anesthesia. Most agents work by combining with the sodium-potassium pumping mechanism, causing a temporary depolarization of the nerve sheath, thus blocking transmission of subsequent impulses. There are two types of local agents: amides (Lidocaine, Mepivacaine) and esters (Novocaine) and related products. The esters are shorter acting, cause higher incidences of allergic reaction, and are metabolized by the tissue esterases. The amides are considered essentially allergy free; they are metabolized in the liver and excreted by the kidney. They are nontoxic in dosages of 5 to 7 mg per kg per hour and provide up to four hours of anesthesia at this dosage. A solution of 0.5 percent is fully effective. Allergic reactions to Lidocaine are extremely rare. Allergic reactions to the preservatives added to the anesthetics occur, however, as well as vasovagal reactions due to the epinephrine. However, these too are rare.

Local anesthesia is frequently used in conjunction with epinephrine for the latter's vasoconstrictive effect. This is an aid to hemostasis and increases the safety margin by slowing the systemic absorption of the anesthetic. Epinephrine should be used cautiously in appendages, such as the fingertips or penis. In some circumstances epinephrine has been blamed for necrosis in these areas. This has probably occurred when circumferential blocks caused mechanical damage to the artery which, in turn, caused intense vasospasm. Concentrations of 1:200,000 or 1:400,000 epinephrine are sufficient for vasoconstriction. Occasionally, hyaluronidase is added to the anesthetic to decrease tissue swelling and to aid in anesthetic diffusion.

Small (30 gauge) needles decrease the pain of injection. The puncture site can be made through skin or through the wound. If injection is made through a mucous membrane, prior application of cocaine virtually eliminates the pain of the injection. Generally a "field block" or direct infiltration of the area is performed, although specific nerve trunk blocks are useful in certain situations. An example of the latter is the axillary block used for hand surgery. An infiltration hematoma can develop when blood vessels are torn by the needle during injection. It is unlikely that sufficient anesthetic to be harmful can be injected directly into a small vessel, but keeping the needle tip in motion while injecting is a prudent practice.

Cocaine is one of the oldest anesthetics in medicine and is extremely effective when used topically on mucous membranes. Topical anesthesia, using a 5 percent solution of cocaine, is employed in rhinoplasty. Cocaine shrinks the membranes, provides anesthesia, and is vasoconstrictive; therefore, added epinephrine is not necessary. Cocaine is a very potent drug and should be kept separate from the injectable anesthetic as it is very toxic when injected.

Adequate premedication sedates the patient prior to injections of local anesthetic and lessens the response to pain. For elective cases, patients are usually given 10 to 20 mgm of diazepam orally one hour prior to the procedure. Once in the operating room, an intravenous supplement of diazepam and then low-dose ketamine (0.5 mg per kg) is used just prior to the injection. Ketamine is effective for about five minutes in this dosage. The patient remains responsive to commands but feels no pain. Use of low-dose ketamine has been very helpful in preventing memory of the injection and, in low dosage, hallucinations and unpleasant dreams are rare. Laryngospasm must still be guarded against until the drug has worn off.

Symptoms of overdose of local anesthetics progress from agitation and disorientation to full convulsions. Death can occur from ventilatory or cardiac arrest as a result. Should this occur, treatment consists of instituting supportive measures which increase the cortical seizure threshold. Oxygenation and placing the patient in Trendelenburg position maximize cortical blood flow. Short-acting barbiturates (thiopental, 50 to 100 mg administered intravenously, and diazepam, 2.5 to 10 mg administered intravenously) act directly on cortical centers to elevate the seizure threshold. Ventilatory support following these measures may be necessary.

Sutures

The purpose of sutures is to draw edges of the wound together without devascularizing them so that the wound can be sealed by fibrin, epithelium and collagen (see Chapter 6, Stages of Wound Healing). The problem with external sutures is that they themselves may cause scarring if left in place too long. The use of intradermal sutures is indicated in such cases. Each suture technique has its particular uses.

External marks, or cross-hatching, are a function of the tension of the suture and of the sebaceous activity of the skin. The latter varies according to the patient's age, sex and the anatomical region in question. For example, in an 18-year-old woman with florid acne, suture marks will form on the central face in 24 hours, whereas in a 65-year-old woman with dry skin, suture marks most likely will not form for five to seven days. Areas of less sebaceous activity, such as the leg, take longer for marks to form, and areas of no sebaceous glands, such as the palm of the hand, sole of the foot, or mucosal surfaces, do not form suture marks even if the external sutures are left in place for three to four weeks.

The type of suture utilized is secondary in importance to the technique of wound closure in minimizing scar formation because the critical factor is that tension be placed on deep structures, not on the skin. If the wound closure is without tension, sutures in areas such as the face can be removed as early as two to five days, and suture marks will not form in most circumstances. In practice, a 6-0 synthetic monofilament suture is used to close the skin that is under no tension. If the wound has moderate tension and is slightly gaping, interrupted 5-0 absorbable (subcuticular) sutures may be used for support of the underlying tissue (Fig. 3-2).

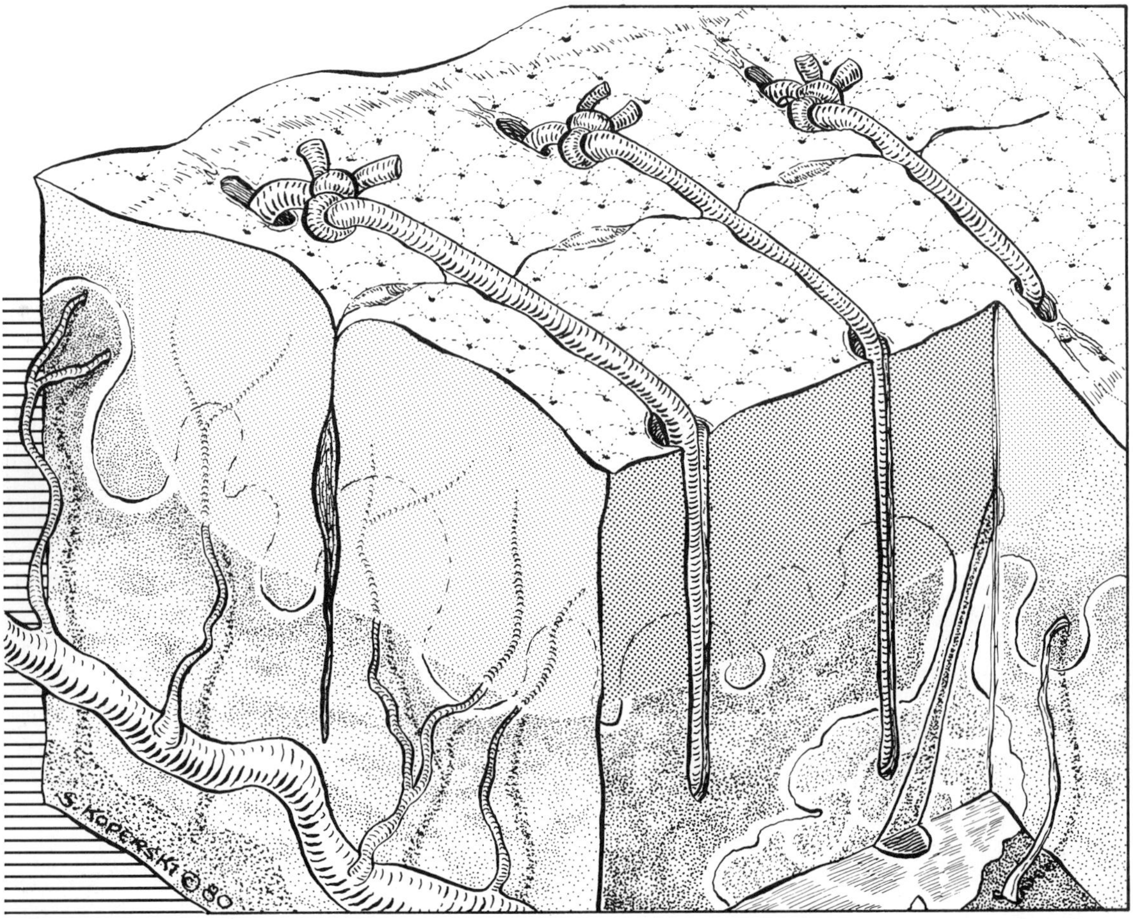

Figure 3-2. **Improper external suture technique.** If an external suture is under undue tension, it will cut through the skin and create additional scar or "cross-hatching." In addition, this causes devascularization (grey area) which leads to infection. If the sutures are left in place too long, the tracks epithelize, leaving tunnels or punctate marks.

Simple interrupted sutures are used for accurate alignment of anatomical areas such as the borders of the lip, eyelid or brow, or for thicker areas of the face such as the chin or malar area. Interrupted sutures should be placed perpendicular to the skin surface equidistant to the edge, the depth and to each other. Adequate depth to the suture is important in order to allow eversion of the skin. If the sutures are placed at an acute angle to the skin surface, the shallow bite allows the skin to roll inward, causing a widened, depressed scar. Placing the sutures equal distances apart allows for an adequate number of sutures, yet does not devascularize the skin edges. When the suture is cut, the length of the "tail" should be equal to the distance between sutures. This will allow a long enough tail for removal, yet will not interfere with placement of the next suture (Fig. 3-3).

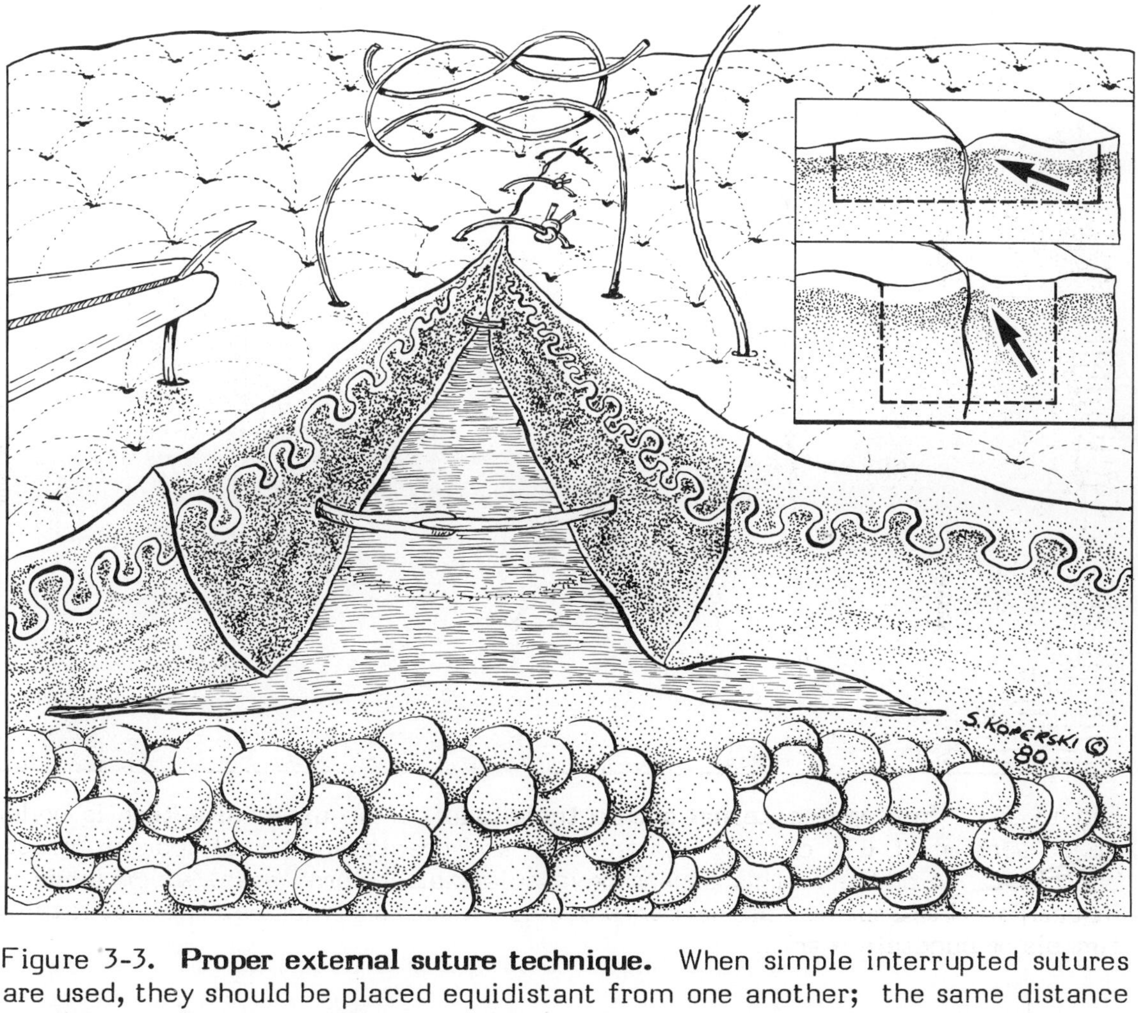

Figure 3-3. **Proper external suture technique.** When simple interrupted sutures are used, they should be placed equidistant from one another; the same distance should be reflected in the suture depth. Graphically, this technique outlines an imaginary row of cubes since suture-to-suture distance and suture depth are linearly equal. The suture needles should enter the skin on a vertical plane in order to allow adequate depth and to permit eversion of the wound edges (lower portion of inset). If a shallow "bite" is taken, there is more horizontal than vertical bite, resulting in unequal forces in the two planes (upper portion of inset). This inverts the wound edges and causes a wider scar because of the interposition of epidermis in the upper dermis.

Sometimes a subcuticular (internal) suture may be used in conjunction with skin tapes. Such a suture may be continuous or interrupted. This technique is especially useful for oily or active acne skin where external sutures are likely to leave epithelial tunnels and suture marks even though removed early (24 to 48 hours). Marks are left on these patients because of the hyperactivity of the underlying sebaceous glands (Fig. 3-4).

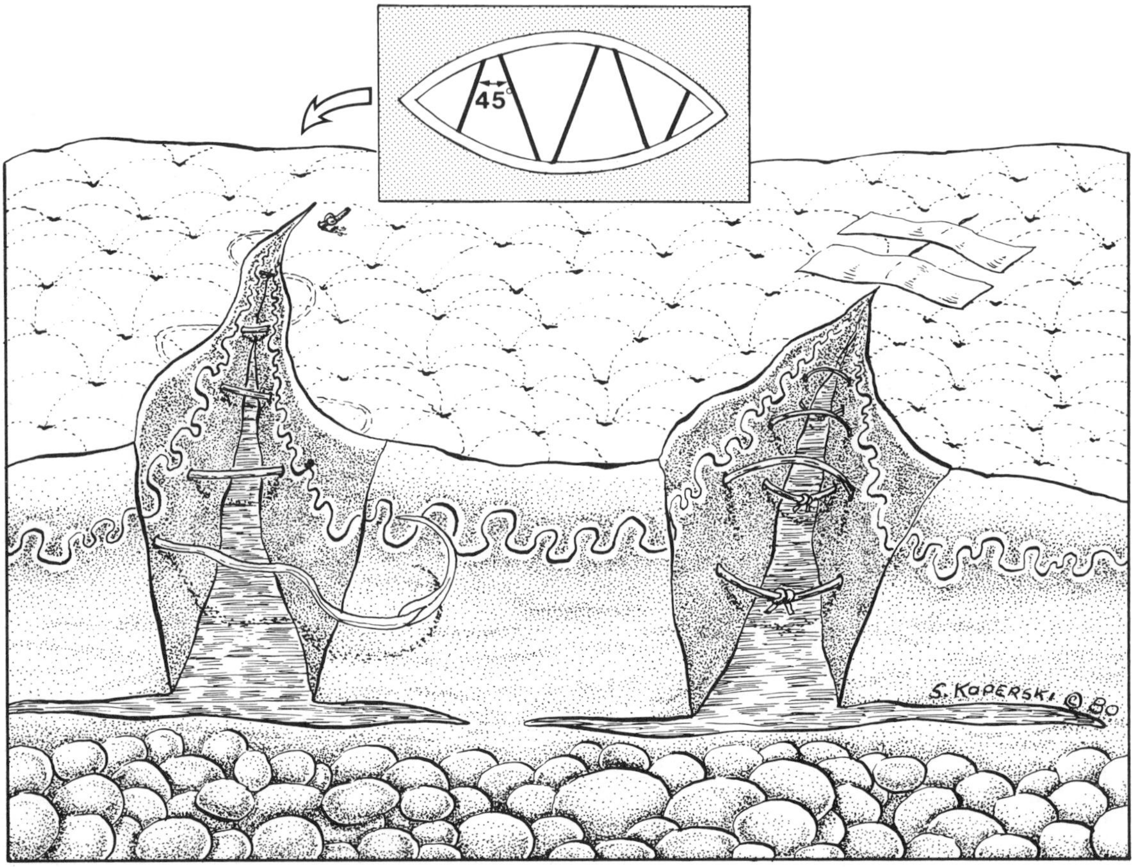

Figure 3-4. **Proper subcuticular suture techniques.** Subcuticular sutures may be either absorbable or nonabsorbable. If a simple interrupted subcuticular suture is used, the knot should be buried (right). If a running subcuticular suture is used, the needle should be placed horizontal to the dermis with opposing bites 45° apart if the wound is straight (inset, left).

In areas of thin dry skin, such as the eyelid or preauricular area, a simple overhand running suture is faster to insert and easier to remove (Fig. 3-5), yet allows accurate coaptation of the edges of the wound because of the thinness of the skin. It does not work well on thicker skin because the edges of the wound tend to invert. Vermilion and other mucosal areas may be closed with external sutures as there are no sebaceous glands in these areas.

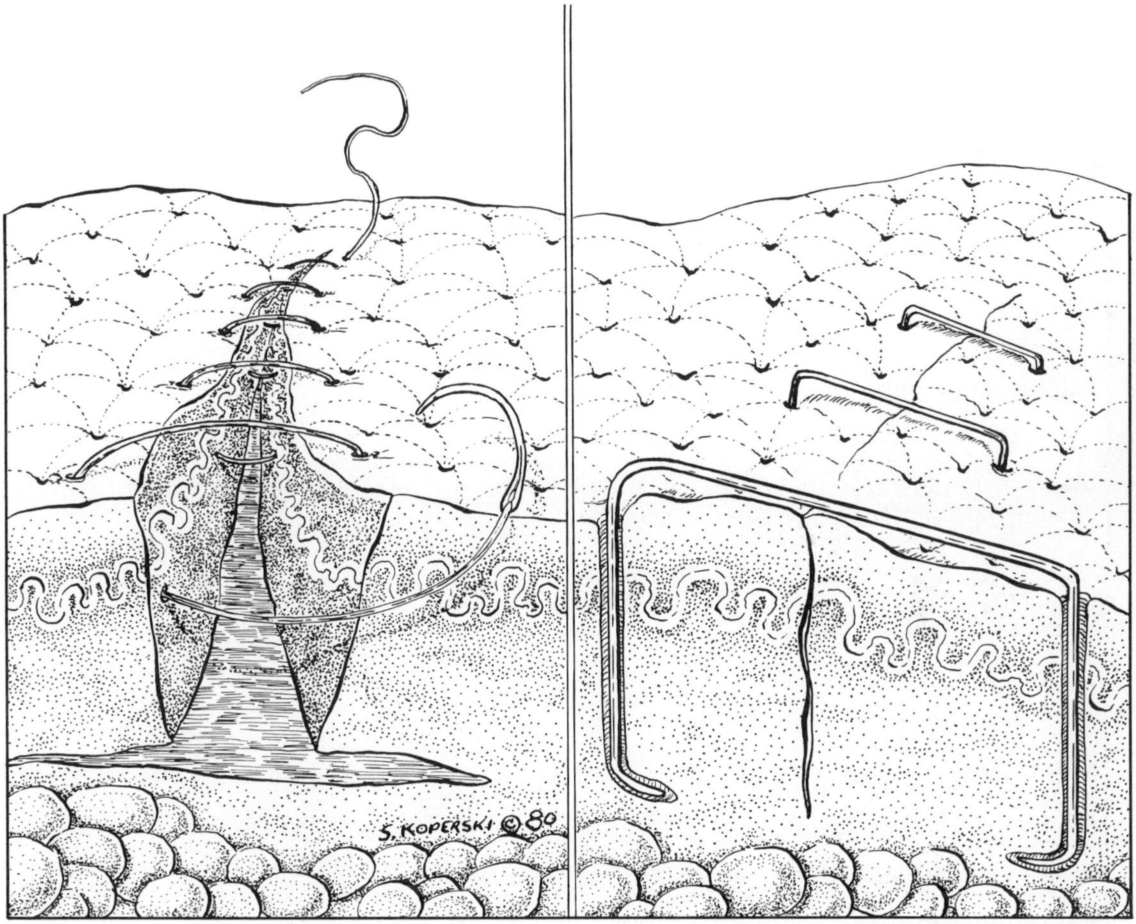

Figure 3-5. **Suiting suture to area of incision.** Left: A simple running suture is useful in areas of thin dry skin with no tension, such as an eyelid. Right: Staples are useful in a variety of locations and, because of their design, do not leave cross-hatched scars. They will, however, leave puncture marks after four to seven days and are most useful in hair-bearing areas where they will not show.

Stitch marks do not form in hair-bearing areas because the hair protects against the possibility of pressure necrosis from the sutures. Interrupted or interlocked sutures or staples are all useful, and these may be left in place for several weeks or longer. The surgeon must take into account the potential baldness pattern of the male patient in the case of elective incisions since a receding hairline may uncover a scar at some future time.

In closing a wound in the trunk or extremities, because of the thicker skin and stronger muscular forces involved, and because of the diminished blood supply vis-a-vis the head and neck, sutures have to be left in place 10 to 14 days or longer. This is also true in wounds with marginal arterial flow, such as flaps or atherosclerotic extremities, and in patients where slow healing is anticipated. To prevent suture marks in these circumstances, external sutures are not used. The subcutaneous tissues are closed with 3-0 absorbable sutures, either interrupted or continuous subcuticular, and the skin closed with sterile tapes.

Staples are useful in large wounds because of the speed of closure. They do not leave cross-hatching marks, but they may leave puncture dots, which usually fade with time. Because the staples do not connect under the skin, epithelial tunnels do not form.

Postoperative Care

The most important aspects of postoperative care are the reduction of pain and the immobilization of the affected part in order to prevent hemorrhage. Resting and elevation of the affected part help to reduce edema.

There is little pain associated with most plastic surgery procedures. If excessive pain develops, it may represent a hematoma formation under a skin flap, and the area should be inspected for this possibility. Mild analgesics at night are all that most patients require.

Dressings are used to help immobilize the area and to provide slight pressure. They should not obscure the area from observation. Excessive pressure may cause necrosis, especially over undermined areas where blood and nerve supply have been compromised.

Postoperative nausea must be controlled because retching can increase the chances of bleeding. Careful selection of preoperative medications, light anesthetics and postoperative antihistamines help to reduce this possibility.

A patient should not be confined to bed if this can be avoided. It is best to encourage early ambulation because a prolonged confinement reduces muscular strength and increases the chance of venous thrombosis.

Summary

The use of small instruments, accurate approximation of structures without tension, and small sutures are the three basic rules of good plastic surgical technique. The type of suture used is less important than ensuring a loose closure which will permit early removal of the sutures. Subcuticular sutures are used where long-term sutures are indicated. Local anesthesia is appropriate for a range of procedures, especially in the emergency setting. The essential elements in postoperative care are reduction of pain, immobilization of the affected part, and early ambulation.

CHAPTER 4

Wound Care

The admonition from the Hippocratic oath, "Above all, do no harm," covers many aspects of medicine, but the warning is especially applicable to the management of wounds. The importance of this concept is well illustrated by an accidental discovery during the 16th Century. It was common practice at that time to employ boiling oil to cauterize battle wounds. Paré ran out of supplies for this treatment during the Battle of Torino and was unable to cauterize the wounds of many of the soldiers. To his amazement, considerably less infection and sepsis resulted.

This is obvious today, but the idea was revolutionary in the 16th Century. The oil cauterization caused significant tissue necrosis, creating a culture material for subsequent bacterial infection. This chance discovery represented a major contribution to proper wound management. Today, in some respects, we are still using "boiling oil," albeit in more subtle, and not readily apparent, forms.

Acute Wounds

Anything placed in a wound with the intention of killing bacterial growth may tend to kill the tissue cells as well. For example, some years ago 0.5 percent silver nitrate solution was used with a great deal of success in preventing sepsis in large burn wounds. Yet it was clinically observed that only small amounts of evaporation could change the concentration of the solution to 1.0 percent, causing the subsequent skin grafts to grow poorly.

This finding was supported by tissue culture work that had been done in the late 1930s, in which the effectiveness of antiseptics was tested against various bacteria in tissue culture. At 0.5 percent concentration, the silver nitrate solution allowed cells of a chick embryo heart to proliferate, yet impeded bacterial growth. At 1.0 percent concentration, the silver nitrate solution impeded both the growth of the chicken heart embryo and of the bacteria. At higher concentrations, the solution killed both the bacteria and the embryo cells.

Antibiotics and Wound Irrigation

Many different solutions are used to irrigate wounds. The safest is lactated Ringer's solution warmed to body temperature. This is a physiologically balanced solution which will not damage cells chemically or osmotically. Wound irrigation with lactated Ringer's solution provides for safe physiological flushing of the wound, decreasing both the number of bacteria and the amount of cellular debris.

Antibiotics applied to a wound are of questionable value, except in two specific circumstances: for drainage of a closed cavity and for an open wound with a persistent streptococcal contamination.

In contaminated cavities where the skin and soft tissue are closed but the entire depth of the wound cannot be closed, a system employing irrigation solutions of appropriate antibiotics, complete with a suction drain, should be established. This treatment may be used to sterilize a joint surface or to save a contaminated prosthesis.

The use of prophylactic systemic antibiotics to ensure clean elective procedures is not of proven benefit, and there is a danger that overuse will produce a resistant bacterial strain. This happened in the 1950s when a resistant "hospital Staphylococcus" emerged because of the widespread prophylactic use of penicillin. If the wound is potentially contaminated, systemic antibiotics are helpful, but only if used briefly during the period of greatest exposure. This method achieves a blood level during the surgery when the tissue is being manipulated, yet minimizes the risk of developing resistant organisms. This is helpful when operating on the mouth or near the anus or in cases of trauma, particularly after an animal bite.

In practice, 1 g of a cephalosporin is given intravenously 30 to 60 minutes prior to the surgery, and 500 mg is given intravenously following surgery every 6 hours for 24 hours; or, alternatively, penicillin G, 1 million units initially followed by 500,000 units every 6 hours for 24 hours. Systemic antibiotics are prophylactically necessary for those patients undergoing surgery who have rheumatic heart disease or artificial heart valves.

In the case of a granulating wound prior to skin grafting, there must be no beta-hemolytic Streptococcus present because proteolytic enzymes of the bacteria will dissolve the graft. Occasionally, systemic antibiotics will not eradicate the Streptococcus; in that case, gauze sponges soaked in a solution of streptomycin, 1 g per 500 cc of dextrose solution, should be applied to the wound four times a day.

Mechanical Factors

The debridement of necrotic tissue and foreign material will hasten healing. In enlarged wounds, where there is a question of the viability of large tissue parts, a fluorescein test may be helpful. This drug is given intravenously after a test dose has been administered. After 20 minutes, the tissue is tested for fluorescence with a Wood's light (an ultraviolet spectrum). The tissue that does not fluoresce is not viable and must be debrided. A urinary catheter and systemic fluid replacement are required because of the drug's potent diuretic effect.

Fluorescein has been used in many situations where accurate debridement is necessary. These include diagnosing the extent of necrosis following subcutaneous adriamycin injection and certain degloving injuries of the extremities. In addition, fluorescein is commonly used to assess the viability of reconstructive flaps.

Reliable indicators of tissue viability which lend themselves to clinical inspection are the color, edge bleeding, and temperature of the tissue. A flap or partially avulsed skin should be of normal skin color, without any hint of cyanosis, or greyish-blue discoloration. Cyanosis should be distinguished from the coloration caused by bruising of the flap by trauma or from arterial spasm brought about by cold, epinephrine or low blood pressure. Arterial spasm may be reversed by topical vasodilators such as Xylocaine or Marcaine and by applying warm compresses. Isoxsuprine has been helpful in preventing arterial spasm but has been more effective when the patient is treated 10 to 14 days prior to the surgery.

Back bleeding from the dermal edge of the flap is a reliable indicator of viability. The blood should be bright red and should reappear in less than a second when the flap edge is wiped with a sponge. The temperature of a flap may not be as reliable an indicator of viability because of transmission of heat from the surrounding normal tissue. However, current experimental work continues to improve precise temperature monitoring of skin flaps, and this may be a reliable factor in the future. Again, it is important to ascertain that the patient is normotensive and normothermic and that the epinephrine or arterial spasm has not intervened (Fig. 4-1).

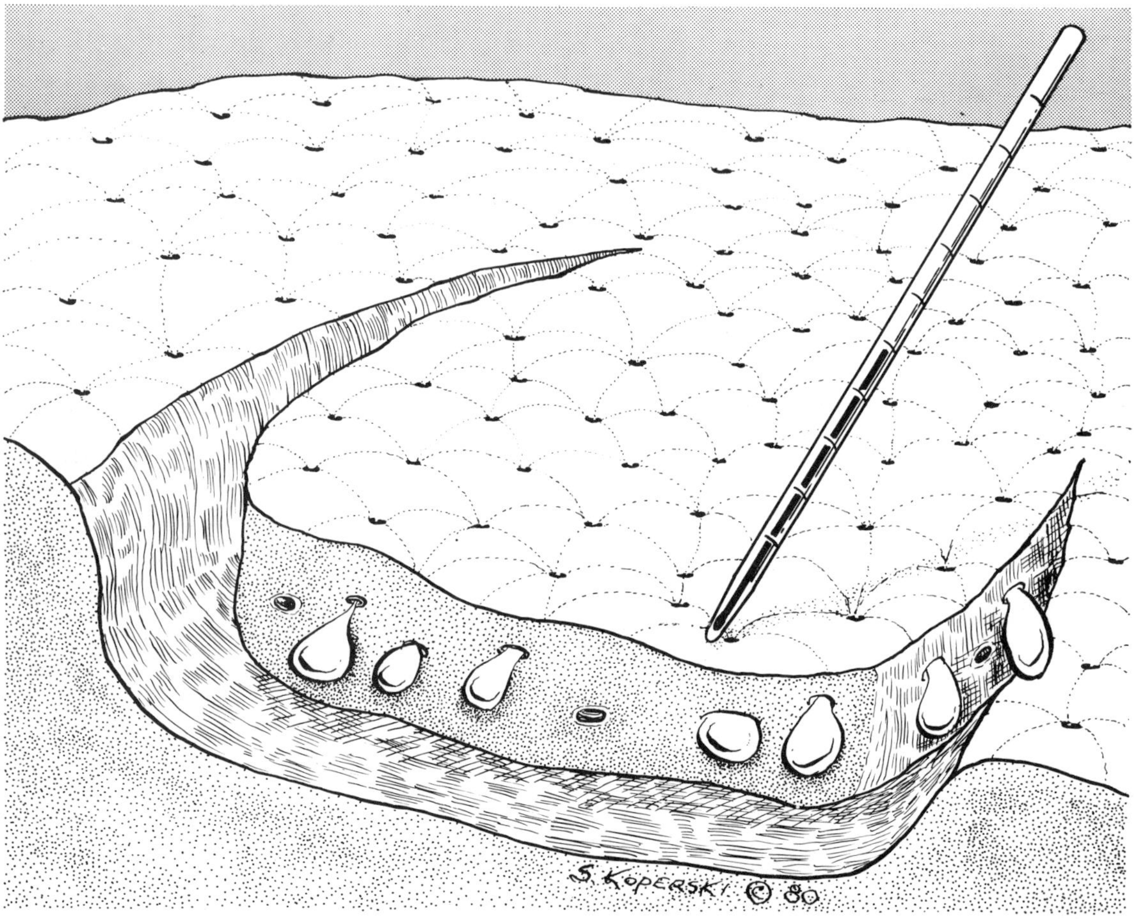

Figure 4-1. **Reliable indicators of tissue viability.** When the cut edge of the tissue is wiped, prompt back bleeding, of well-oxygenated blood, indicates that the tissue will survive. Tissue should be normal skin color, and the blood should be bright red. The temperature of the flap is not a reliable indicator of viability, because warmth may be transmitted from the surrounding tissue.

In the case of exposure of a patient with a large wound to a cold operating room (especially under general anesthesia with accompanying dilatation of the skin vessels), an otherwise viable flap may appear to have poor circulation. This is because of the lower body temperature. It is always a good precaution to use a warming mattress and a rectal or esophageal temperature probe when performing surgery for these patients.

Wound Protection

During surgery the wound must be protected from hot operating room lights, heavy-handed retraction, large crushing instruments, large ligatures, dry tissue environment and damage from high-speed drills. These all contribute to tissue necrosis which provides a culture medium for bacteria. (Good wound management techniques include keeping the wound moist, handling the tissue gently, using water to cool the drill head, clamping only the bleeding vessel, and using small ligature and precise electrocautery.) *

Chronic Wounds

When preparing chronic wounds for closure, it is desirable to have red, flat granulation tissue. The surrounding epithelium should be beginning to proliferate from the wound edges. Clinically, this latter sign is a reliable indication that a chronic wound is ready for closure. If the granulation tissue is too swollen, it can be trimmed mechanically by blade or chemically with silver nitrate. The granulation tissue can also be compressed with pressure from an elastic bandage to reduce its exuberance. It should be emphasized, however, that it is not necessary in all instances to wait for the presence of granulation tissue before closing wounds (Fig. 4-2).

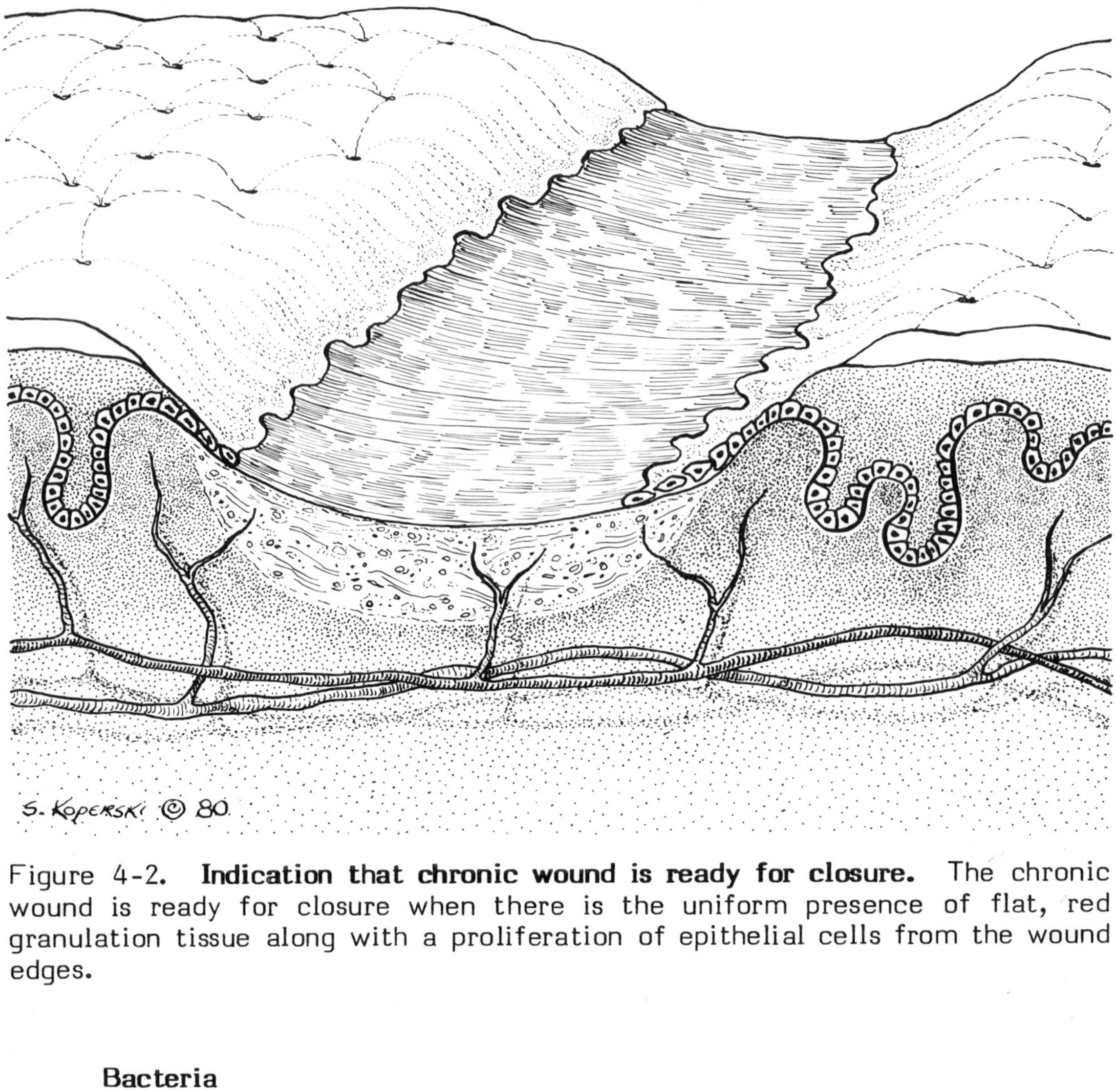

Figure 4-2. **Indication that chronic wound is ready for closure.** The chronic wound is ready for closure when there is the uniform presence of flat, red granulation tissue along with a proliferation of epithelial cells from the wound edges.

Bacteria

Useful laboratory confirmation of the readiness of the wound to be closed is the bacterial count per gram of tissue. If the concentration of bacteria is greater than 10^5 per g, the closure is liable to fail because of infection. (This is not the case, of course, in the mouth or anus where bacterial counts frequently are greater than 10^9.)

Ultimately, a wound is sterilized only by closure, not by antibiotics or dressings. It is rarely necessary, or even possible, to remove all bacteria prior to closing a wound. The presence of common organisms such as E. coli, Pseudomonas, and Staphylococcus are not in themselves a contraindication to closure as long as the concentration is reduced to less than 10^5 per g. (Pseudomonas and

Staphylococcus defeat skin grafts by the exudate they produce.) This exudate of leucocytes and tissue fluid separates the new graft from the wound bed and, hence, from vascularization. Techniques of wound preparation vary according to the organism in question. For Pseudomonas, 1 percent acetic acid compresses tend to reduce the number of organisms to manageable proportions. For wounds with Staphylococci, full strength Dakin's solution will reduce the concentration.

There is one exception. Beta-hemolytic Streptococcus, because of the production of wound lysins, streptokinase and streptodornase, must be removed from the wound prior to closure. This organism is extremely sensitive to systemic penicillin. If it persists on repeat cultures after treatment, a topical application of streptomycin compresses should be used.

Naturally, anaerobic organisms, such as Clostridium, must be eradicated prior to closure.

Antiseptics

Iodine is a useful topical antiseptic, but in alcohol solution it is too damaging to tissue. Polyvinylpropyl iodine, however, allows slow release of the iodide ion, yet the polyvinylpropyl base is neutral to the tissue. This agent has been useful clinically under plaster casts where dressings cannot be changed frequently.

Saline Dressings

Where dressings can be changed frequently, it is hard to surpass the benefits of moist, isotonic sodium chloride dressings. Plain gauze dressings, saturated with sodium chloride, are wrung out, placed directly on the wound, and allowed to dry. The wick action of the dressing will pull necrotic material into the gauze. The dressings should be replaced every two to four hours. Plain gauze makes the best dressing because absorbent gauzes have inner cotton pads which prevent evaporation. The wound should not be covered with waterproof tape, heavy pads or plastic wrappers because they will prevent the dressing from drying out (Fig. 4-3).

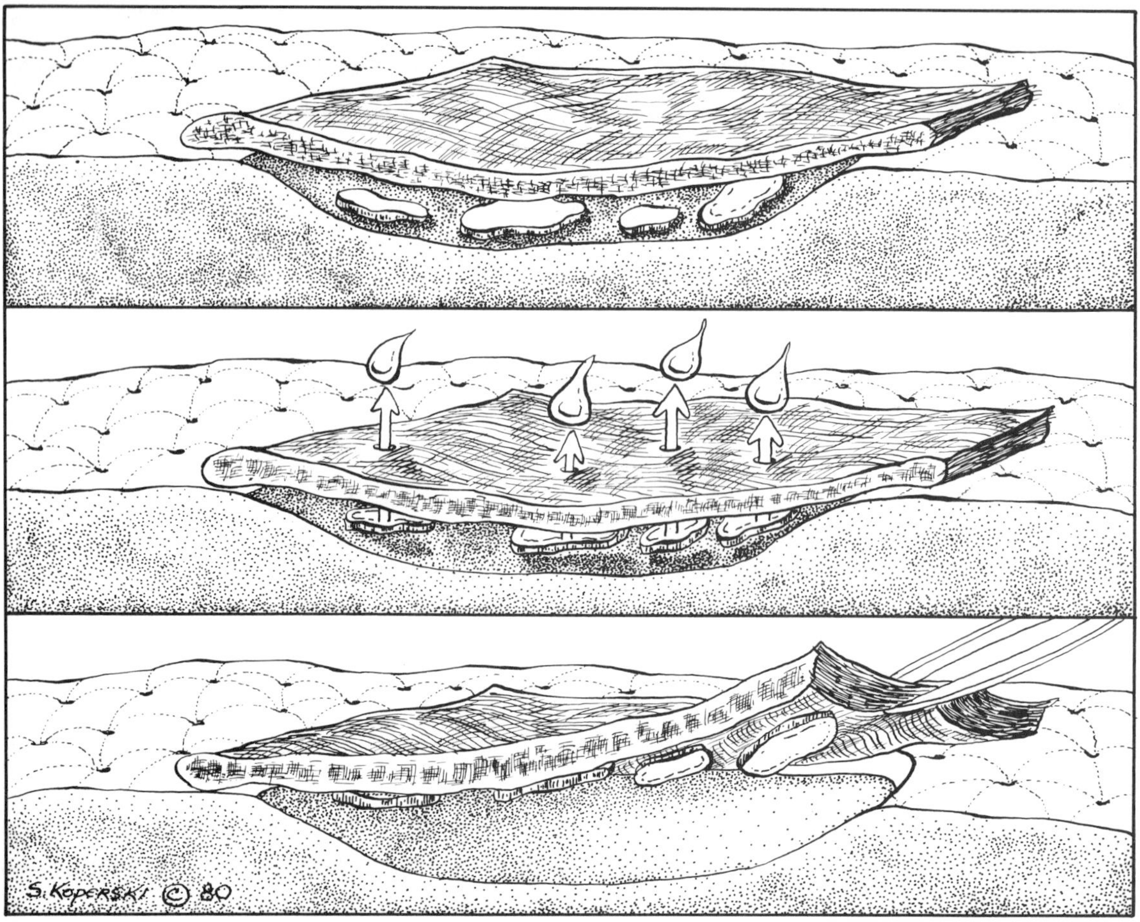

Figure 4-3. **An effective wound dressing.** A saline wet-to-dry dressing using plain gauze is placed on the wound (top). As the solution evaporates, necrotic debris sticks to the gauze (center). When the gauze is dry, it can be stripped off, further helping to debride the wound (bottom).

Although the technique of using wet-to-dry saline compresses with plain gauze is advocated for most wounds, it is sometimes useful to change the environment of a wound from time to time because bacteria accommodate themselves to certain environments. Wounds that are dry and crusty should be kept moist with saline compresses beneath a plastic cover. This helps to liquefy the crust. Most wounds have so much fluid exudate that the wet-to-dry technique is more useful. However, often the adage "If it's wet, dry it, and if it's dry, wet it" is appropriate for chronic wounds. A change from time to time in topical agents also appears to be of benefit in chronic wounds. For example, changing polyvinylpropyl iodine to saline every two to four weeks may effect a dramatic change in the wound.

Ointments

Five percent scarlet red in a petroleum and lanoline base is useful in wounds that are dry, noncrusty and apparently refractory to epithelization. A common example is a small chronic postradiation burn. Scarlet red is an analine dye which was a precursor to the sulpha drugs. This compound has been shown to promote rapid epithelization in these difficult wounds. Since it is a dye it stains fabrics and must be used carefully.

Summary

The basis of proper wound care is to render no harm. Care must be taken not to cause tissue damage by using caustic solutions. The use of physiological solutions for irrigation and delicate instruments for manipulation and careful debridement will properly prepare an acute wound for closure. A chronic wound requires control of the bacterial concentration but, in the final analysis, only closure will sterilize the wound.

CHAPTER 5

Wound Closure

Poor blood supply, infection, or an uncooperative patient are the only legitimate reasons for leaving a wound open. All other wounds, including animal bites, pressure sores and burns, should be closed as early as possible in order to reduce scarring and to improve homeostasis. The bacterial population of a wound doubles every six to eight hours, and if the concentration becomes too high (i.e., greater than 10^5 per g of tissue), clinical infection may result. Because of this, most fresh wounds cannot be closed after six to eight hours. Wounds of the head and neck, however, because of the rich vascular supply, resist infection and may be closed as late as 12 hours after wounding.

Some clinical examples illustrate this concept: A wound of the palm of the hand that involves a tendon must be repaired immediately because of the relative avascularity of the tendon and its poor resistance to infection. If immediate repair of the tendon is not possible, it is better to close the skin immediately and repair the tendon several weeks later, after the wound has become sterilized. By contrast, a wound on a lower extremity in an older patient with impaired circulation is better served by delayed closure if it cannot be closed in the first few hours following injury. The use of antibiotics has extended the length of time a wound can be left open, depending on the condition of the wound. For example, a clean knife wound sustained at home should be closed within 8 hours but a surgical wound can be left open for 16 hours, whereas a dirty crush wound sustained in the street may best be treated left open initially, even if seen very early.

Types of Wound Closure

Clinically, there are three ways of closing a wound short of providing additional tissue in the form of flaps or grafts (Fig. 5-1):

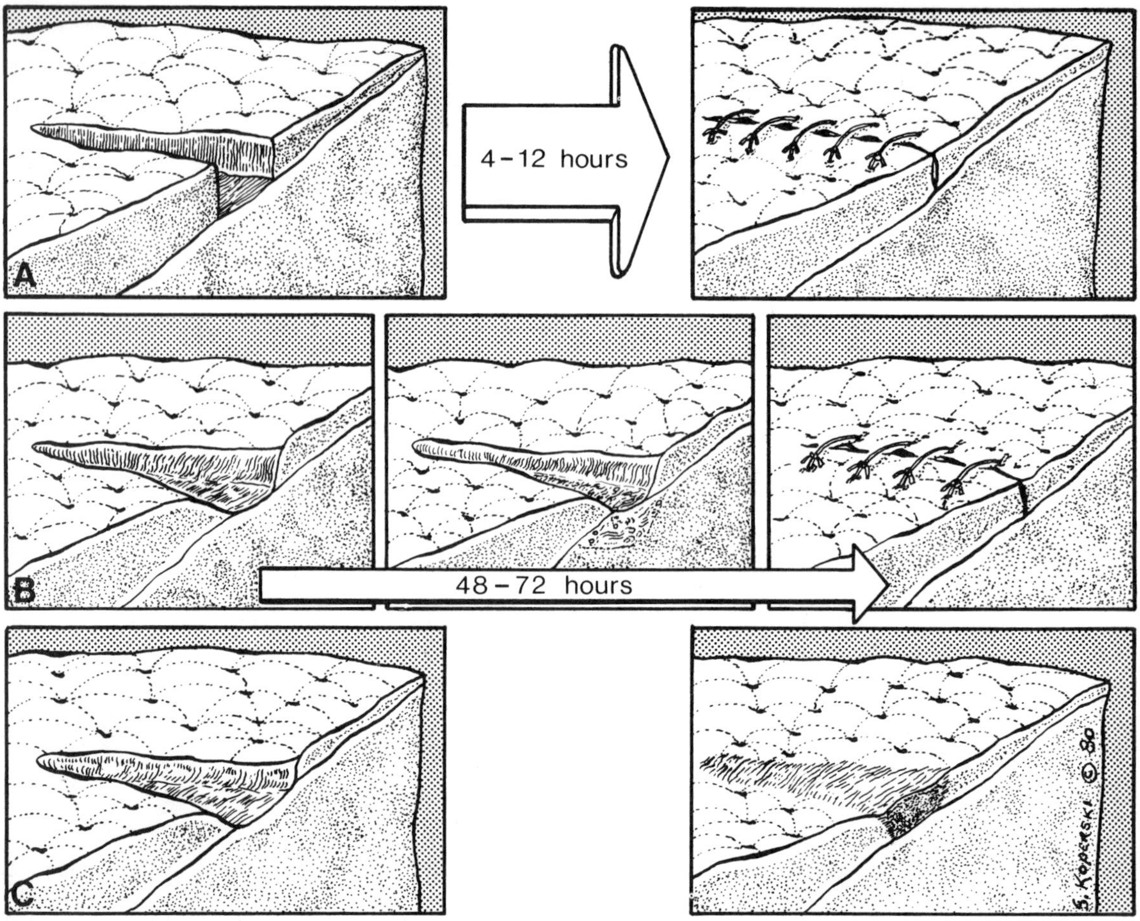

Figure 5-1. **The three types of wound closure.** In primary closure, the wound is closed up to 12 hours after wounding (A). This can only be done for clean lacerations or surgical wounds. Delayed primary closure is wound closure two to three days after wounding (B). It is used in wounds where contamination is suspected, yet overt infection is not present. Wound closure by secondary intention relies completely upon wound contracture and epithelization (C). This results in a wider scar but is useful in small wounds or in acute infections.

- Primary. The wound is closed by sutures within a few hours of injury, usually within 4 to 12 hours.
- Delayed primary. The wound is closed by sutures after a waiting period of from 48 to 72 hours, sometimes longer. This allows the lymphatics to seal and white blood cells and other host defenses to mobilize. The technique is used in wounds with gross contamination or in wounds not seen in the initial four- to eight-hour period.
- Secondary intention. Allowing the wound to granulate and epithelize spontaneously constitutes healing by secondary intention. This is

rarely indicated except in a small wound that had been abscessed, such as a boil or pilonidal cyst. Allowing a large wound to granulate and close spontaneously only prolongs the morbidity and increases the subsequent scar tissues. However, the morbidity of surgery must also be weighed when making these decisions.

Most wounds encountered in plastic surgery are elective and are closed primarily. The key to successful closure is a lack of tension on the wound edges, as excessive tension leads to a conspicuous scar and may predispose the patient to an infection. The statement, "The wound got infected," may actually indicate a poor wound closure technique; that is to say, the wound may have become devascularized by tight closure, causing infection as a secondary phenomenon. It has been shown that tissue pressures exceeding the actual mean arterial pressure will stop skin circulation. Even a lesser degree of pressure, 20 to 40 mm Hg, will cause skin degeneration and prevent wound healing.

If the wound cannot be closed without tension, tissue must be added by either a flap or a graft. These methods are used if the edges of the wound cannot be drawn together easily without ischemic changes.

Before discussing the addition of tissue, however, it is necessary to provide an understanding of how the blood is supplied to the skin. This supply has two major sources: (1) perforating vessels from the underlying musculature, and (2) direct cutaneous vessels.

Perforating musculocutaneous arteries supply each individual muscle and the skin that overlies it. They connect to the segmental vascular system by perforations through the muscles. These vessels begin deep in the superficial fascia of the muscle and end in the subdermal arterial plexus.

Direct cutaneous vessels course in the subcutaneous plane superficial to the muscular fascia. These vessels supply specific areas of skin and end in the subdermal arterial plexus. They do not perforate a muscle. Direct cutaneous arteries supply larger areas of skin than do the musculocutaneous arteries. Direct cutaneous arteries are usually accompanied by paired venous comitans, while perforating vessels are usually not accompanied by veins.

Flaps

A flap is a section of tissue that retains its blood supply during the transfer. This allows for the transfer of thicker tissue than does a graft, because of the accompanying subcutaneous tissue. As a result of this thickness, a flap contracts less than a graft. Flaps most commonly consist of skin and fat but may include muscle or other tissue. Flaps can be classified in various ways; however, the simplest classification begins by placing all flaps into one of two categories according to their source of vascular supply. They are random flaps and axial flaps. Random flaps have an irregular and uncertain pattern to the arteriovenous system. Axial flaps incorporate at least one major identifiable artery and vein.

The classifications are further divided according to whether tissue adjacent to the wound is utilized (local flap) or tissue is from another area (distant flap). Random flaps can also be classified by descriptive terms such as rotation, interpolation and bipedicle. These and other subgroups are described below (Table 5-1). Important subheadings of axial flaps are also included.

Table 5-1. Classification of Flaps

Random	Local	Advancement Rotation Bipedicle Interpolation
	Distant	Direct (i.e., cross-leg) Jump Tube
Axial	Local Distant	Musculocutaneous Cutaneous Free

Random Flaps

Because random flaps contain an irregular and uncertain pattern to the arteriovenous system, they are limited in size and flexibility. For safety, the random flap length cannot exceed twice its width and a one-to-one ratio, i.e., it is an almost infallible rule that the base be as wide as the length. If longer flaps are needed, the flap elevation must be delayed (Fig. 5-2).

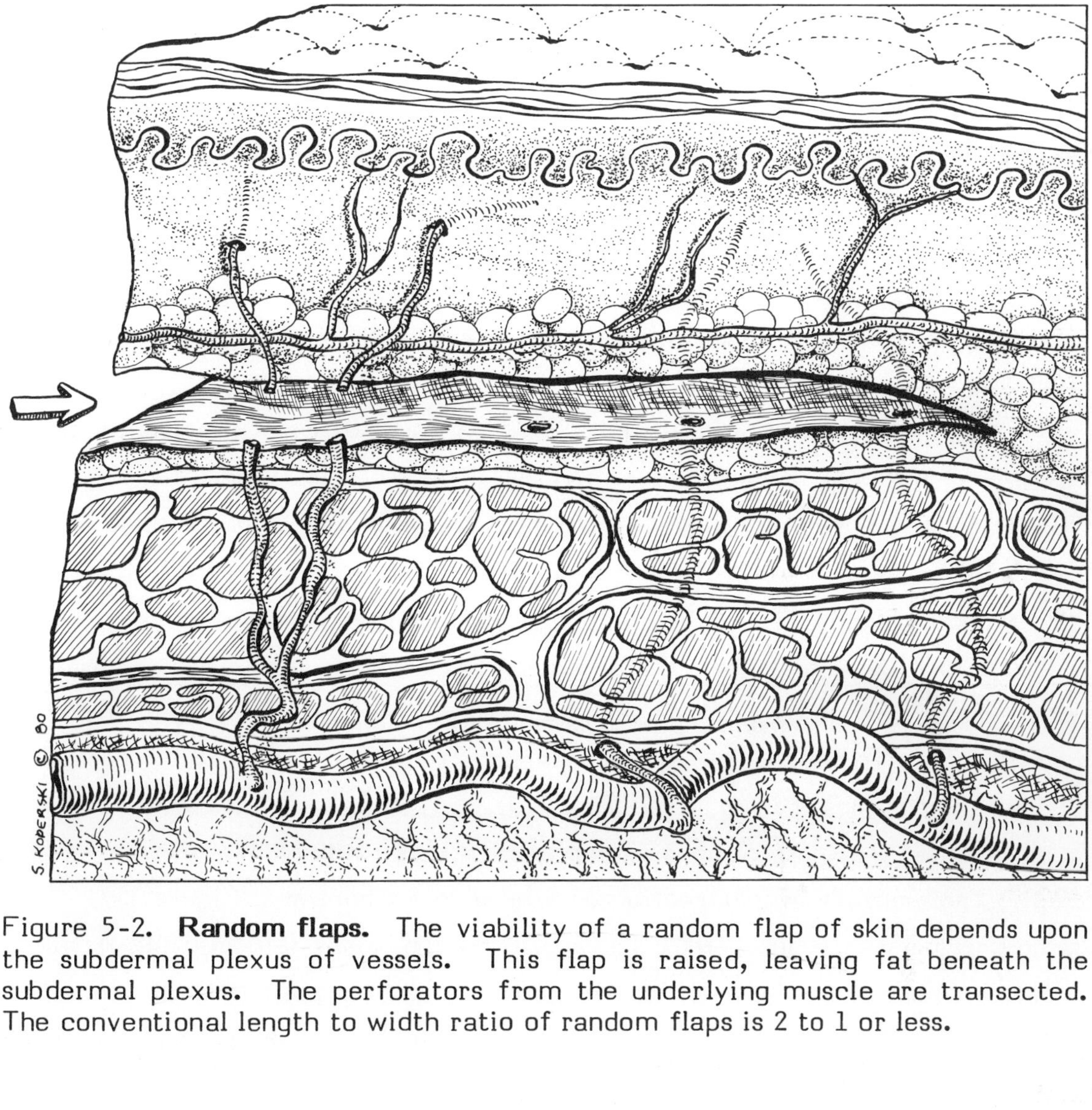

Figure 5-2. **Random flaps.** The viability of a random flap of skin depends upon the subdermal plexus of vessels. This flap is raised, leaving fat beneath the subdermal plexus. The perforators from the underlying muscle are transected. The conventional length to width ratio of random flaps is 2 to 1 or less.

It has long been observed that if a flap is elevated (i.e., surgically lifted) in several stages, greater flap length is possible than if a flap is elevated and transferred as a single procedure. A staged delay of the flap accomplishes two goals: it sympathectomizes the flap, dilating the blood vessel, and it orientates the blood flow along the long axis of the flap. The stimulus for this latter phenomenon is believed to be the period of ischemia following division of part of the blood supply; this phenomenon is at its maximum 10 days following a delay.

The most common type of random flap is the advancement flap which is used to close a simple wound. Here the wound edges are undermined and the attachments to the underlying fascia divided, permitting advancement of the tissue and approximation without tension. If undermining is not sufficient, tissue can be rotated in from the sides of the wound (rotation flap). This maneuver creates a donor site which may be closed primarily or skin grafted. A rotation flap is commonly used to close sacral pressure sores. Another example of a random flap is the bipedicle flap which is used to close a scalp defect or a trochanteric pressure ulcer. These flaps utilize a bipolar vascular system as opposed to the unipolar design of the other random flaps. There are other variations on the rotation flap theme, such as a sliding flap or interpolation flap, but basically they should all be thought of as random flaps and the descriptive subheadings are not important.

Local tissue is always preferred as a flap source because the color and texture of the skin match that of the defect. If local tissue is insufficient, however, random flaps can be transferred from other areas of the body. These distant flaps can be transferred either directly or in stages. An example of the direct transfer of a distant random flap is the cross-leg flap. A skin flap is raised on one leg and set into the defect on the opposite leg. The legs are held together for up to two weeks while the flap gains a new blood supply from the recipient leg. After that time, the attachment of the flap to the donor leg is divided and the legs are separated (Fig. 5-3).

One of the most famous examples of direct transfer of a distant random flap is Tagliacozzi's reconstruction of a nose (see Chapter 1, Figure 1-1). This famous Renaissance surgeon raised a flap on the upper arm, applied it to the nose, and maintained the position with a splint. During the period of immobilization, a new blood supply entered the flap from the recipient area. When this process was complete, the flap was divided. Hand injuries in which skin and soft tissue are lost can be covered directly with a flap from the groin or abdominal wall and the flap subsequently divided.

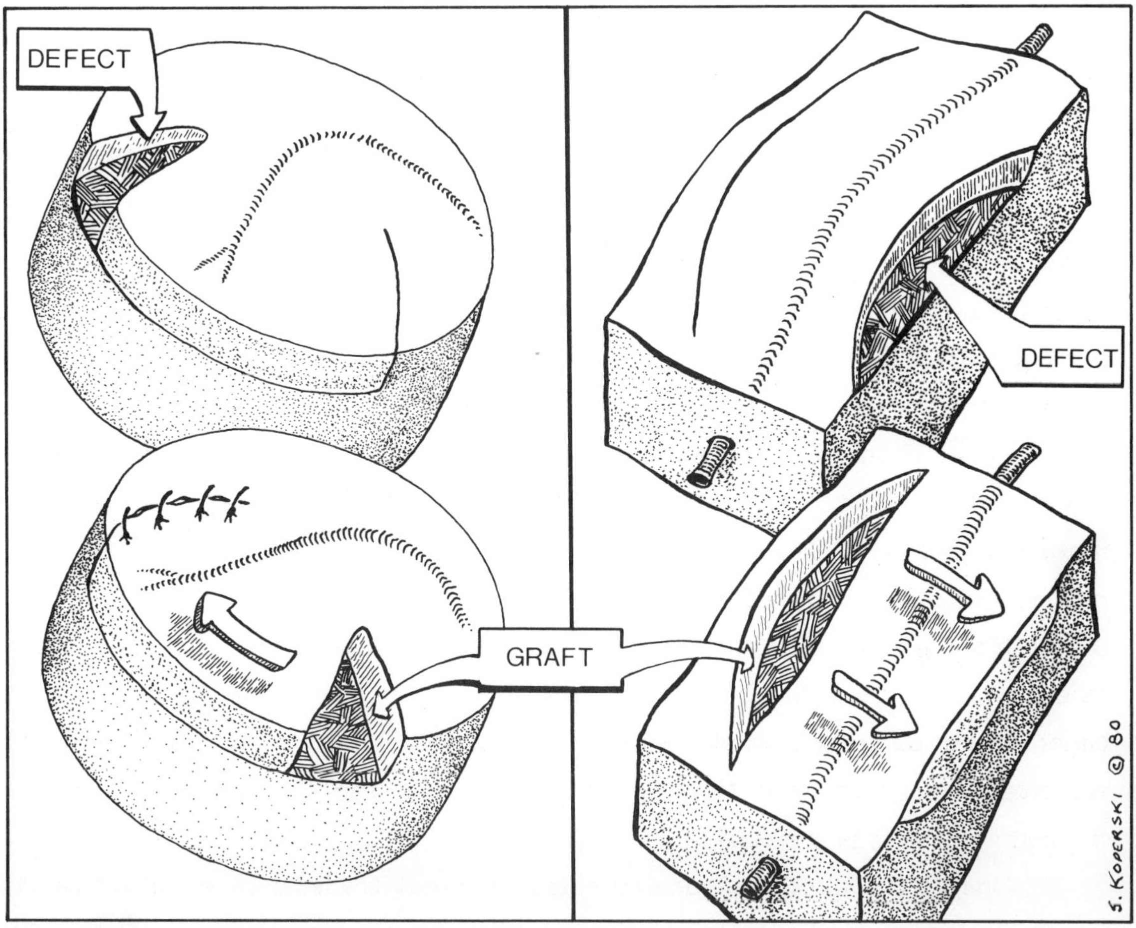

Figure 5-3. **Variations of the random flap.** A rotation flap depends upon one vascular pole (as illustrated by the striped line, left), whereas a bidpedical flap utilizes vessels at each end (right). (The arrows indicate the difference in direction of tissue shift in these two types of flaps.) Although the donor defects are usually grafted in the trunk area (bottom left, right), facial rotation flaps can frequently be closed without a graft.

Jump flaps are distant random flaps that are transferred in a series of staged procedures. They are rarely used today because of the length of time required for the reconstruction. Musculocutaneous flaps (described later in this chapter) generally are more useful. An example of a jump flap is a flap using the hand as a carrier to transplant tissue from one part of the body to another. Such a flap is elevated and placed on the wrist. After two weeks, the flap is severed from its original site and placed in the area to be covered. The flap will survive by means of the blood vessels that have grown into the flap from the wrist. When the new vasculature has entered the flap through the wound margins, the attachments to the wrist carrier can be transected (Fig. 5-4).

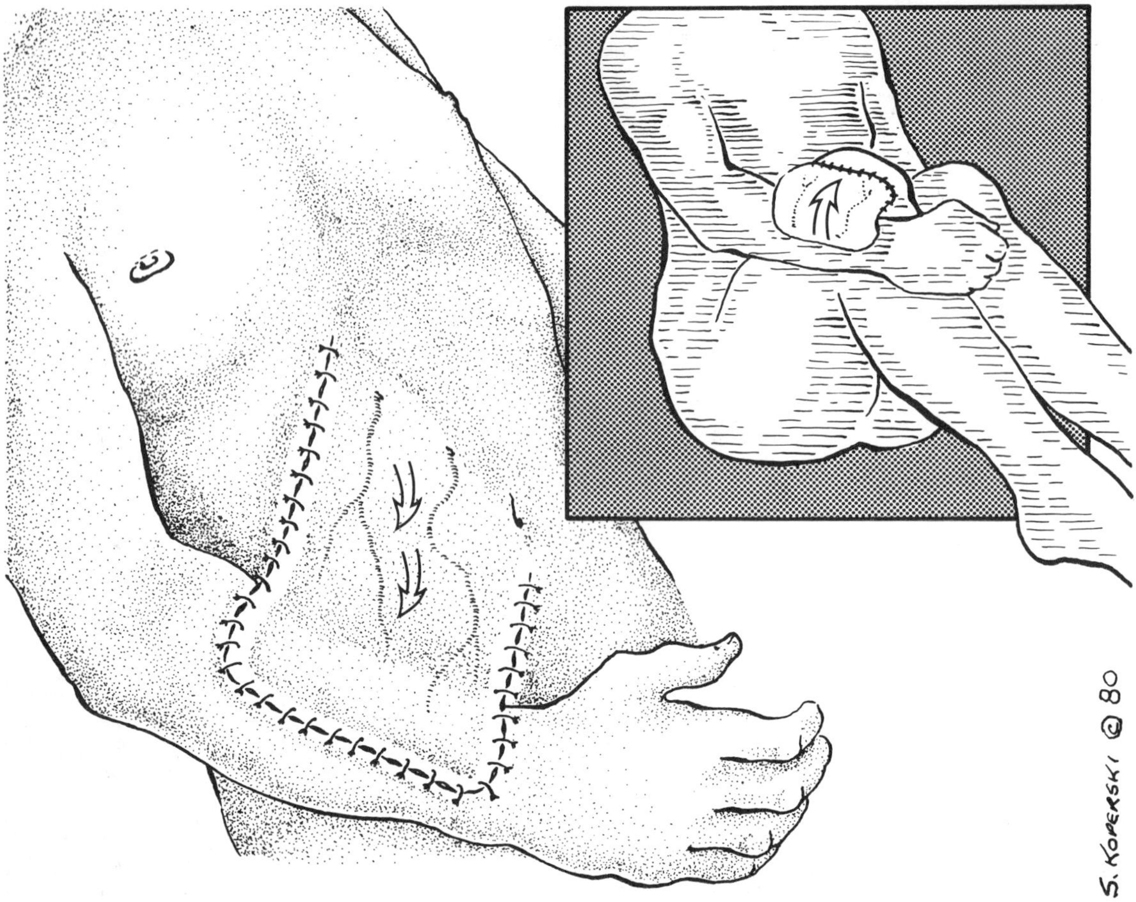

Figure 5-4. **Jump flap.** A jump flap relies upon an intermediary (in this case the patient's arm) for carrying the tissue from one site to another (in this case from the abdomen to the knee). It is important to note that the vascular supply will be entering the flap initially from the abdomen (arrow, left), but after transfer will enter the flap through the scar tissue from the wrist (arrow, right). After two weeks, the arm can be detached from the knee, and the flap will survive on the blood supply from the nose. These flaps, although less commonly utilized today because of the newer musculocutaneous flaps, are reliable in certain locations and can transfer large blocks of tissue rapidly.

Axial Flaps

As previously explained, axial flaps incorporate at least one identifiable artery and vein running the distance of the flap. These flaps can be much longer than random flaps and are not limited by the length to width ratio demanded of random flaps, but by the anatomy of the specific vascular supply. The size of an axial flap can be increased by adding a random flap to it and employing a delay procedure. An axial flap alone generally requires no delay (Fig. 5-5).

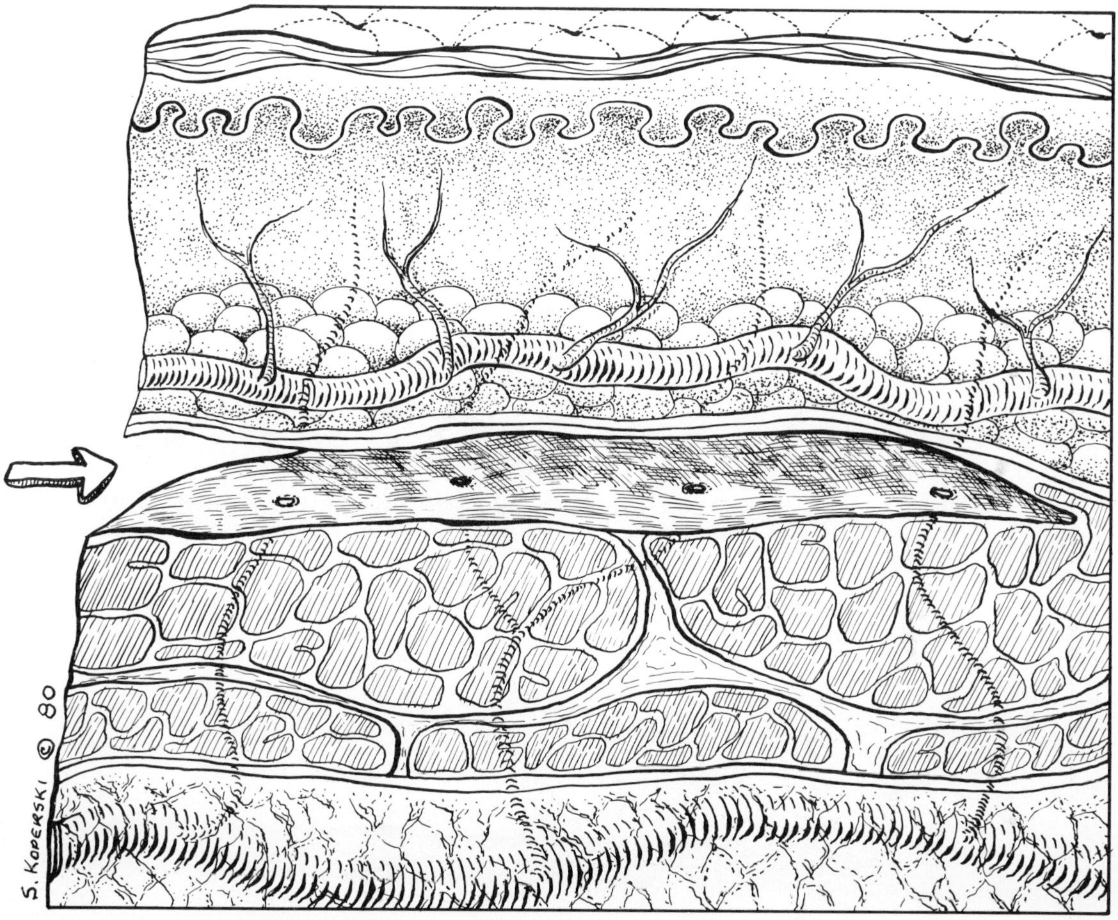

Figure 5-5. **Axial flap.** The axial flap differs from the random flap in that it contains a major, recognized arteriovenous system, such as the superficial temporal artery and vein just beneath the skin, in addition to the subdermal plexus. These flaps are usually raised at the level just beneath the fascia. In scalp wounds, this larger blood supply may allow a length to width ratio of up to 8 to 1, in some areas, without delay procedure.

There are a limited number of types of axial flaps. The best known are the forehead flap, utilizing the superficial temporal artery, and the groin flap which is supplied by the superficial circumflex iliac artery. Axial flaps will survive on their nutrient vascular pedicle alone. If the rest of the cutaneous attachments to the donor site are severed, an island flap results. Island flaps have a much greater arc of rotation because of the narrow pedicle (Fig. 5-6).

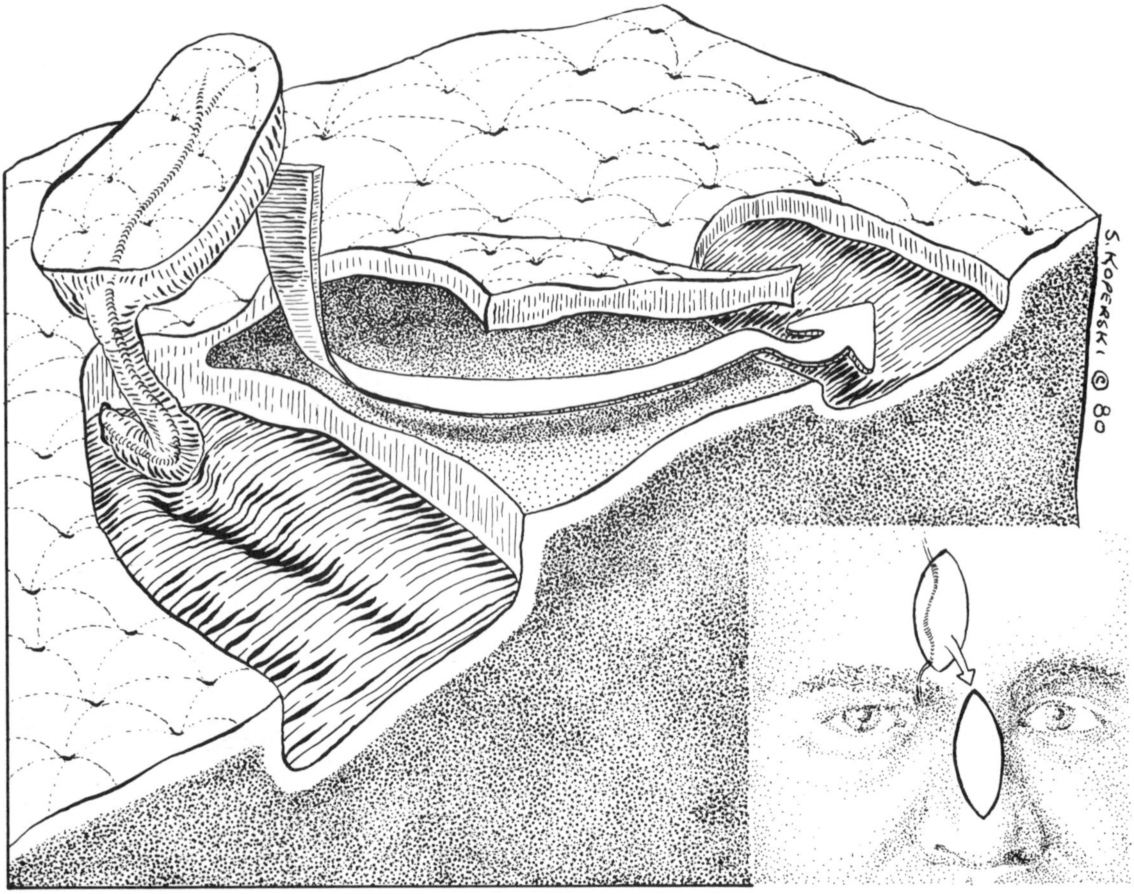

Figure 5-6. **Island flap.** An island flap is really a "peninsula" attached by an axial vessel which is moved subcutaneously. One of the most useful flaps is forehead to nose, utilizing the supraorbital and/or supratrochlear vessels (inset).

Musculocutaneous flaps employ the system of muscle-perforating vessels to sustain the skin portion of the flap. For years, surgeons complained about perforating arteries when working on skin flaps. It was not until the 1970s that reconstructive surgeons realized that the skin could reliably be transferred by utilizing the underlying musculature. The muscle can be isolated on its blood supply (in fact, a deep axial pattern) and rotated into a defect with or without the overlying skin attached. While there are only a few recognized types of axial skin flaps, there are a great number of musculocutaneous axial flaps available for clinical use (Fig. 5-7).

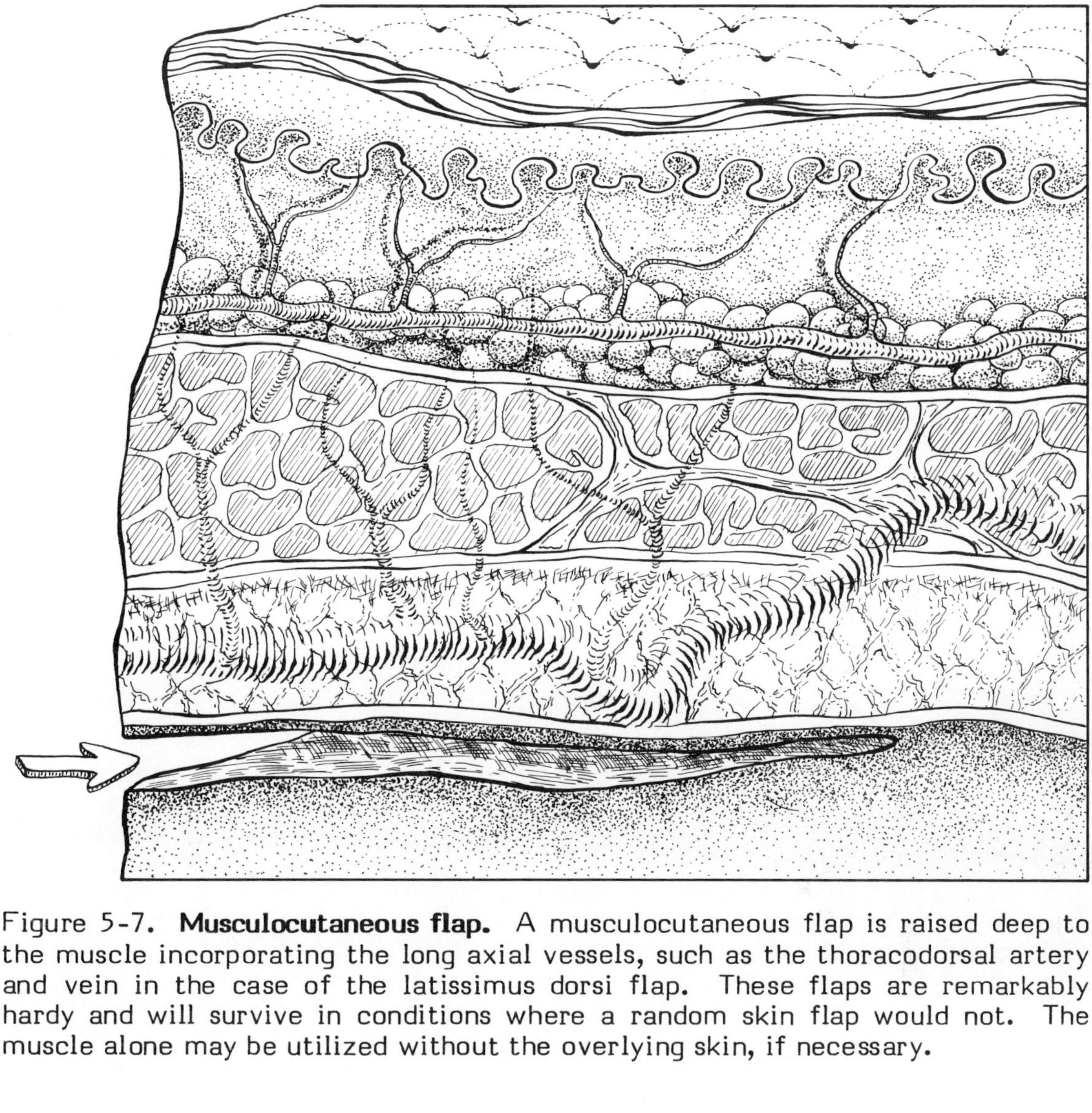

Figure 5-7. **Musculocutaneous flap.** A musculocutaneous flap is raised deep to the muscle incorporating the long axial vessels, such as the thoracodorsal artery and vein in the case of the latissimus dorsi flap. These flaps are remarkably hardy and will survive in conditions where a random skin flap would not. The muscle alone may be utilized without the overlying skin, if necessary.

The most useful musculocutaneous axial flaps have been those of the latissimus dorsi muscle utilized in breast reconstruction, the tensor fascia lata flap used for groin and buttock reconstruction, and the gracilis flap for perineal areas. The medial gastrocnemius flap has been used for wounds of the lower extremity, and the rectus femoris musculocutaneous flap has been used for abdominal reconstructions. These flaps are based on known neurovascular supply and are as reliable as axial pattern cutaneous flaps. With most of these reconstructions, there is little measurable functional deficit associated with muscle transfer.

Individual muscle axial flaps without the overlying skin can be used to close a wound. These muscle flaps can then be grafted with skin immediately. An example of this is the use of the gracilis muscle to reconstruct the perineum.

Free Flaps. These flaps are an exception to the strict definition of a flap as their blood supply is temporarily detached during transfer. They can be axial skin flaps or musculocutaneous axial flaps, and are promptly attached to a vessel in its new location by microsurgery (Fig. 5-8). Microvascular techniques have made it possible to transfer large blocks of tissue to axial vessels of from 0.5 to 2 mm in diameter with a high degree of success. The procedures are lengthy and require a surgical team with special training (see Chapter 16).

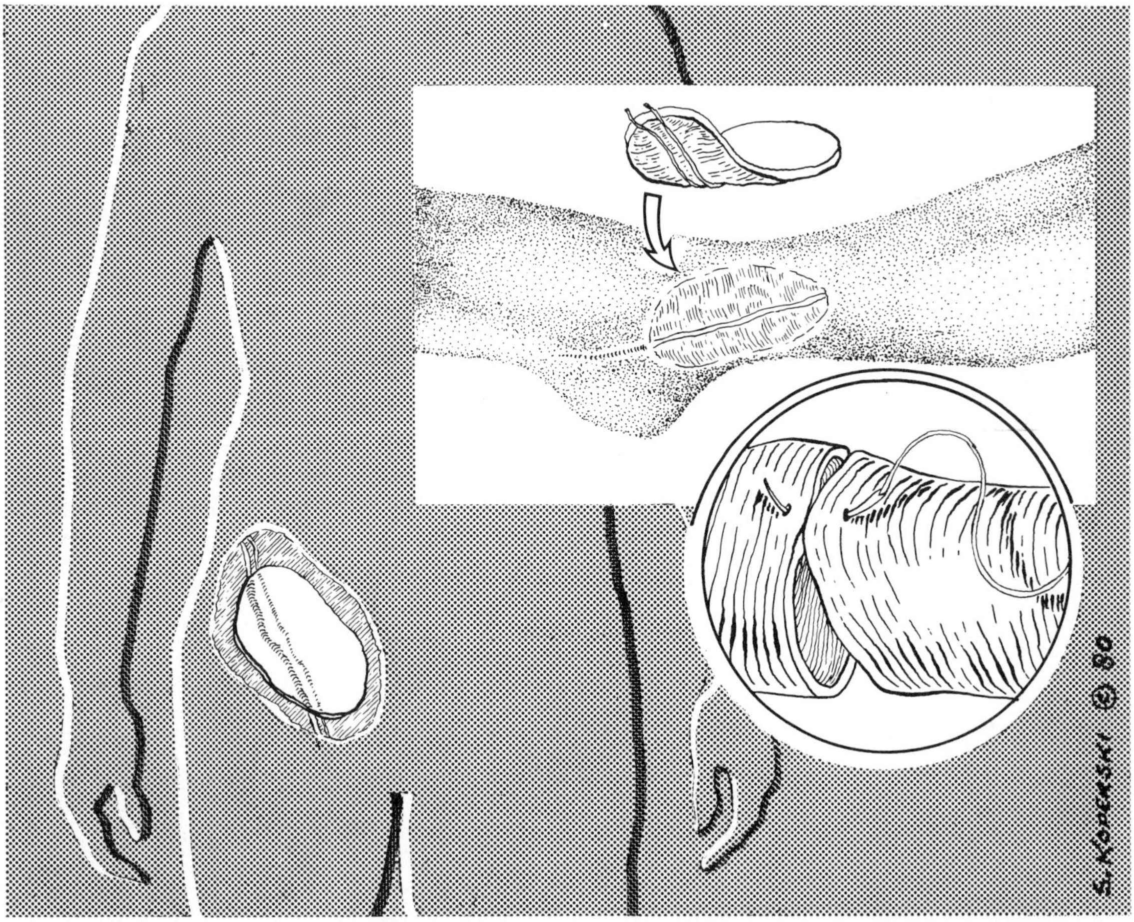

Figure 5-8. **Free flap.** A free flap transfers large blocks of tissue at a distance in one operation utilizing microsurgical anastomosis (circular inset). The groin flap utilizing the superficial circumflex iliac artery and vein (torso) is one example. In this case, the groin free flap is anastomosed to the anterior tibial artery (rectangular inset). The donor site can often be closed without a skin graft.

Any axial skin flap or musculocutaneous flap with a suitable nutrient artery can be used as a free flap. A free flap is most commonly used when other forms of reconstruction are not possible. For example, if a standard musculocutaneous flap, such as the gastrocnemius and soleus, may not sufficiently cover the defect, a free flap may be indicated. This is especially true if the patient is obese or is middle-aged, as a cross-leg flap can be hazardous because of the possibility of thrombophlebitis or pulmonary embolus. In this circumstance, a free flap may be the only way to salvage the extremity. Free flaps and myocutaneous flaps are developments of the 1970s and have dramatically increased reconstructive options. The older skin flaps are not without their usefulness, but their applications are less frequent today.

Grafts

In contradistinction to a flap, a graft is a section of tissue that has been detached from its blood supply during transfer and, therefore, must depend entirely upon the recipient area for its nourishment. Almost any type of tissue can be used for a graft and can even be taken from other species.

Grafts, like flaps, can be classified in various ways. The broadest classification is based upon the graft source. An autograft is a graft from the same individual. An allograft is a graft from a different individual of the same species (for example, a graft from mother to son). A xenograft is a graft from one species to another. Although in immune-deficient individuals allografts and xenografts may take and survive temporarily until the immune system recovers, the permanent take of a graft can only occur with an autograft or, in the case of identical twins, an allograft.

Skin Grafts

The most common form of graft is a skin graft. This may be a full thickness skin graft (FTSG), in which case it includes the epidermis and the entire dermis with its skin appendages, or it may be a split thickness skin graft (STSG). The latter includes the epidermis and only part of the dermis. STSGs are divided into thick and thin split thickness grafts depending upon whether they are taken from the reticular (thick) or papillary (thin) dermis (Fig. 5-9).

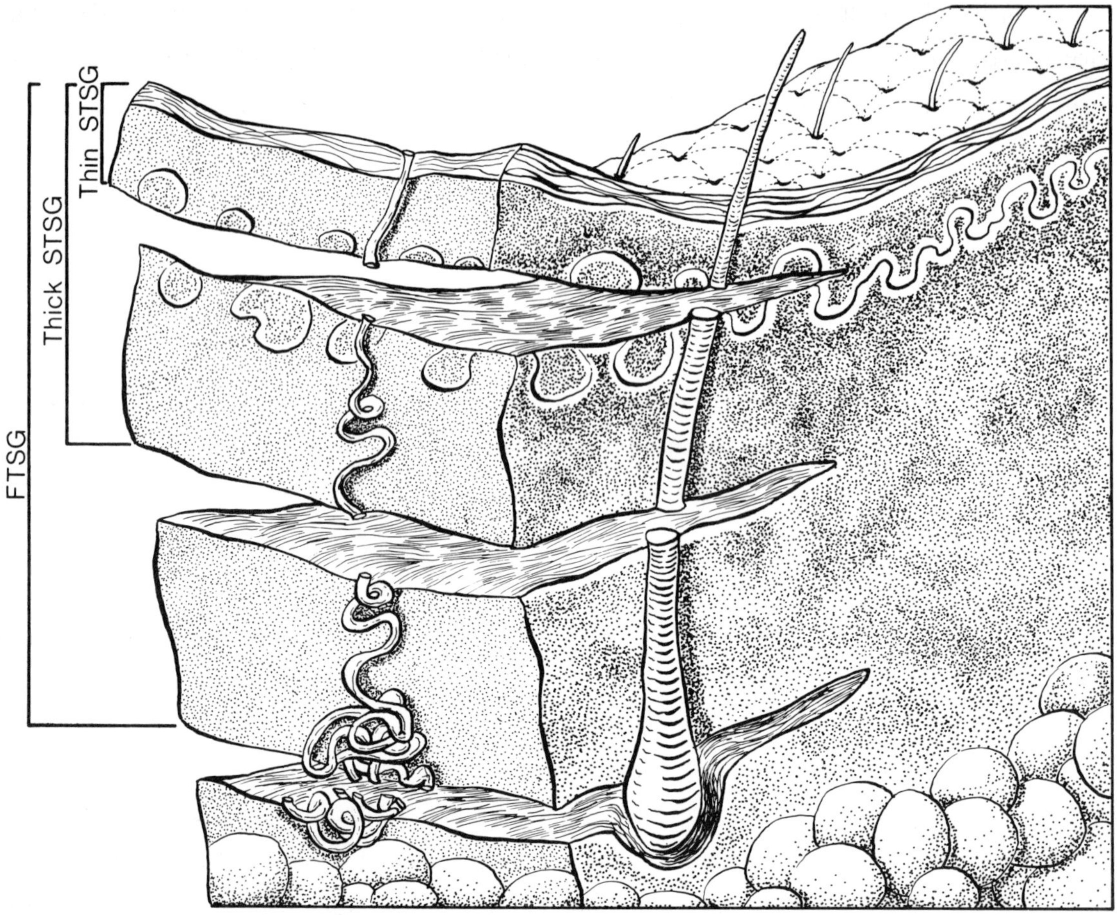

Figure 5-9. **Thin split, thick split and full thickness grafts.** Note that FTSGs transplant sweat glands and hair roots, whereas the STSGs do not. Donor sites for split thickness grafts will therefore epithelize, whereas donor sites for full thickness grafts require surgical closure because of the absence of these appendages.

Basically, the thicker the graft the better the result both cosmetically and functionally, because the surgeon is replacing more accurately what was lost. Obviously, FTSGs best fit this qualification. Also thick skin contracts less and gives a better color match. However, the size of the required graft will determine the availability of full thickness skin as this donor site must be closed, whereas the STSG donor site epithelizes from the remaining skin appendages.

The best donor areas for FTSGs, because they are readily closed, are the upper eyelids, the area behind the ear, and the groin. Grafts from behind the ear or from the supraclavicular area are best for use on the face because of the better color match.

Split thickness skin is more readily available since the donor site heals spontaneously and, if the harvested skin is thin, the same donor site can be used repeatedly. These grafts are commonly used to close burn wounds. The area to be covered can be increased by meshing the graft for expansion. In this manner, a drum of skin 4 in x 8 in can be used to cover two to three times that area. Expanded grafts have holes which epithelize quickly from the edges of the mesh, but healing leaves a patch-like scar. Because there is less tissue to revascularize, thin skin grafts have a more reliable take than thicker grafts.

The donor sites of STSGs leave a scar, and it is best to hide them, when possible, in an area such as the buttock, hip, lower abdomen or other areas which would be covered by a bathing suit. The anterior thigh is a more comfortable donor area, but it is best reserved for older patients who may not be as concerned about the subsequent scar. The donor sites must be protected from infection. If they are not, they can convert to a full thickness defect. Donor sites are treated with topical dressings like second-degree burns.

Skin Graft Survival. Skin grafts begin survival immediately after placement by absorption of nutrients and fluids from the recipient bed. This process of nourishment is called plasmatic circulation. Following this, there is an anastomosis, called inosculation, between host and graft blood vessels. After three to four days, the graft assumes a pinkish hue indicating revascularization (Fig. 5-10).

Anything that separates the graft from the recipient bed will interfere with the take of the graft. Most commonly, this physical barrier consists of a hematoma. Pressure placed on a skin graft while it is healing prevents anything from disrupting contact with the host bed. Less commonly, infection may cause skin graft loss, particularly a streptococcal infection with its destructive enzymes. Other bacteria rarely interfere with a graft take since the graft itself is bacteriostatic. Occasionally, the surgeon may find it beneficial to take advantage of this bacteriostatic action by applying a xenograft to help clean up a burn wound prior to final grafting.

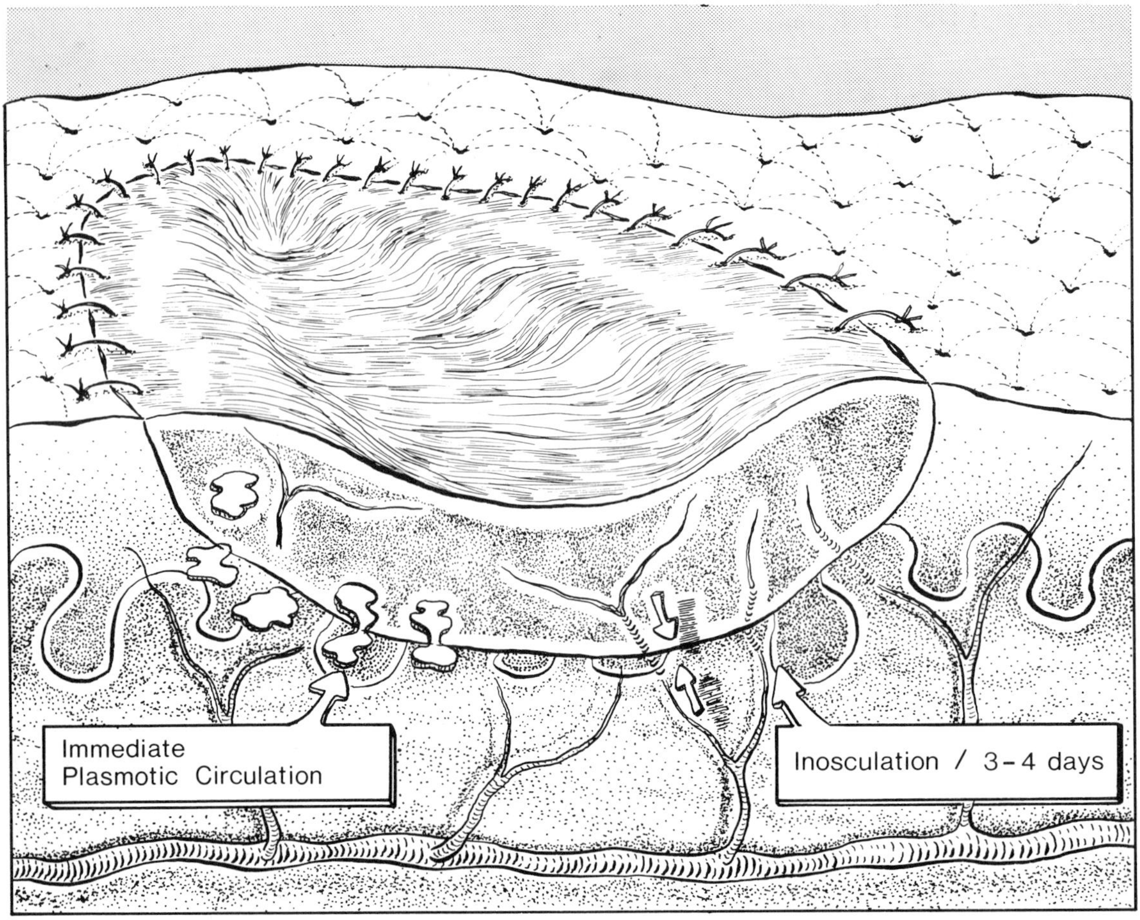

Figure 5-10. **Skin graft survival.** A graft of skin survives initially by plasmotic circulation. However, it should be noted that skin will live by itself for several days if cooled and kept in a sterile moist environment. The vessels in the bed of the wound spontaneously anastomose with existing vessels in the graft within three to four days. This is called inosculation. If a graft is separated from the recipient bed by a hematoma, the graft will not survive because of the blockage of this revascularization.

Composite Grafts

A composite graft is a graft of two or more tissues such as a graft of dermis and fat used to fill a contour defect under intact skin. When using a dermal fat graft, the surgeon removes the epidermis from the donor site and places the dermis and fat in a subcutaneous pocket at the graft site. The fat is revascularized through the dermis and provides bulk for filling the defect. A composite graft of intact skin and cartilage is used to fill small defects on the ear or the rim of the nose. These grafts cannot generally be larger than 1 cm square because the center will not then vascularize. For such grafts, the typical donor site is the ear lobe.

Other Grafts

Most tissues, including blood vessels, nerves and whole organs such as the kidney, can be used as grafts. Cartilage grafts are useful for contour defects such as defects of the nasal dorsum or chin. The donor site is commonly the nasal septum or the rib. Rib cartilage can also be used for rebuilding an ear.

Bone grafts, too, can be used for contour defects and also to provide fusion in fractures. Onlay bone grafts are employed to fill out facial contours, to provide stability in craniofacial surgery, and for cosmetic repair of facial fractures. Bone grafts are commonly taken from ribs or from the iliac crest.

The palmaris longus tendon provides a donor site for replacing injured finger tendons. Removing the tendon leaves no functional deficit. The plantaris tendon in the leg is another potential donor site for hand reconstruction.

Flaps vs. Grafts

The anatomical replacement of a lost or damaged part with minimal scarring and morbidity is the goal of wound closure. Whenever more extensive procedures are required, scar morbidity is added; therefore, the simplest procedure consistent with proper wound care should always be selected. Closing a laceration by undermining and advancing tissue, in essence a flap technique, is an example of this concept in its purest form. Flaps are preferable to grafts because they provide thicker tissue. For this same reason, FTSGs are preferable to STSGs.

Flaps are used to fill deeper defects, to provide contour, or to establish a new blood supply to damaged tissue. They are necessary to cover bone, tendon, or prosthetic material. Flaps are also indicated where there is radiation injury. In such wounds, there is a progressive thickening of the blood vessel walls and eventual ulceration from devascularization. These wounds cannot be grafted with skin due to the poor vascular supply. Flaps bringing their own rich blood supplies are required for closure.

Summary

Early closure of most wounds reduces morbidity. Closure without tension is the key to preventing devascularization, a condition which often leads to infection and scarring. If a wound cannot be closed directly, tissue is added either by a local or distant graft or flap. A flap provides better coverage as it is thicker, contracts less, and has a more normal appearance. If a graft is used, a full thickness graft is preferred, donor site permitting, because it has better color match, contracts less, and provides hair follicles and sweat glands.

CHAPTER 6

Wound Healing

The result of injury and subsequent wound healing is a scar. Factors that influence the process of wound healing also influence the final physical appearance of the scar. Plastic surgeons are often consulted about wounds that fail to heal or that have healed with noticeable deformity. It is essential that the physician be aware of the basic events in wound healing and the factors that can influence them.

Stages of Wound Healing

The wound heals by means of a series of vascular and cellular events culminating in the formation of collagen which provides the tensile strength of the scar tissue. These events can be separated into four stages: (1) vascular, (2) epithelial, (3) dermal, and (4) maturation. Stages 3 and 4 are associated with collagen formation. The vascular stage represents the initial response to the injury and occurs within seconds of its inception. The epithelial stage begins in 24 to 48 hours. The dermal stage commences after 5 to 7 days, with the maturation stage beginning 15 days after onset of injury and continuing for as long as 18 months.

These four stages are identifiable in all wounds but differ in intensity, depending upon the type of wound closure employed. A wound that is closed primarily will heal by normal collagen deposition and with minimal epithelization and minimal contraction. By comparison, a wound closed by secondary intention requires a similar amount of collagen deposition but requires greater epithelization and wound contracture to seal the surface. These events are common to the healing of all body tissues, but they proceed more rapidly in the healing of skin than they do in the healing of bone or tendon.

Vascular Stage

Following injury, the local vascular bed responds with immediate vasoconstriction followed within seconds by vasodilatation. Circulating leukocytes adhere to the vessel wall, diapedese through the basement membrane, and enter the interstitial space where they phagocytose debris and bacteria. The vascular response and subsequent separation of the endothelium are caused by histamine, serotin, kinins, leucotoxins and norepinephrine (Fig. 6-1).

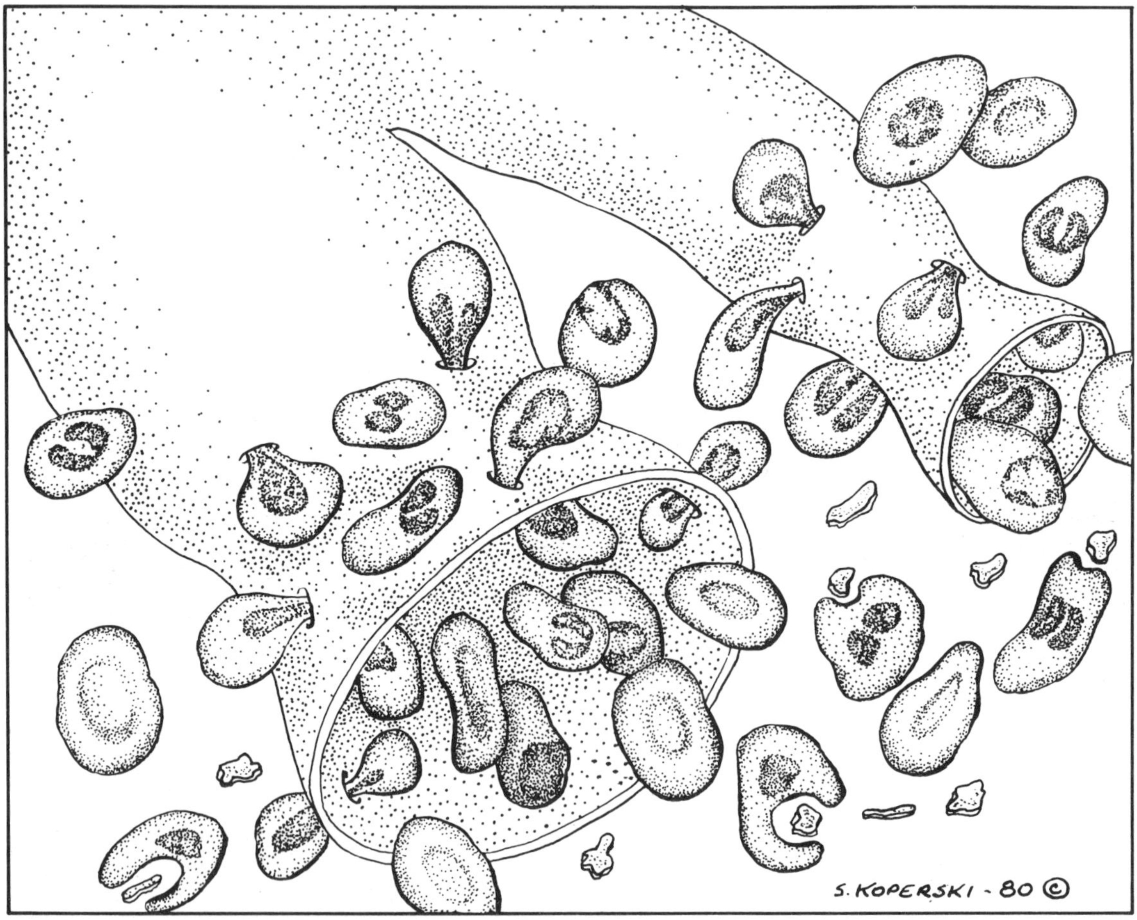

Figure 6-1. **White cells enter interstitial space by two routes: leakage from cut end of vessel or by diapedesis through vessel wall.** The cut end of the vessel quickly seals by spasm or clot, leaving diapedesis as the main route through which phagocytes enter.

Plasma coagulation factors and fibrinogen enter the wound through the injured blood vessels. Coagulation is initiated in large measure by platelet agglutination. The normal vascular endothelium is nonthrombogenic, but when it is injured the subendothelial collagen is exposed, causing the platelets to adhere. Within minutes, a fibrin mesh is formed at the cut end of the vessel. This fibrin screen attracts more platelets, and their developing pseudopods contract the fibrin mesh to form a firmer plug, sealing the end of the blood vessel. The resultant fibrin mesh contributes to wound healing by providing a trellis which guides the proliferating fibroblasts and capillary buds into the wound (Fig. 6-2).

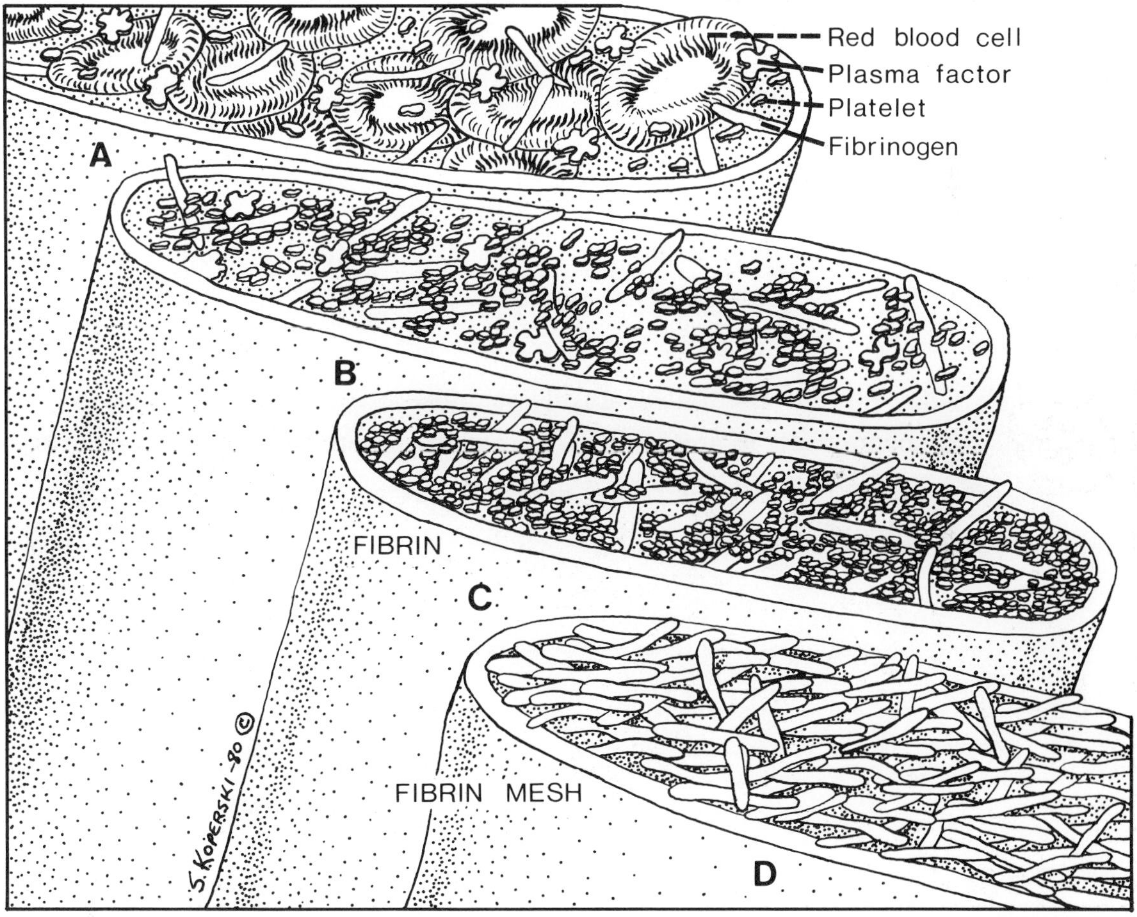

Figure 6-2. **Steps in clotting.** Damage to the vessel endothelium initiates the clot mechanism (A). Platelets become more adherent to the vessel wall and to each other (B). Fibrinogen converts to fibrin within minutes (C) and fibrin forms a screen which attracts more platelets forming the fibrin clot (D).

Epithelial Stage

In normal skin, low levels of mitotic activity occur in the basal layer of the epidermis at rest when basal epinephrine and glucocorticoid levels are low. In response to injury, however, the basalar cells of the dermis within 2 mm of the injury site increase their mitosis rate up to 40 times the normal. This mitotic activity spreads from the basalar layer to the stratum spongiosum. The stimulus for this increased activity may be as slight as the removal of a piece of adhesive tape from the skin.

Two chemical agents produced by the epidermal cells influence this response: chalones and collagenase. Chalones are produced by the outer layer of the epidermis and serve to inhibit basalar mitoses. When these outer cells are lost through injury, the inhibitory factor is absent and mitotic levels increase. Epidermal collagenase regulates the amount of dermal collagen present by breaking down immature collagen as new collagen is produced. Injury causes the release of collagenase which also serves to facilitate migration of new epidermal cells from the wound edge.

Aided by the wound collagenase, sheets of epidermal cells at the wound margin migrate into the depths of the wound. Using the fibrin mesh trellis as a guide, a ring of epidermal cells converges toward the center of the wound beneath the fibrin clot. This migration, led by cells within a ruffled membrane, ceases only upon contact inhibition. This occurs when the leading cells are completely surrounded by neighboring epidermal cells. Contact inhibition then returns the mitotic rate to normal (Fig. 6-3).

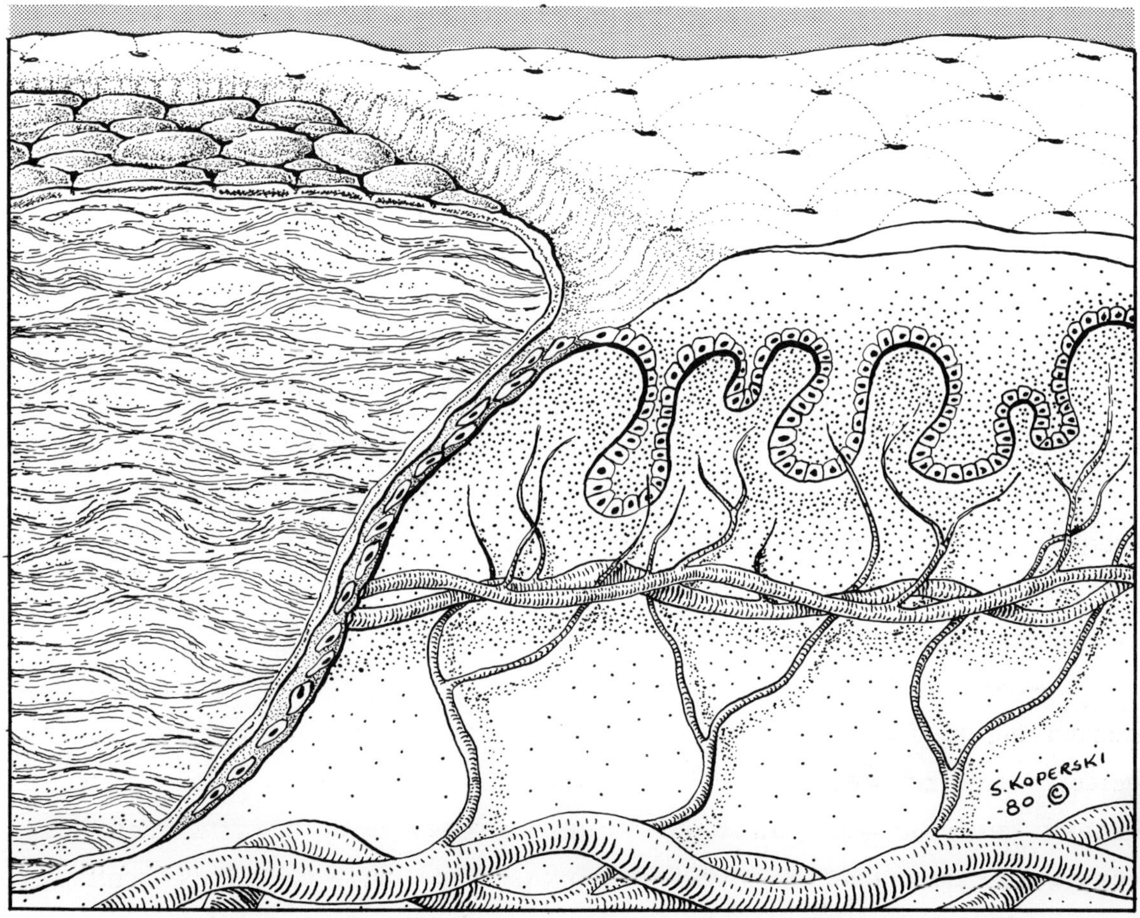

Figure 6-3. **Sheets of epidermal cells migrate from wound edges beneath clot.** This process begins in 24 to 48 hours and ceases only upon contact inhibition. It seals the wound but provides little tensile strength.

It is presumed that the sheets of epidermal cells follow this deep course to avoid dehydration. Clinically, it is known that wounds kept moist epithelize more rapidly. Topical scarlet red ointment increases the basal mitosis rate and hence epithelization. Some investigators believe that topical vitamin A increases epithelization as well.

The process of epithelization can close a clean incised wound in 48 to 72 hours, but epithelization provides little tensile strength. These healed wounds are fragile, and the thin epithelial layer is easily disrupted by minor trauma. In addition, this type of coverage possesses no potential for sweat or sebaceous activity because there is no dermis.

From the clinical point of view, this means that suture tracks can epithelize very rapidly, leaving small cysts or tunnels, especially in certain areas including the face. A subcuticular suture does not always prevent this because the suture may pierce the basilar layer of the epidermis without surfacing, causing small cysts. This is especially true in the case of the eyelid (Fig. 6-4).

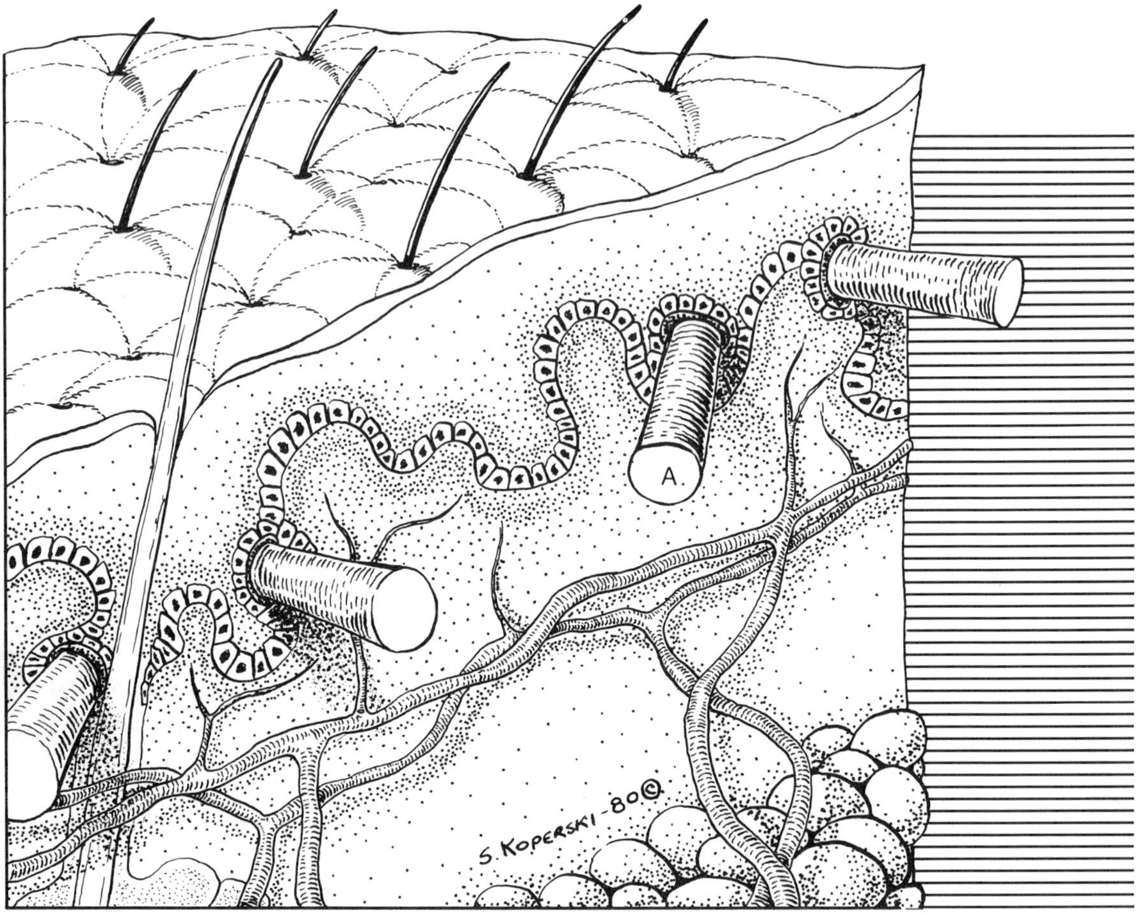

Figure 6-4. **Cyst formation.** Even subcuticular sutures (A) may cause cysts when they pierce epithelial structures such as rete pegs. In such a case, mitosis of the epidermal cell is stimulated and, if the suture is left in place for two to four days, epithelial tunnels may develop around it.

Dermal Stage

The onset of the dermal stage is marked by the production of new collagen. Collagen is what holds us together and what contributes strength to wound tissue. It is produced by a variety of cells, including epidermal and smooth muscle cells, but the tensile strength of a wound comes from the collagen produced by fibroblasts of the dermis.

Five distinct types of collagen have been identified. Types I and III are the most important of these. Type I is found in rigid structures such as bone which has 100 percent type I collagen. Type III is distensible and is present in blood vessels, which include 65 percent type III and 35 percent type I collagen.

Youthful skin is made up of 80 percent type I collagen and 20 percent type III collagen. As skin ages, however, the percentage composition of type III collagen increases dramatically. This helps explain the increased distensibility of aging skin. The extremely distensible skin of Ehlers-Danlos syndrome is composed mainly of type III collagen.

Dermal collagen is a macromolecular protein composed of three polypeptide chains in a helical configuration. The molecule is 3,000 angstroms (Å) long and has a molecular weight of 3 million daltons (D). Each chain is composed of more than 1,000 amino acids held together by covalent bonds. Cross linkages between amino acid chains result in the fiber formation which gives collagen its strength. These fibers align with each other every 640 Å. This occurs under the influence of adenosine triphosphate (ATP), given the proper temperature and pH.

A 1 mm fiber of mature collagen can support up to 40 kg. The tensile strength of a wound increases rapidly at the end of a week and peaks at 42 days (Fig. 6-5). It has been postulated that human beings contain one long chain of collagen arranged in coils. Intact collagen can stretch by uncoiling, but after certain physical limits are reached further expansion can only occur by rupture of the coil. A clinical example of this is seen in the stretch marks left by the rapidly expanding skin of pregnancy. These marks represent scars from the rupture of dermal collagen (Fig. 6-6).

Collagen is synthesized by locally recruited, undifferentiated mesenchymal cells which are modified into fibroblasts. These fibroblasts appear in the wound three days following injury. They migrate over the fibrin trellis, using their ruffled membranes to contact other fibroblasts. They may pause or move off in another direction until eventually they are surrounded on all sides by other fibroblasts. (This action is similar to that described earlier for epidermal cells.) At this time motion ceases, and in about five or six days the cells have begun to synthesize collagen.

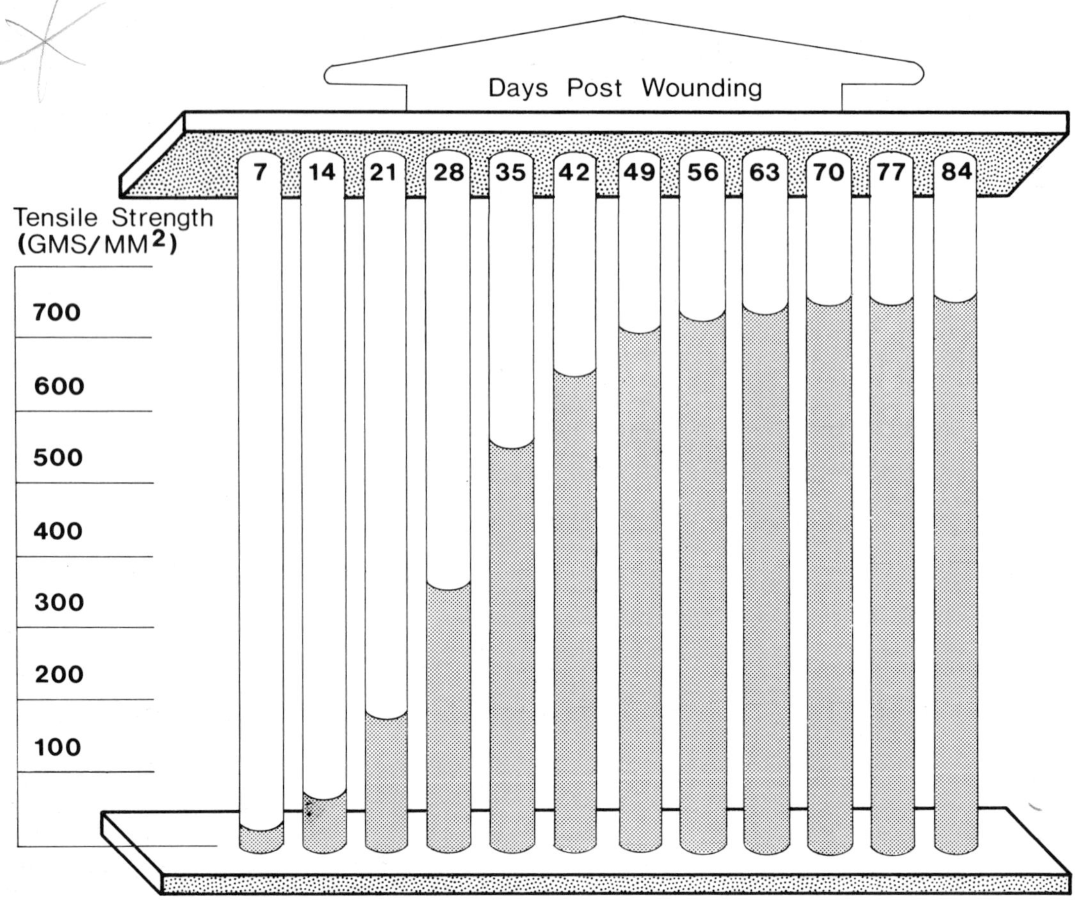

Figure 6-5. **Tensile strength development.** Although it begins to develop at seven days after wounding, tensile strength essentially reaches its peak at 49 days after wounding. Tensile strength is the result of cross linkages of collagen.

Classical studies of wound tensile strength have demonstrated that the wound does not increase in strength for about seven days following wounding. This delay, known as the lag phase, is a period of quiescence preceding collagen synthesis. It is now known that, during this interval, changes are taking place in the composition of the mucopolysaccharides and protein polysaccharides of the ground substance. While the precise nature of these changes is not known, it is believed that the proper biochemical environment is being created in the substrate at this time in order to ensure the orderly manufacture and orientation of new collagen fibers. This period of metabolic activity, prior to collagen elaboration, is now called the substrate phase.

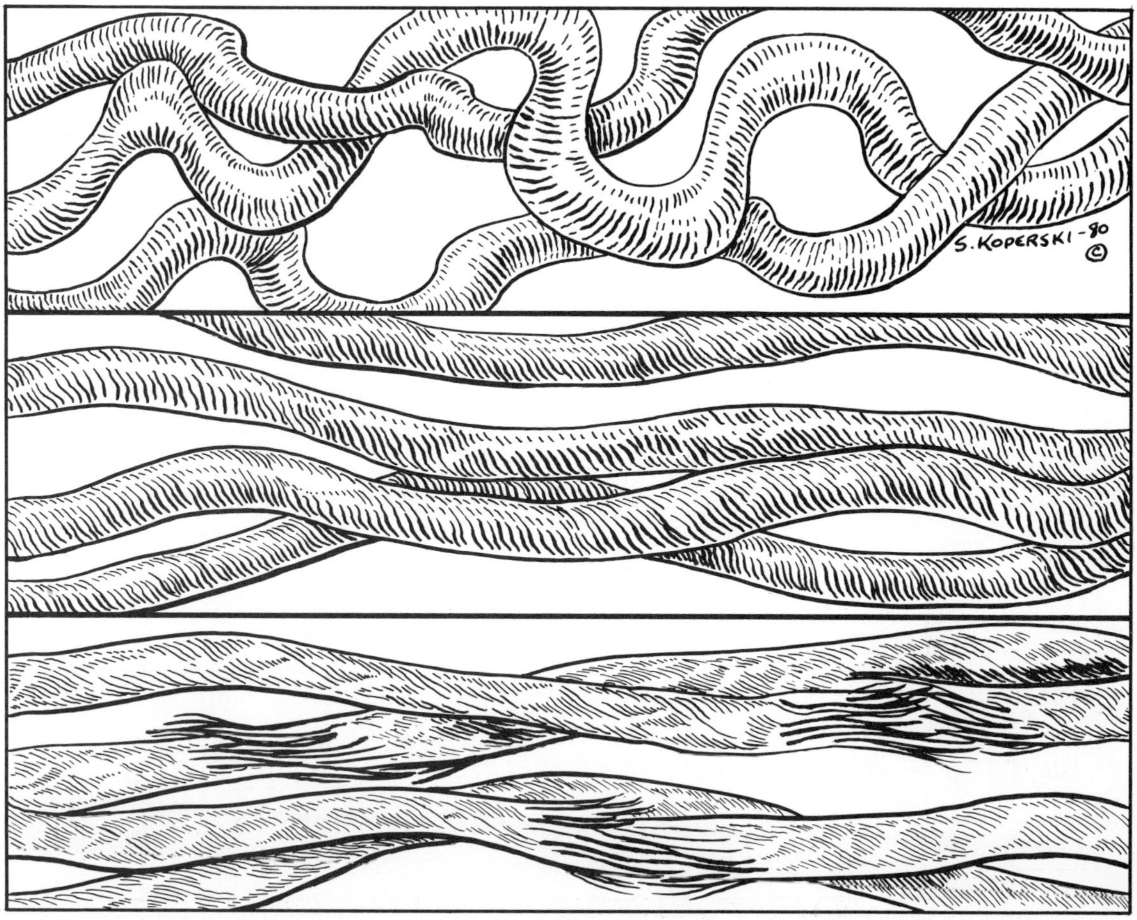

Figure 6-6. **Collagen can be subjected to only limited strain.** It has been likened to a continuous, coiled ball of yarn (top). It can stretch to a certain extent (center), but beyond those limits, further expansion can only occur through rupture of the fibers (bottom).

Phases of Collagen Synthesis (Table 6-1). Collagen synthesis is developed in two phases: intracellular and extracellular.

The intracellular phase begins within the fibroblast nucleus. Large molecules of ribonucleic acid (RNA) are synthesized from desoxyribonucleic acid (DNA) and secreted from the nucleus into the cytoplasm as messenger RNA. With the messenger RNA as the template, long amino acid chains are synthesized at the ribosome complexes by the sequential addition of amino acids from the cytoplasm. Three alpha chains associate in a loose triple helix, while these molecules are still within the fibroblast, to form protocollagen (Fig. 6-7).

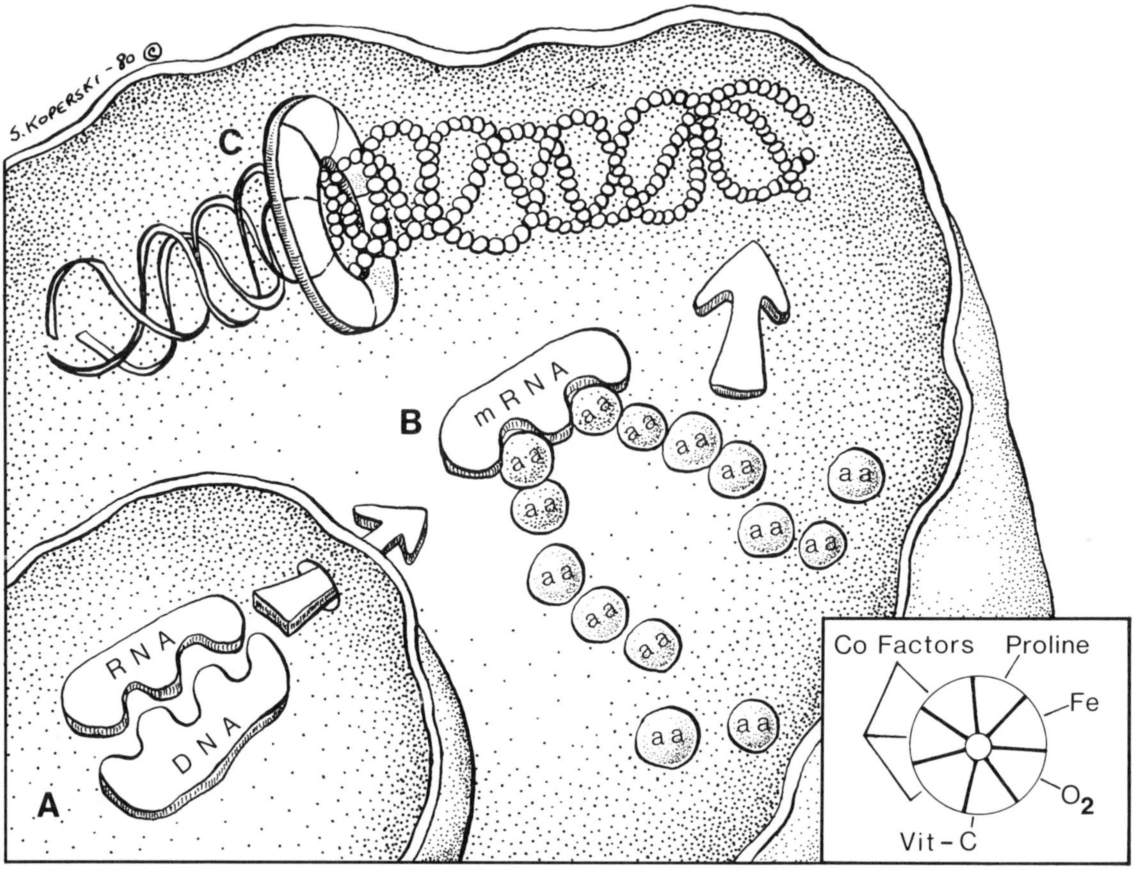

Figure 6-7. **Collagen formation begins in the fibroblast nucleus.** The intracellular formation of collagen begins in the nucleus with the formation of messenger RNA from DNA (A). After extrusion to the cytoplasm, messenger RNA (B) functions as a template for the association of the amino acids to produce protocollagen (C). The necessary cofactors for this intracellular reaction are shown in the inset.

Protocollagen must be modified, prior to extrusion from the cell, by the hydroxylation of proline and lysine amino acid radicals. Protocollagen, proline, and lysine hydroxylases, as well as several cofactors including ascorbic acid, alpha-ketoglutorate, iron, and oxygen, play a role in this modification. Scurvy, a disease caused by a deficiency of vitamin C, results in immature, unhydroxylated protocollagen which lacks tensile strength.

Table 6-1. Collagen Metabolism Synthesis

DERMAL STAGE		MATURATION STAGE
Intracellular Phase	Extracellular Phase (cross linkage formation)	(remodeling)
Requires:	Requires:	Requires:
Ascorbic acid Iron Ketoglutarate Protein Oxygen	Monoamine oxidase for oxidative deamination of lysine	pH Temperature ATP Diminished rate of collagen production

The extracellular phase begins when hydroxylated protocollagen, now called tropocollagen, is extruded into the extracellular space by the microtubules of the cell membrane. Tropocollagen is water soluble. Covalent bonds must be formed between adjacent helixes before mature, water insoluble collagen fibers are formed. These stable cross linkages require removal of several terminal amino acid groups by monoamine oxidase which deaminates lysine. Several factors can influence the creation of stable cross linkages between tropocollagen molecules. Beta-aminoproprionitrile (BAPN) and penicillamine combine with moniamine oxidase preventing its action. The presence of BAPN results in a state called lathyrism in which there are no cross-linked collagen fibers, leading to ruptured blood vessels and viscera. Unstable cross linkages can also be traced to a copper deficiency (Fig. 6-8).

As cross linkages are formed, tensile strength and burst strength of the wound increase. Development continues until the 17th to 21st day when a tensile strength of 120 to 180 g per square millimeter has been reached. During this period, while the wound continues to be metabolically active, the maturation stage commences.

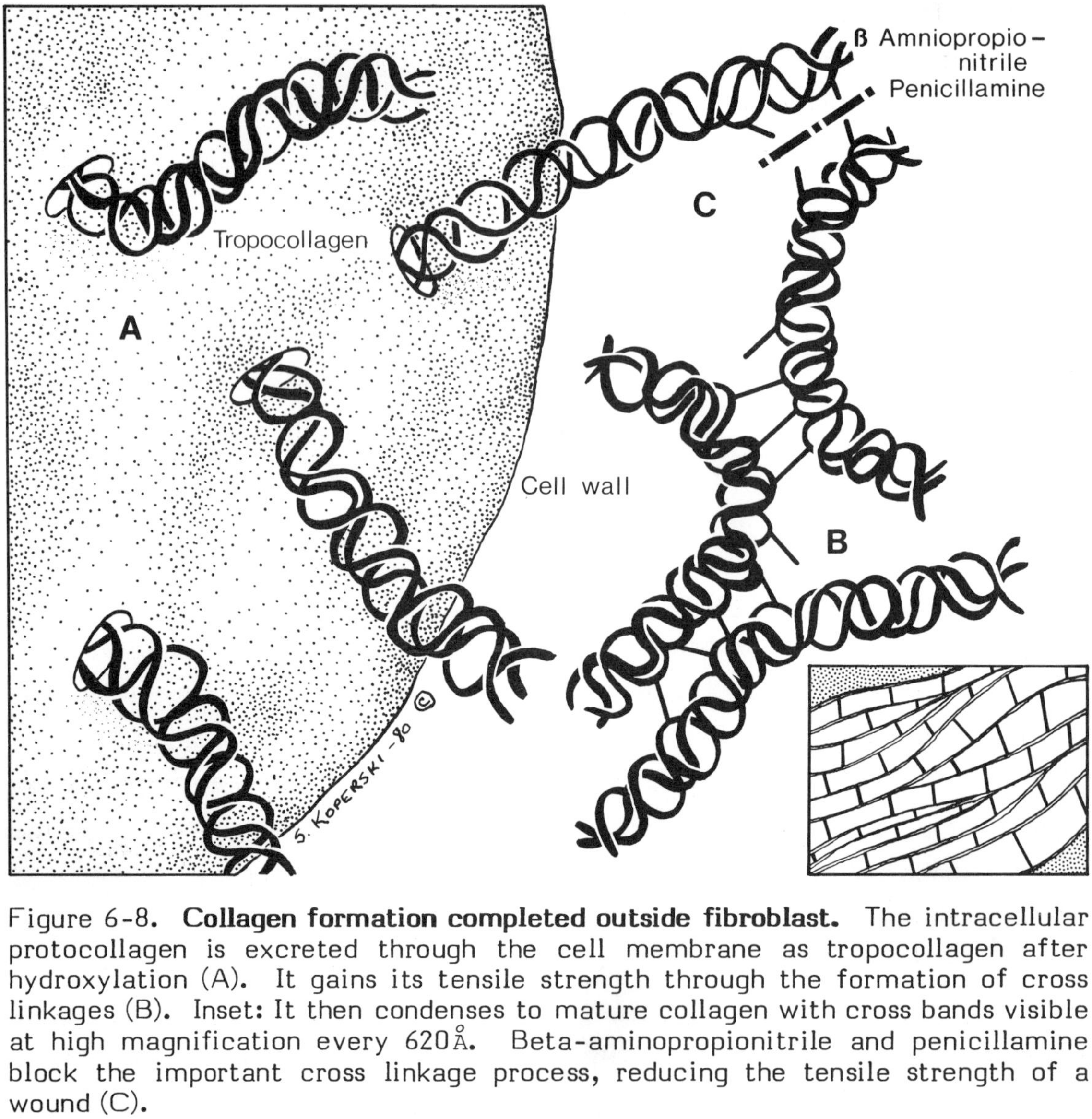

Figure 6-8. **Collagen formation completed outside fibroblast.** The intracellular protocollagen is excreted through the cell membrane as tropocollagen after hydroxylation (A). It gains its tensile strength through the formation of cross linkages (B). Inset: It then condenses to mature collagen with cross bands visible at high magnification every 620Å. Beta-aminopropionitrile and penicillamine block the important cross linkage process, reducing the tensile strength of a wound (C).

Maturation Stage (Wound Remodeling)

During the maturation stage, the scar contracts in all dimensions and additional water is squeezed out of the extracellular space. The collagen becomes more dense, the fibroblast population diminishes, and many vascular channels are obliterated. During the active maturation stage, the scar is red and raised. As the collagen becomes more dense and the vascular supply is compressed, the mature scar becomes flatter, thinner and paler.

Finally, in normally healing scars, a balance between production of collagen by fibroblasts and degradation of collagen by epidermal collagenase is reached. The rate of collagen production and degradation is high for about six months but diminishes greatly after that. Scars that remain active after that period may be hypertrophic scars or keloids. A hypertrophic scar is a raised, reddish mound that fails to mature. A keloid is a benign tumor of collagen fibers. In both types of wound there is an imbalance between collagen synthesis and degradation.

Two ways in which the surgeon can control the flatness of a scar are by applying pressure up to six months and by orienting the incision in the proper direction. Pressure can be applied by adhesive tape or elastic bandage and can be very light. The pressure must be applied during the early weeks of healing as it will have little effect after the scar has already arisen. The direction of the scar is controlled by the initial incision or by subsequent revision (see Chapter 7).

Systemic Factors in Collagen Production

The healing of a skin laceration is effected by a synthesis of fibrous proteinization and epithelization. The systemic factors necessary for the intracellular production of collagen include proper proteins, vitamin C, iron, oxygen, and alpha-ketoglutarate. These substances are used by the hydroxylase enzymes for the hydroxylation of proline. Factors which may suppress the intracellular formation of collagen include x-irradiation and high dosages of certain antibiotics which interfere with DNA coding (Table 6-2).

Steroids suppress the hydroxylation reaction, but this effect can be reversed with vitamin A. The cellular secretion of collagen may be blocked by colchicine which disrupts the functioning of the cellular microtubules. It is important for the collagen to be unwrapped prior to the cross-linkage process and fibril formation. In Ehlers-Danlos syndrome, this step never takes place and weak connective tissue results.

Proper control of collagen production, secretion and cross linkage is a practical clinical problem and is essential in avoiding keloids, abdominal adhesions, strictures and tendon adhesions. Animal experiments with agents that promote proper healing have been promising. However, side effects (e.g., ruptured aneurysms in the case of BAPN) can be serious.

Table 6-2. Collagen Suppression

DERMAL STAGE: Intracellular Phase	DERMAL STAGE: Extracellular Phase (cross linkage formation)	MATURATION STAGE (remodeling)
Suppressed by:	Suppressed by:	Influenced by:
Actino-puromycins (interfere with DNA code)	Beta-aminopropionitrile (BAPN)	Direction of the scar, tension
Steroids (suppress hydroxylation of proline)	Penicillamine (both above combine with monoamine oxidase, preventing its function)	Pressure on the scar
Radiation (suppresses all cellular activity)		Collagenase (tissue collagenase remodels, bacterial collagenase fragments)
Colchicine (disrupts secretion of collagen)		

Wound Contraction

An unclosed square wound in an experimental animal will contract at the rate of 0.74 mm per day and form a stellar shape. This occurs for approximately 12 days (exact length of time depending on the laxity of the surrounding tissue), and the tissue then ceases to change.

There is evidence that the fibroblasts remaining in the wound bed are the main agents responsible for wound contracture. Some evidence for this is found in guinea pigs with scurvy as the wound contracts even though no collagen is formed. Under certain circumstances, fibroblasts differentiate into myofibroblasts which resemble those found in smooth muscle tissue. These cells are responsive to agents that stimulate or inhibit smooth muscle contracture. There are two theories as to how these myofibroblasts function. One theory hypothesizes that they pull the wound edges as they migrate toward the center; the other says that they migrate to the center and contract upon reaching there. In either case, this process helps to close a wound (Fig. 6-9).

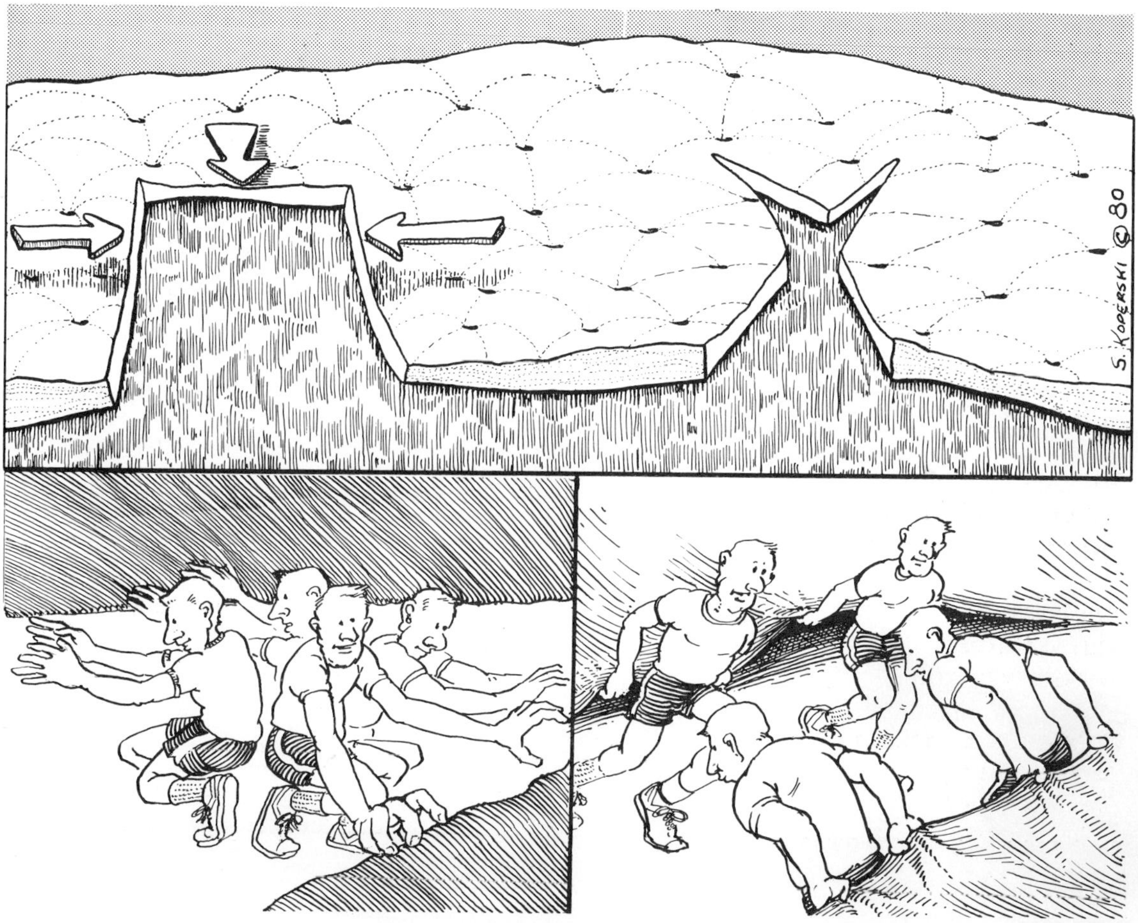

Figure 6-9. **Forces of contraction in wound bed.** When a 1 cm square is made experimentally and the wound allowed to heal by secondary intention, it results in a star-shaped wound (top). There are two theories as to how this wound contraction occurs: Either myofibroblasts reach the center of a wound and then pull the wound edges together (lower left) or they pull the wound edges with them as they migrate toward the center (lower right). In either case, the wound will be drawn in, reducing its size. The limit of this contraction depends upon the looseness of the adjacent tissue.

Wound contracture also occurs beneath skin grafts, especially when the grafts are placed on granulation tissue. This phenomenon is useful in clinical situations, since wound contracture can be encouraged by the temporary application of a thin skin graft. The contraction creates a smaller defect which can often be closed primarily at a later time.

Summary

There are four interrelated stages of wound healing: vascular, epithelial, dermal and maturation. After a brief, initial vascular stage, epithelization seals the surface (epithelial stage). The dermal collagen provides wound strength which begins building at about 7 days and increases for up to 42 days (dermal stage). Dermal collagen is produced by the wound fibroblasts and, once formed, matures for six months or a year (maturation stage), after which the turnover of collagen occurs at a slower rate.

Primary wound closure results in less collagen formation and, hence, less scarring.

CHAPTER 7

Placement of Incisions and Scar Revisions

The most important consideration in achieving a minimal scar is the direction of the original incision. The location of the incision on the body and the age of the patient make some difference, but the type of suture, wound closure, and dressing are only minor modifying factors provided they are effected with reasonable care.

Inherent Properties of Skin

The function of the skin is to regulate body temperature, to provide a barrier against loss of body fluids, and, through its nerve endings, to act as an auxiliary sensor for the brain. Skin and its appendages represent one of the largest organs of the human body. The skin consists of two very different layers: the epidermis and the dermis.

The epidermis consists wholly of epidermal cells and pigment-forming cells called melanocytes. The epidermis also acts as a conduit for the dermal appendages: sweat, sebaceous, and apocrine glands, and hair follicles. Epithelium regenerates by cellular proliferation from mitosis of cells in the basilar epithelium.

Pigmentatory skin changes may occur from epidermal injury, but scarring is a function of collagen formation and will not take place if the epidermis alone is injured. The "S" shape of the rete pegs probably contributes to the distensibility of the skin.

The dermis consists of an endless mesh of collagen fibers intertwined with elastin, skin appendages, nerves, fibroblasts, and blood vessels. The dermis heals by collagen formation, which explains why the dermis must be penetrated for scar tissue to form. In the unstretched state, the collagen fibers in young patients are convoluted, much like meshwork in three dimensions. These fibers become less convoluted with advancing age. As the skin is stretched these convolutions lengthen until the collagen assumes the form of parallel strings and resists further extension. Greater convolution permits a younger patient's skin to stretch further than an older patient's skin.

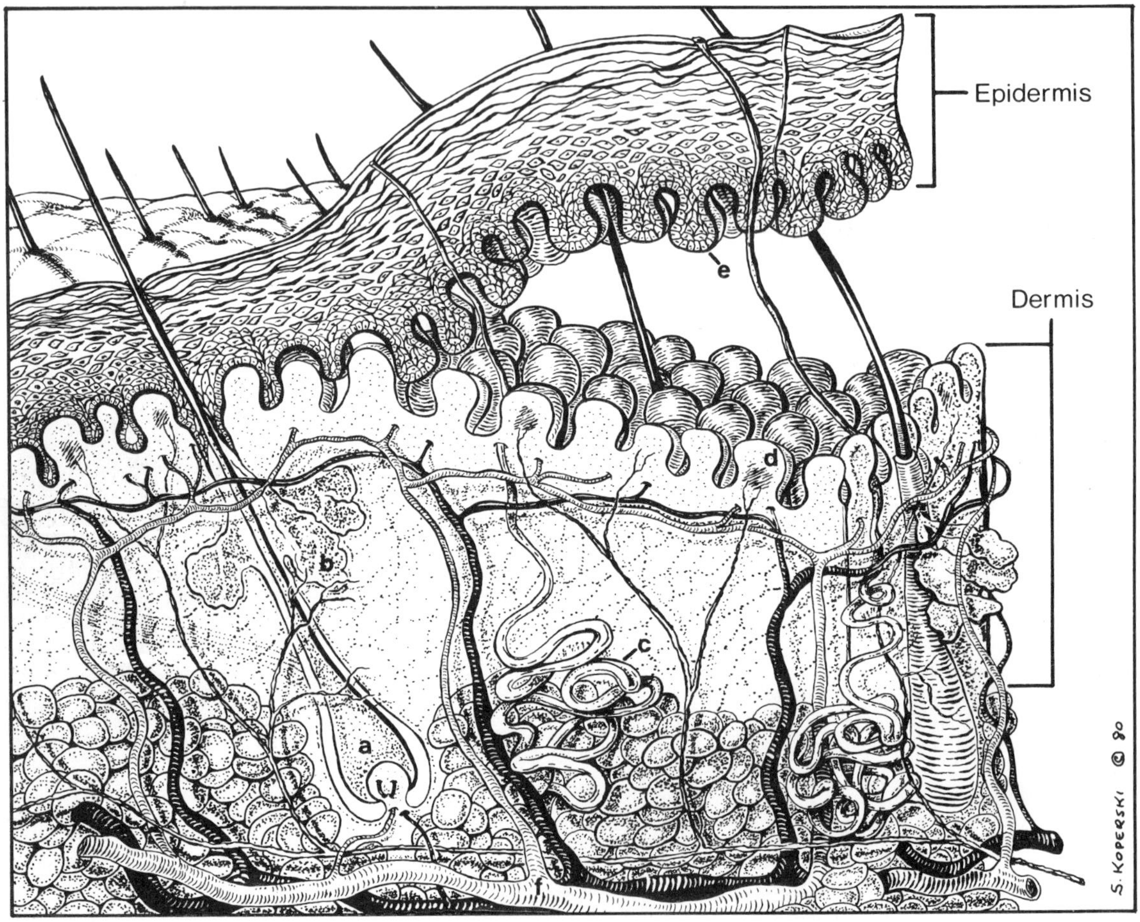

Figure 7-1. **Cross section of human skin showing dermal and epidermal layers.** Note that the hair follicles and sweat glands originate in the subcutaneous fat near the subdermal plexus. a, hair follicle; b, sebaceous gland; c, sweat gland; d, nerve ending; e, rete peg; f, blood vessel.

It is the elastic fibers that return the skin to its relaxed state as collagen fibers themselves have no powers of retraction. The inherent tension of the skin in the relaxed position is partially a function of the internal pull of the elastic fibers and partially a function of the external force of gravity pulling on the skin. (For example, the grativational pull on the shoulder skin has been likened to the pull which water exerts on a wet suit on a coat hanger.) Elastic fibers lose their elastic properties with age, and, therefore, the skin loses its retractibility. This explains both the skin laxity and the decrease in skin tension seen in elderly patients.

Sebaceous glands contribute to scar formation because of their capacity to regenerate the epidermis. If the sebaceous glands are hypertrophied in teenage patients with acne or in older patients with acne rosacea, the epidermis closes very rapidly. This can cause suture tracts and trenching or grooving of the scar. These glands are useful, however, in dermabrasions because they permit a deeper planing of the skin in those areas with thick sebaceous glands. Sebaceous glands decrease in size with age (Fig. 7-1).

Clinical Applications of Skin Variations

Older skin is thin and dry and forms a less noticeable scar. This is because there is less skin tension, less sebaceous activity, and therefore less collagen required to knit the scar together.

Location of the incision on the body is also an important factor. Scars are less apparent in areas of thin skin such as the eyelid, areola, ear, genitalia, conjunctiva, and vermilion. Areas without sebaceous glands and with a thick keratin layer, such as the sole of the foot and the palm of the hand, will not form prominent suture marks. Areas of thicker skin are usually associated with sebaceous gland activity. These areas, such as the back, nose, forehead, and cheek, are particularly prone to suture mark formation, and it is best to use subcuticular sutures for closure in these areas.

The tension of the skin, as determined by location and age, influences the appearance of the scar. Growth, as well as the presence of more resilient elastic fibers, adds to the greater skin tension of children. In all individuals, areas of the presternal, deltoid, and upper back are under greater tension because of gravity and because of the powerful muscular movement. The head and neck heal faster than the leg, in part because of circulatory differences. Heredity is an additional factor in scar formation; some families form large scars, and keloids are more common in individuals with pigmented skin.

Angle of Incision

An incision perpendicular to the dermis is easier to close and hence causes the least scarring. A beveled incision is difficult to approximate accurately and is used electively only in certain circumstances. Generally, in the emergency setting we do not incise beveled wounds unless they are very traumatized or dirty. It is best to fit the pieces together and perform any necessary revisions later when a fuller assessment of any other problems can be undertaken.

Beveled incisions are preferable, however, in hair-bearing areas such as the brow or scalp in order to preserve the hair roots. Many scars in the scalp which appear to be wide are really areas of alopecia surrounding the scar and are caused by incisions which transect hair follicles (Fig. 7-2).

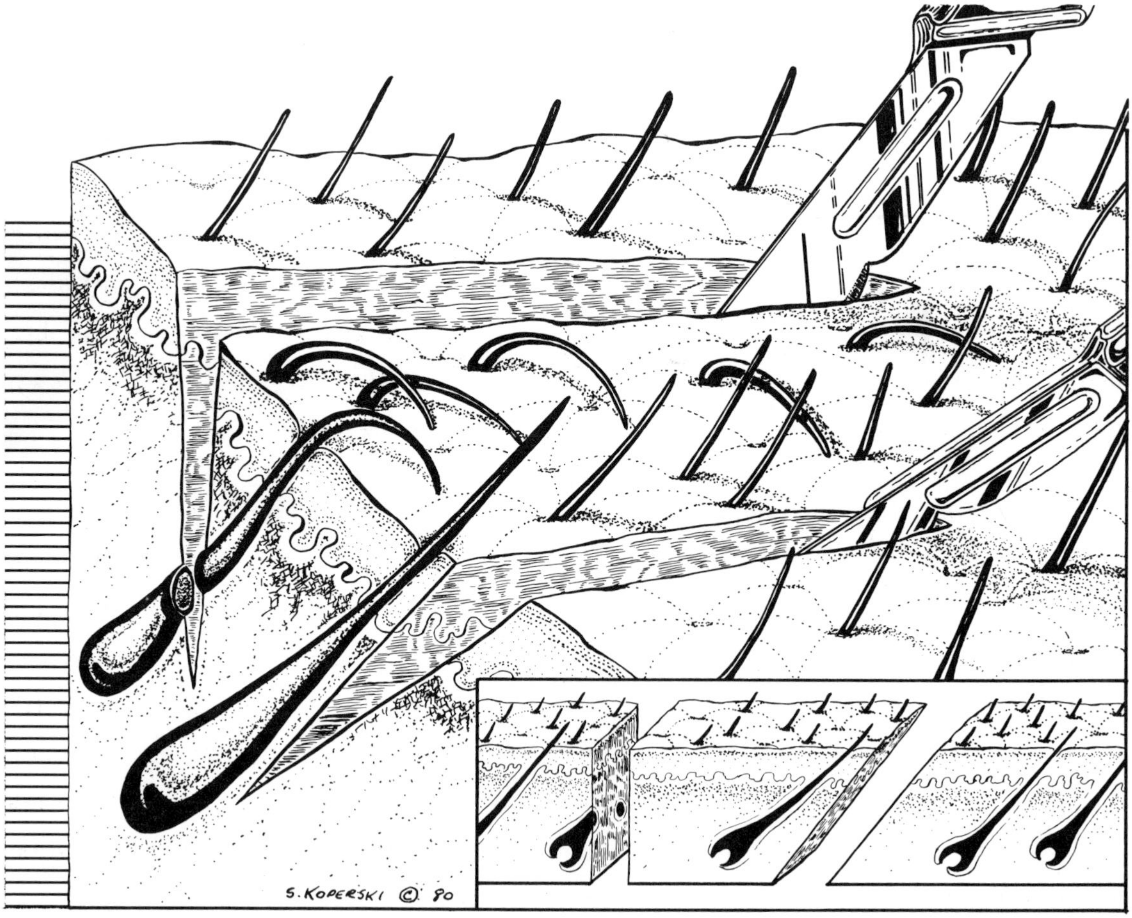

Figure 7-2. **Beveled incision used to preserve hair roots in hair-bearing areas.** If a hair root is damaged by a vertical incision, the subsequent scar appears wider than it actually is owing to the area of alopecia surrounding the scar (inset). Beveled incisions are typically used within the scalp or eyebrow.

Direction of Incision

It cannot be overemphasized that the single most important factor in creating a minimal scar is the direction of the original incision. A plethora of diagrams exists on how to make incisions for specific anatomical regions. There are, however, just three directional principles for permitting the surgeon to create a minimal scar:

- The incision should be at right angles to direction of muscle pull, or
- The scar should be allowed to bend, or
- There are certain privileged anatomical regions that follow their own directional rules.

Many scars have been mistakenly called keloids that are really hypertrophic scars. These latter result from excess skin tension, which in most patients is due to directional errors in making the skin incision. In some patients, it is due to inherent skin tension from gravity (especially around the shoulders) or from the skin's own elastic tissue. This latter cause of a hypertrophic scar is usually seen only in younger individuals because of their active and stronger dermal elastic fibers. A scar revision which lengthens a hypertrophic scar and relieves the skin tension will create a subsequent scar which is flatter if it is the result of a directional error. Pressure on the scar will correct those hypertrophic scars due to inherent skin tension.

Incisions At Right Angles to the Direction of Muscle Pull

Placing an incision perpendicular to the direction of major muscle pull prevents most hypertrophic scars. (This is because the skin expands and contracts according to the flexion and extension of muscle groups.) Effective contracture of the scar occurs more in its length than in its width, thus shortening the scar; therefore, an incision parallel to the direction of muscle pull causes a checkrein on the muscle extension. To strengthen the scar and prevent rupture, nature responds by depositing increased amounts of collagen, resulting in a raised, red, active hypertrophic scar (Fig. 7-3).

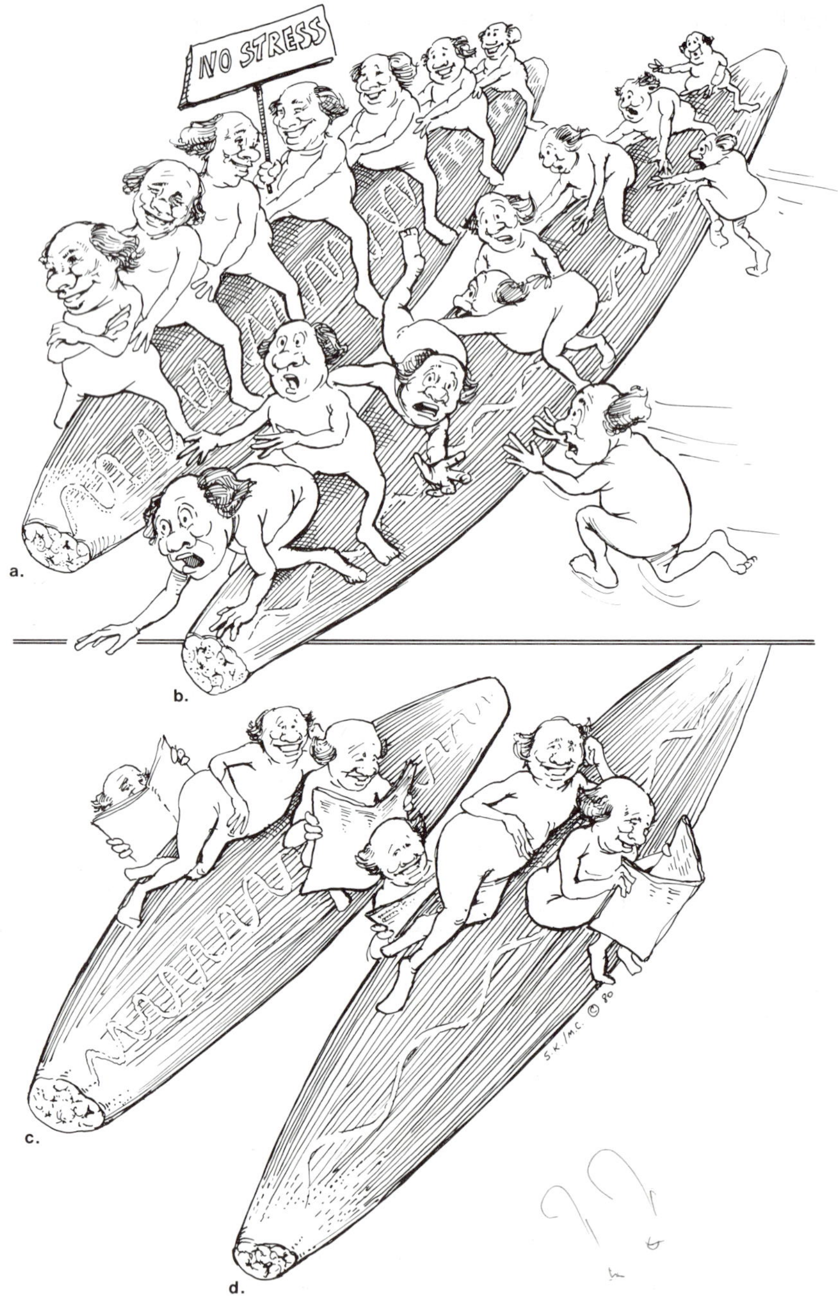

Figure 7-3. **Direction of muscle pull dictates direction of incision.** Where practical, the incision is placed at right angles to the direction of underlying muscle pull. The figures in the illustration represent collagen formation. If the incision is made parallel to the direction of muscle pull, collagen will be quiescent as long as the muscle remains inactive (a). However, as the muscle stretches the scar, additional collagen will be formed to prevent the scar from rupturing (b). This causes a hypertrophic scar. When the incision is made at right angles to the direction of muscle pull, the scar is not stretched regardless of whether or not the muscle is stretched (c) or contracted (d). Hence, additional collagen formation is not stimulated and a hypertrophic scar due to direction of incision does not form.

These lines of incision often correspond to skin creases which are formed by muscle pull and are more obvious on the older patient. Skin lines can be ascertained by having the patient contract underlying muscles. This maneuver is particularly useful on the face where skin line direction so often changes.

In the younger patient, the skin has not yet been creased by muscle pull and knowledge of the underlying anatomy is necessary. For example, if a lesion is to be removed from the forehead, a transverse incision would be made at right angles to the underlying frontalis muscle. Around the lip, a radial incision would be made perpendicular to the obicularis oris line of muscle pull. For a lesion of the cheek, an oblique incision would assume the correct direction because of action of the oral levators and the zygomaticus (Fig. 7-4).

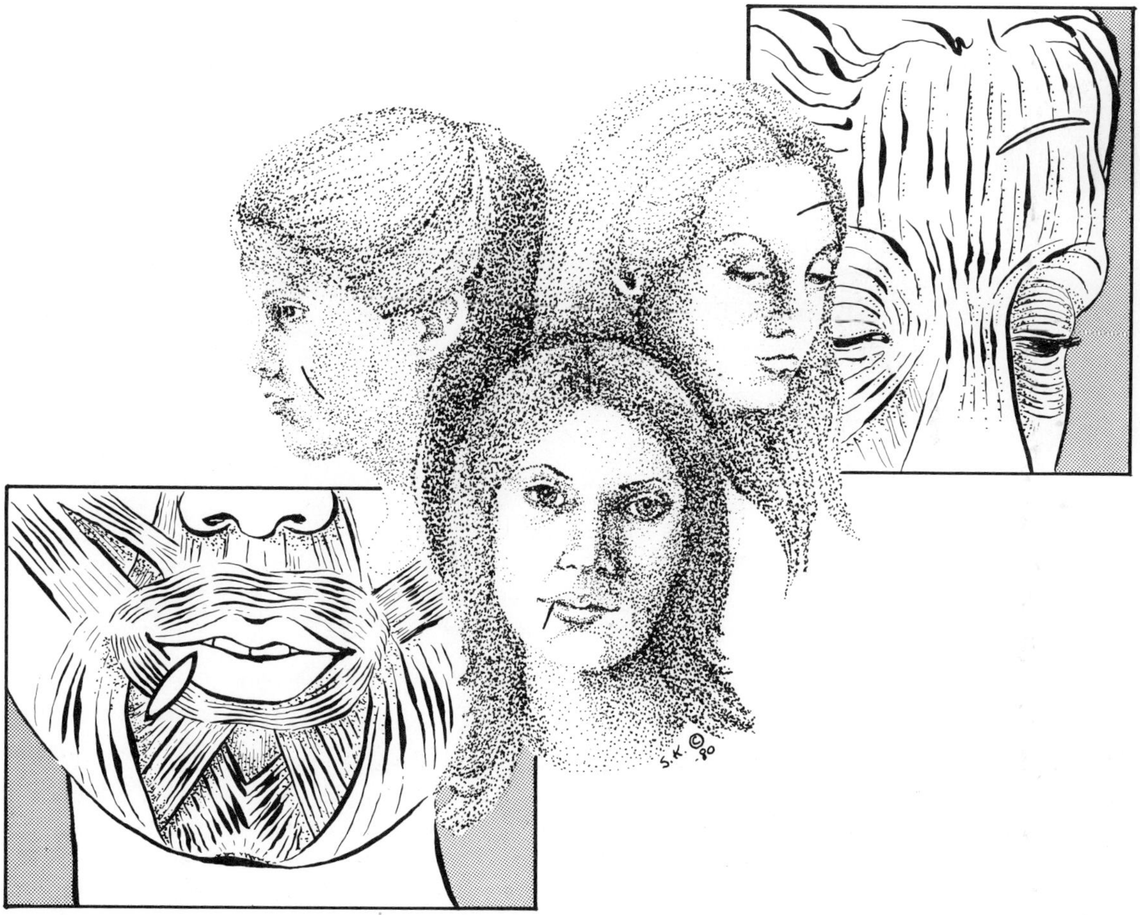

Figure 7-4. **Lines of incision in specific facial areas.** On the forehead the proper direction is horizontal because of the vertical pull of the frontalis muscle. Near the lip the direction is radial because of the circular configuration of the orbicularis oris muscle. Incisions on the cheek would be made at right angles to the levators of the mouth and to the zygomaticus.

In certain anatomical locations, such as edges or rims, wedge incisions are useful. These are made in a stairstep pattern to prevent notch deformity from scar contracture. As an alternative, a Z-plasty over the rim could be applied to break up the scar (Fig. 7-5).

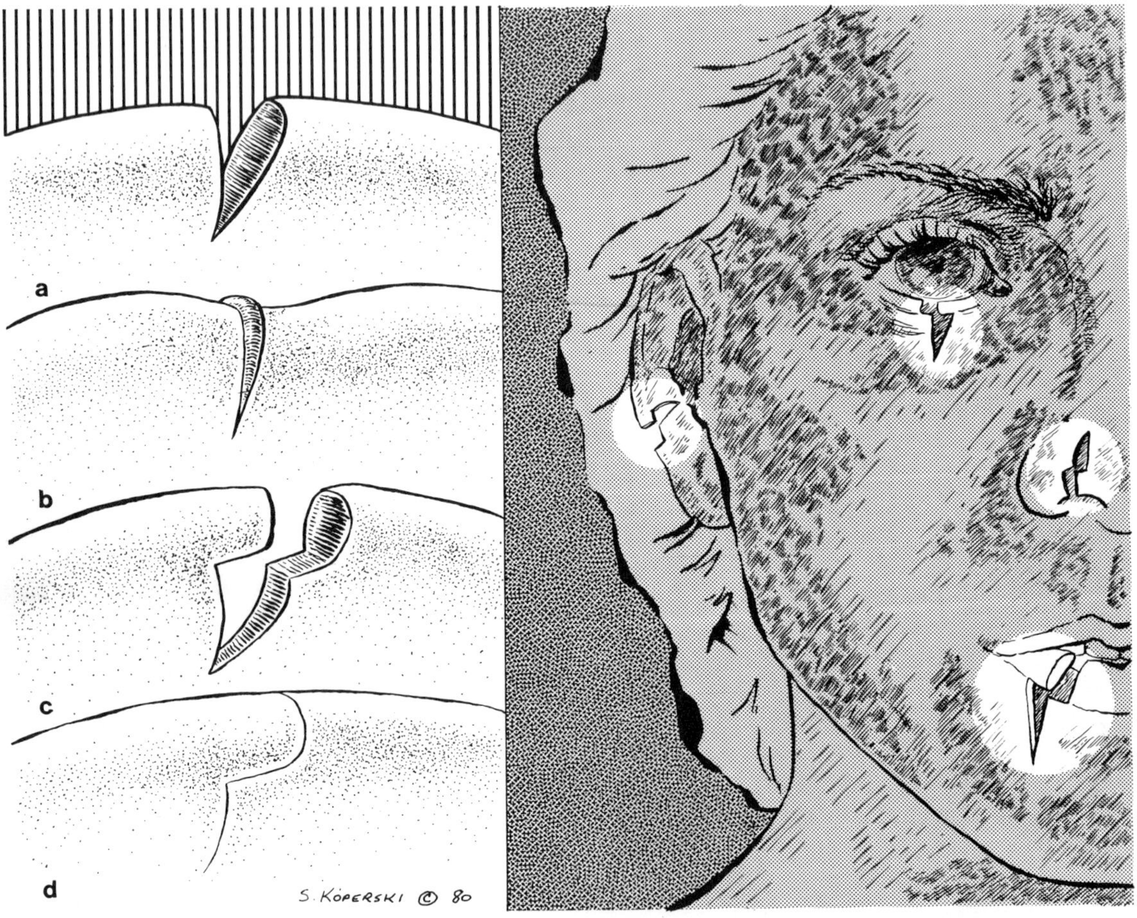

Figure 7-5. **Stepping incisions around a rim.** When a scar contracts around a rim, it tends to cause a dent because of the end-to-end scar contracture or "bow string effect" (upper left, a and b). Breaking the scar by stepping the incision prevents this deformity (lower left, c and d). Right: Proper step incision in the ear, eyelid, nasal ala and lip.

Skin distensibility permits body movement, and this distensibility occurs more in one direction of the skin than another. Pinching the skin together in various directions will demonstrate the dominant skin creases. This maneuver is particularly useful in determining the correct direction of an incision over the midportion of the extremities where there is no demonstrable muscle creasing of the skin.

Bending the Scar

In the Axis of a Joint. Since a scar shortens along its length and since a mature scar has little stretch, its direction around a joint becomes critical. For example, if a scar on the flexor surface is directed across skin creases parallel to the muscle force, it will contract along its length and limit extension of the joint. Incisions made in the axis of the joint cannot do this because the scar pivots rather than lengthening or shortening with joint motion (Fig. 7-6).

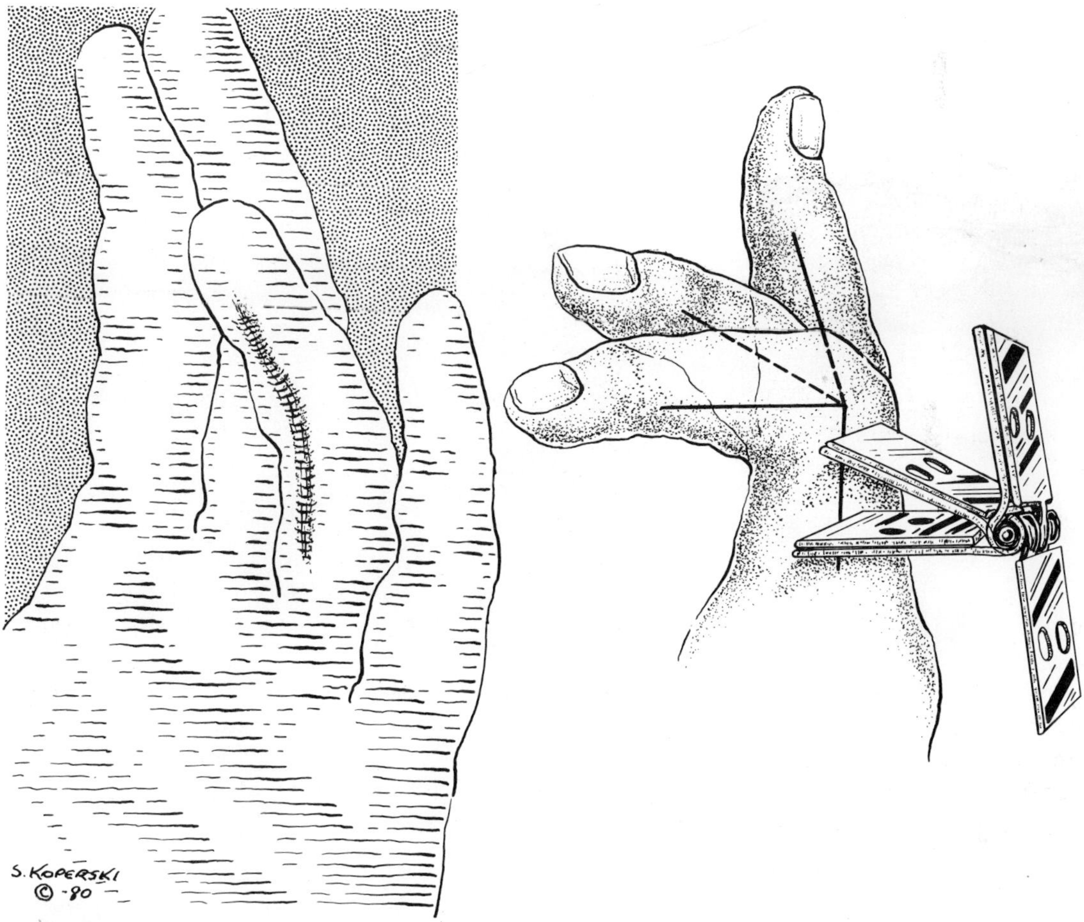

Figure 7-6 **Incisions involving joints.** In areas of a joint where there is flexion and extension but no lateral motion, a lateral incision along the long axis of the bone adjacent to the joint permits the scar to bend like a door hinge (right). This procedure prevents the hypertrophic scarring which will occur if the incision is made straight across skin creases marking joints (left).

Providing Spring to the Scar. Some areas of the body present difficult problems of surgical exposure. The volar aspect of the finger is difficult to reach from a lateral incision in the long axis of the finger joint. In such areas undulating incisions or scar-lengthening incisions are useful. For example, to cross a flexor crease the surgeon may use a Z-shaped incision or close the straight line incision with a Z-plasty. This type of incision provides spring to the scar by allowing it to bend when the joint extends (Fig. 7-7).

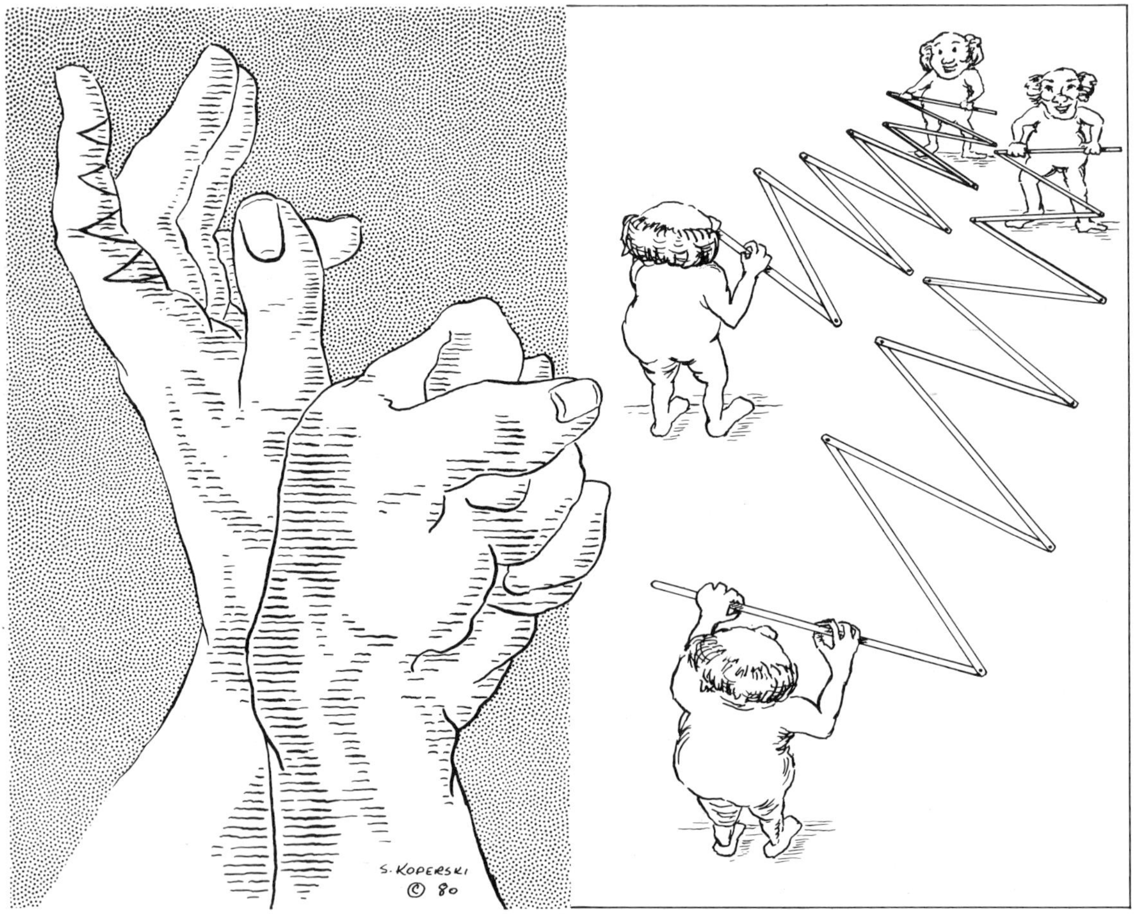

Figure 7-7. **Bending the incision.** When the scar area is subject to the force of flexion and extension yet the incision must be made across skin creases, the incision must bend, otherwise a hypertrophic scar will develop. A zigzag incision produces a scar which can stretch with an accordion effect.

A variation of this technique is useful in excision of small irregular lesions. It has been dubbed a "haptoplasty" because of the seemingly haphazard line of excision. This method minimizes the scar by utilizing all the tiny pieces of normal skin available. In addition, the scar appears shorter because some of the limbs are hidden in skin creases (Fig. 7-8).

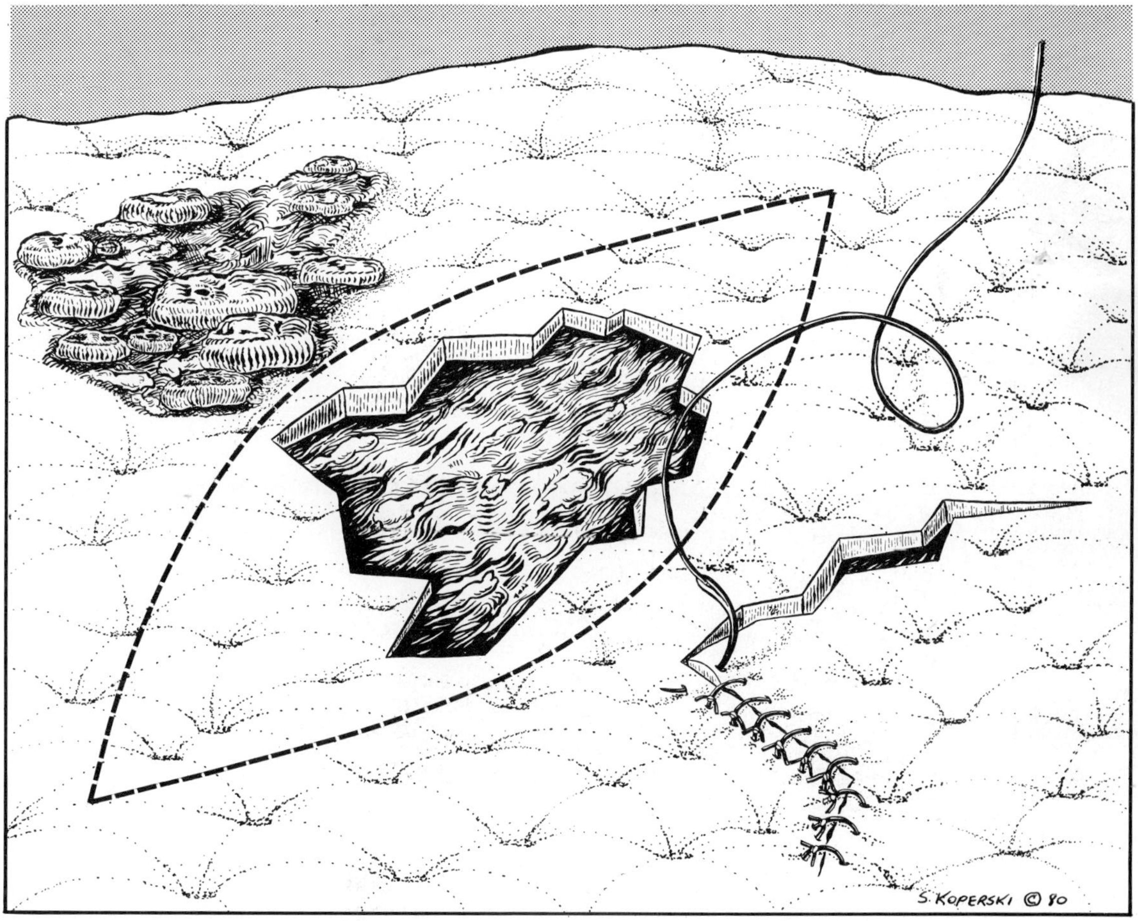

Figure 7-8. **Excising a benign lesion by skimming borders ("haptoplasty").** The procedure preserves tissue which can often be fitted together in a broken line. This makes the scar appear shorter; provides a bend, which is often desirable; and preserves tissue. Left: The original lesion. Center: The defect made by skimming the lesion. The dotted line of the center illustration shows the amount of tissue which would have have to be removed if a standard fusiform excision technique were used. Right: The pieces from the haptoplasty are fitted together, producing a shorter, bent scar.

Privileged Anatomical Regions

There are certain areas of the body that do not follow the above rules about incision placement. Interestingly enough, these areas do correspond to Langer's lines (see "Langer's Lines" which follows in this chapter), which otherwise are not useful for placing incisions. Such areas are listed below:

Sternum. Incisions placed along the long axis of the body minimize the scar although the muscle pull is in both transverse and vertical directions. Transverse scars crossing the midline in the sternal or xyphoid areas are always hypertrophic. Therefore, incisions here must be vertical.

Dorsum of Finger or Toe. As long as the joint is not crossed, an incision straight down the dorsum of a finger or toe will heal well. If the joint is crossed, the scar must be made as discussed previously in this chapter under "Bending the Scar."

Scalp, Brow. The muscle influences here are minimal. As long as the incision is beveled, a good scar will result. In males one must take into account the possibility of future baldness and plan accordingly.

Areola. Scars in and around the areola heal well because of the thin skin.

Genitalia. As in the eyelid, the thinness of the skin generally allows for a good scar. Hypertrophic scars are rare because the elasticity of this skin allows room for directional error.

Ear. The skin over the ear is so thin that incisions usually heal well. Step incisions have to be used around the edges, otherwise a notch will form from contracture of the scar around a bend. The natural attachment lines of the ear to the head are utilized effectively in rhytidectomy incisions.

Langer's Lines

In the 19th Century, Karl Langer expanded upon Dupuytren's observation that a puncture wound of the skin produces oval rather than round wounds. He conducted a series of studies which led to descriptions of the inherent forces of tension, elasticity, and compression within the skin. Langer traced the basis of tension to a mesh of fibers whose parallel bundles were of unequal length, causing the skin to give more in one direction than in another.

This led to the famous drawings of skin tensions published in the 1860s. Langer noted that wounds made at right angles to skin tension lines gape more than wounds parallel to skin tension lines. However, "Langer's lines," as they have come to be called, do not always correspond to elective incision lines, probably due to the direction of the underlying muscle pull, a factor which Langer did not study in his experiment. We have found that the three directional principles (incision at right angle to muscle pull, bending, and attention to privileged anatomical regions) correlate better with clinical experience than does the distribution of Langer's lines (Fig. 7-9).

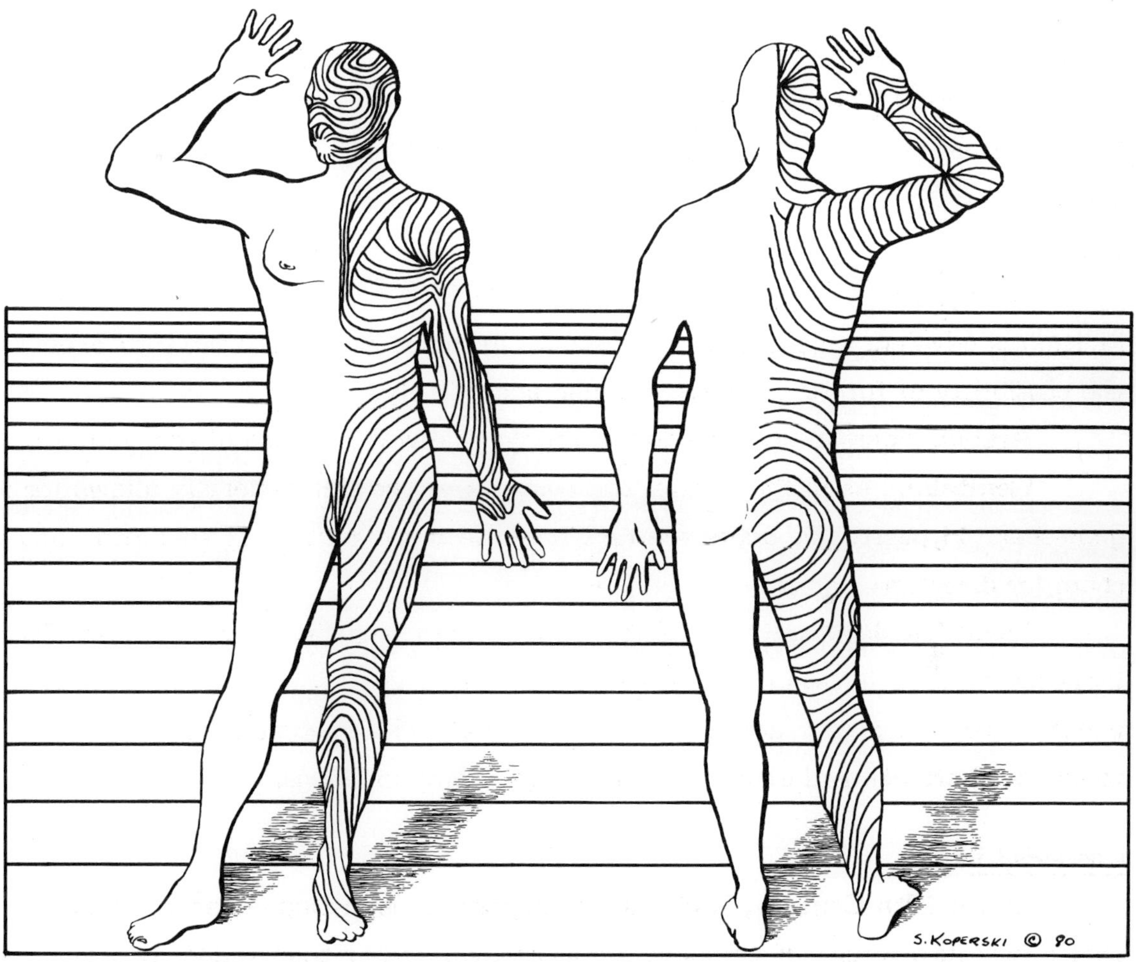

Figure 7-9. **Langer's Lines.** Lines of skin tension as described by Karl Langer correspond to proper incision lines in certain privileged anatomical areas. The lines are not clinically useful for determining the direction of incision in other areas because the effect of underlying muscle pull was not taken into consideration in Langer's experiments. These lines may be useful, however, in flap rotation because they indicate the line of inherent skin tension.

Scar Revisions

A scar revision should achieve cosmetic and functional improvement over the original scar, although a straight line revision alone may not always produce this objective. It is imperative to ascertain why it was that the original scar failed. Four considerations must be kept in mind: type of skin, type of incision, type of closure, and timing of revision.

Type of Skin

Pigmented skin, active sebaceous glands, the increased inherent skin tension of youth, and a family history of large scars all produce a predisposition toward a suboptimal scar. Some of these factors can be influenced by the surgeon. Deferring a scar revision until after a spurt of growth is helpful when treating a younger patient. Control of acne or drying of oily skin is also helpful. Avoidance of pigment-producing factors, such as birth control pills or sunlight, may lessen hyperpigmentation in a maturing scar.

Type of Incision

If the original scar does not correspond to the optimal direction as outlined previously, the scar can be reoriented by a revision. A bend can be placed in the scar by either a Z-plasty or a W-plasty technique. A Z-plasty consists of two lateral rotation flaps which make use of loose lateral tissue to elongate the scar and change its direction. The Z-plasty technique is particularly useful for repairing functional defects where the release of scar contractures is required (Fig. 7-10).

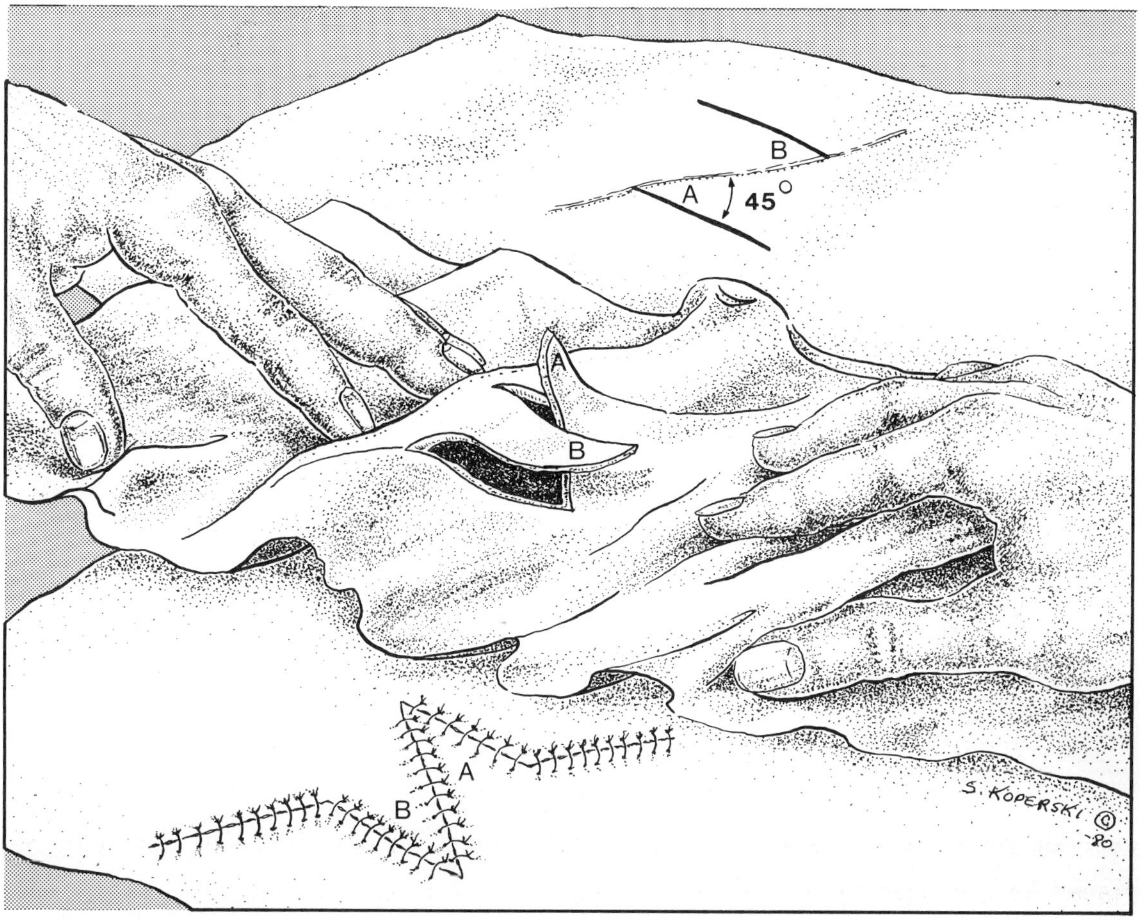

Figure 7-10. **Formation of a Z-plasty.** Top: Parallel lines are incised at an angle of about 45° from the scar line and the scar is excised. Middle: The flap points are interchanged, drawing in the lateral tissue. Bottom: The closure. Note that flap B is now where flap A began. The technique effectively lengthens the original scar by about 50 percent and adds a spring to the scar line. A Z-plasty generally is more useful for functional purposes, i.e., a severe scar contracture.

A W-plasty consists of two lateral advancement flaps closed in a broken line which provides spring to the scar. A W-plasty also changes the scar direction, but, because smaller flaps are utilized, it produces a more aesthetic scar. However, this technique rarely provides enough tissue for correction of functional deficits. The W-plasty relies heavily on loose lateral tissue because more normal tissue is discarded than with a Z-plasty. The former is most useful on the face where a scar may cross normal skin lines (Fig. 7-11).

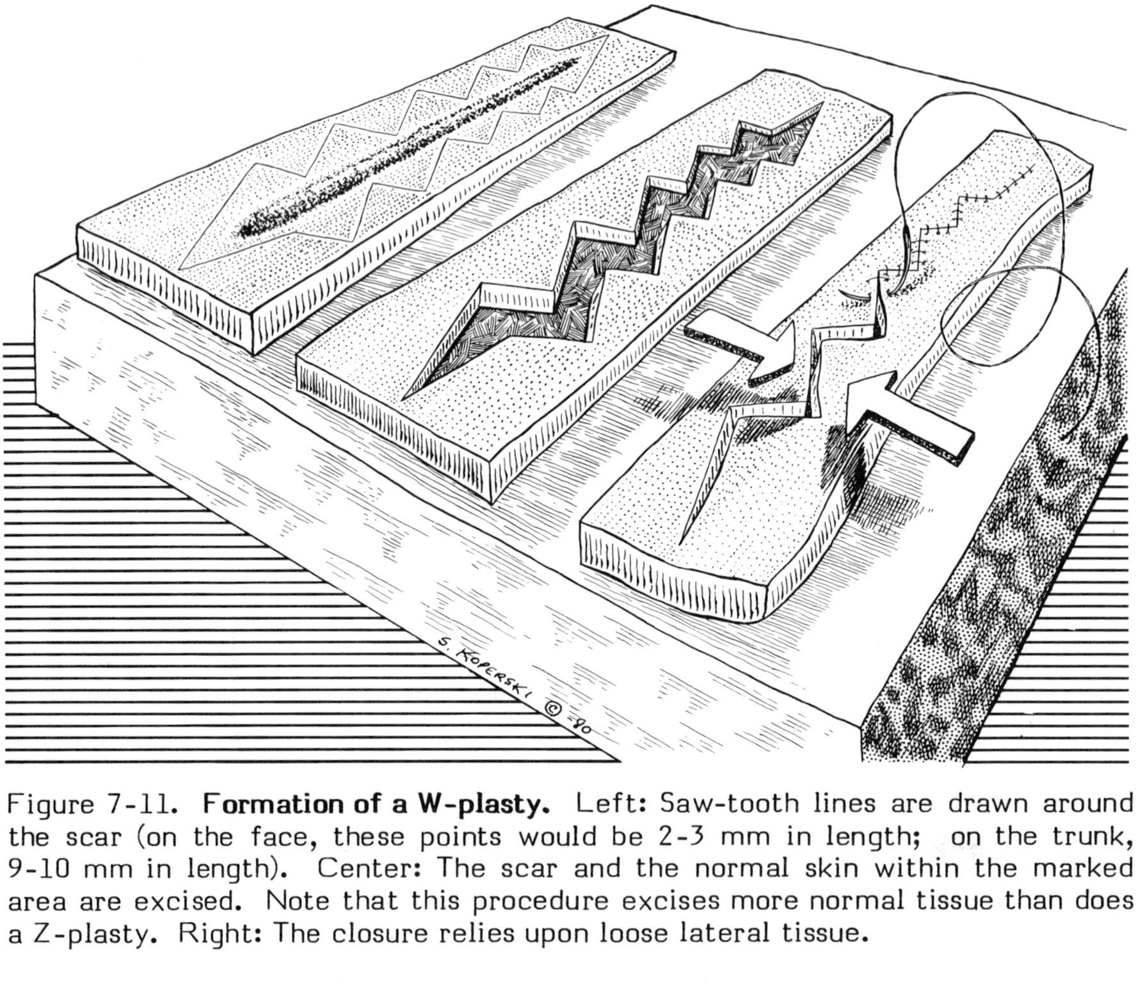

Figure 7-11. **Formation of a W-plasty.** Left: Saw-tooth lines are drawn around the scar (on the face, these points would be 2-3 mm in length; on the trunk, 9-10 mm in length). Center: The scar and the normal skin within the marked area are excised. Note that this procedure excises more normal tissue than does a Z-plasty. Right: The closure relies upon loose lateral tissue.

An additional factor to be considered in a scar revision is the optical illusion of a shorter scar length caused by bending the scar. Following Z- or W-plasty, some of the cross limbs of the W or Z can be placed in skin creases, thus making them less noticeable.

Type of Closure

If the skin is closed under tension, particularly in the trunk, revisions may result in thinner scars because with time the adjacent skin will stretch and reduce the tension. In emergency conditions where the skin healing may have been impaired due to crushing or subclinical infection, or where dirt has produced a tattoo, revision of these areas may help produce a better scar. If the skin edges are not accurately approximated, notching can result. This can be seen particularly if eyebrows or vermilion borders are mismatched. In the case of misalignment of borders, simple realignment will improve the appearance. If the initial closure was crude, simply excising the scar and initial wound suture marks with careful reapproximation can produce a good result.

Timing of Surgery

Unless there is a gross functional deformity, such as contracture of an eyelid, impairment of joint motion, or a hypertrophic scar, a revision should be undertaken only after the wound is mature. This can vary from 3 to 18 months, depending upon the location of the wound and the type of skin involved. Reliable clinical indications are color and softness. A mature scar will have few blood vessels and will be pale. Also the scar and surrounding tissue will be free of edema and will be soft.

Hypertrophic Scars and Keloids

A hypertrophic scar, as has been pointed out, results from increased tension. There are two types: those that form from inherent skin tension, particularly in younger patients, and those that form from a directional error in the incision. Hypertrophic scars appear as firm, raised, reddish mounds. They are wide scars that fail to regress and mature. They do not outgrow the confines of the original scar.

A change in scar direction will resolve the hypertrophic scar problem when improper direction is the villain. In some cases where general skin tension is a problem and if evidence of hypertrophic scarring is detected, the problem can be resolved by gentle pressure on the scar until maturity. This is done by applying skin tapes or compression bandages and massage to the wound for six months or more.

A keloid is a benign tumor of collagen which will recur regardless of treatment. Keloids occur most frequently in members of the Negro race and in dark complected Caucasians. There is a definite hereditary predisposition to their occurrence. Keloids and hypertrophic scars are similar in appearance, but keloids may outgrow the limits of the surgical trauma and invade normal tissues.

Keloids are often seen in areas of increased skin tension, such as the sternum and deltoid, where they are difficult to differentiate from hypertrophic scars. However, a raised scar in areas of no tension, especially one that does not violate directional principles, most likely is a true keloid. They can be found, for instance, in an ear lobe after ear piercing or in a transverse scar of an abdomen. These keloid scars are frequently "ropy" in appearance in contrast to the hypertrophic scars which are usually smoother. Although some histologists can differentiate between keloids and hypertrophic scars on the basis of tissue culture, in our opinion the diagnosis can best be made in a clinical setting. Frequently pruritis, mild pain, and hyperesthesia are associated with keloids.

The precise cause of keloid formation is unclear. There is a biochemical loss of regulation of the synthesis and degradation of collagen. An unusual type of fibroblast found only in keloid scars may be responsible for the derangement. The greatest mistake a surgeon can make is to completely excise the tumor as most keloids will recur in larger form, since the wound has been enlarged by this new incision. Proper treatment consists of intralesional excision in which a rim of tumor is purposely left. In this case, a wrinkled scar must be accepted (Fig. 7-12).

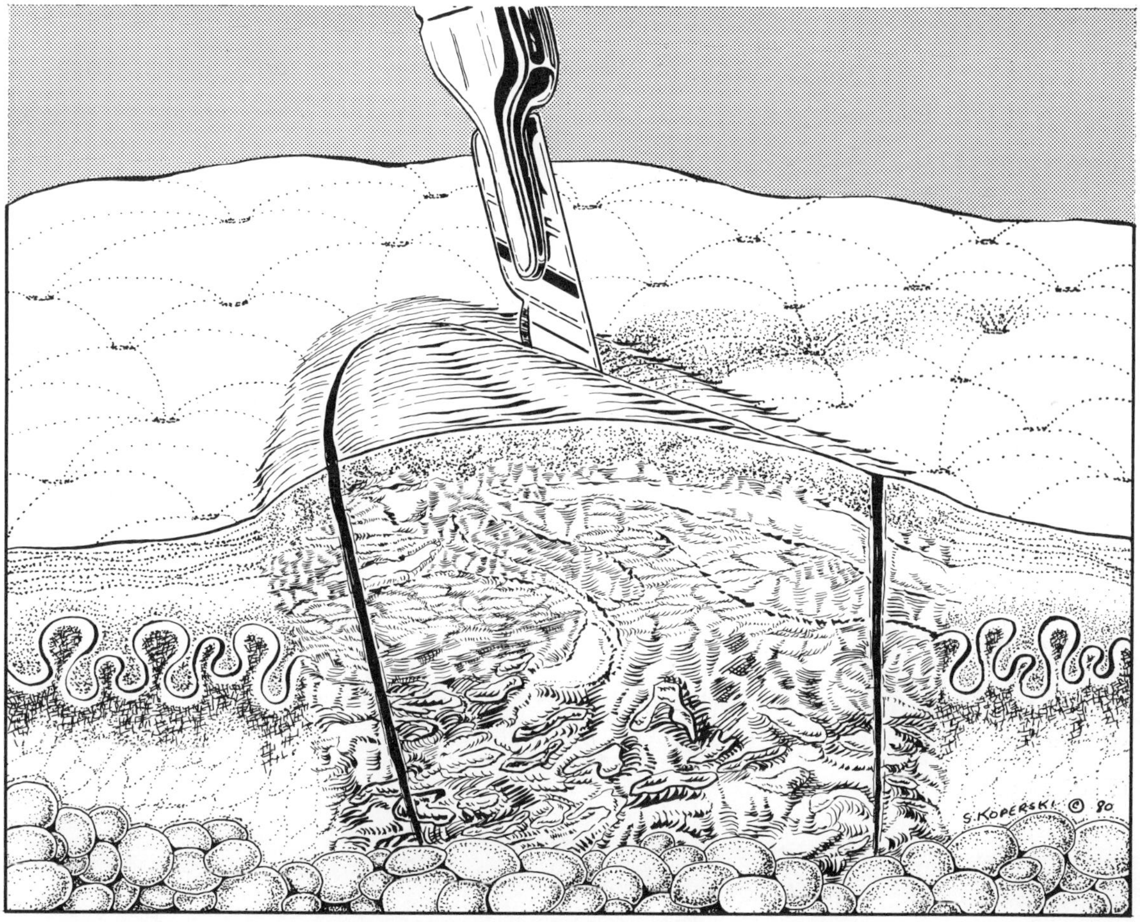

Figure 7-12. **Excising a keloid.** It is of paramount importance that the excision of a keloid be intralesional. The technique purposely leaves a small rim of keloid tissue although it slightly compromises the result. Total excision would cause the scar tissue to become further enlarged when the keloid recurs.

Constant postoperative pressure and injection of the remaining tumor with steroids will minimize recurrence. Radiation is useful for keloids in areas, such as the ear lobes, that can be well shielded. However, radiation may carry a risk factor in younger individuals.

Particularly difficult decisions are required when dealing with those scars which are a combination of keloids and tension-induced hypertrophy. Very careful clinical judgment must be made in these cases.

Dermabrasion

Dermabrasion consists of planing or sanding the skin with a rotating burr or brush. The epidermis is removed, and the abrasion is carried into the underlying dermis, mechanically creating a superficial second-degree burn. In this manner, elevated scars and irregularities in the dermis are removed. The epithelial layer is regenerated from skin appendages such as sweat glands and hair follicles, and it leaves a smoother surface when healed. Because of the mechanical forces involved, dermabrasion is more effective for scars than is a chemical peel (see Chapter 8, "Chemical Peel").

Dermabrasion offers considerable improvement for shallow depressions, such as acne scars, or the points of W-plasty flaps which are accentuated when oblique lighting casts shadows on those areas. It is also helpful in some raised scars or deep rhytids. The technique is less helpful for deep "ice pick" acne scars or enlarged pores because it cannot go deeply enough to erase them (Fig. 7-13).

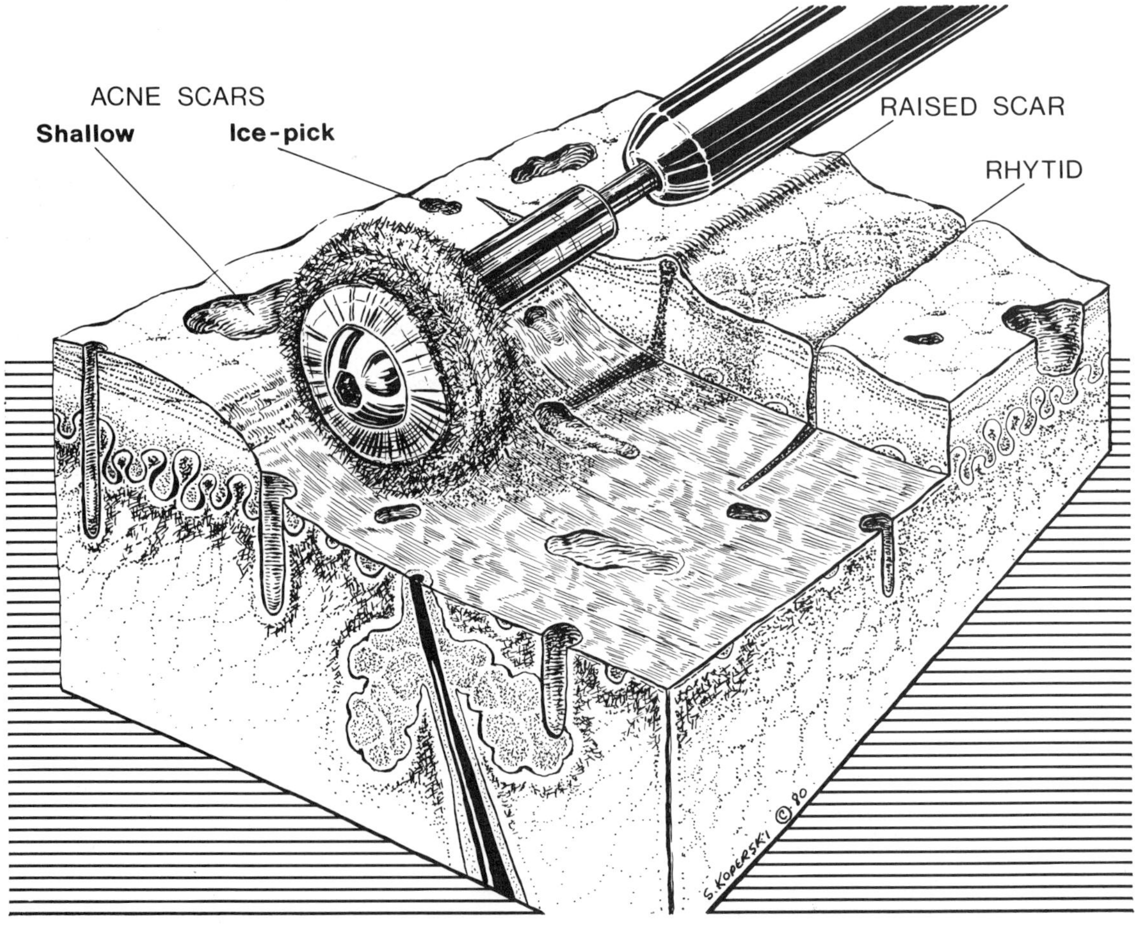

Figure 7-13. **Dermabrasion.** The epidermis and upper dermis are mechanically removed, creating the equivalent of a superficial burn. The epidermis regenerates from the remaining rete pegs, the hair follicles, and sweat glands. Dermabrasion helps to smooth superficial scars such as shallow acne scars and raised scars. It will help smooth some rhytids but not improve "ice pick" acne scars because they run too deep. Planing to that level would cause a deep burn.

Dermabrasion creates the equivalent of a second-degree burn and requires protection from a subsequent infection which can convert this superficial burn into a deeper burn. The area epithelizes within five to seven days. Some skin pigments are removed, leaving the dermabraded area lighter in color than the surrounding skin. Direct exposure to sunlight may exaggerate pigment discrepancies and should be prevented by sun screening agents and by the avoidance of estrogen or progesterone preparations such as birth control pills. These stimulate tyrosine production, leading to increased melanin formation.

Summary

The final appearance of a scar is influenced by a combination of three factors: direction of incision, type of skin, and type of closure.

Reasonable attention must be exercised in the care and suturing of a dermal wound. However, it is the direction of the original incision that is the major determinant of a fine scar. This direction can be determined anywhere in the body by following three basic principles: placing the incision at right angles to muscle pull, bending the scar, and taking into consideration the special requirements of certain anatomical regions.

Scar revisions may be useful: (1) for correction of directional errors, (2) in dealing with wide scars previously closed under tension, (3) after emergency wounds have healed, (4) when anatomical areas are mismatched, (5) for correction of functional impairment, and (6) in situations involving raised dermis.

The assumption that a revision will always improve a scar is an unsound one. Clinical judgment must be utilized in distinguishing between a hypertrophic scar and a keloid because the treatment for each of these conditions is entirely different.

II. Clinical Entities

CHAPTER 8

Aesthetic Surgery

Three considerations should be taken into account when counseling a patient regarding an aesthetic procedure: the patient's general health, the patient's psychological make-up, and the type of surgery involved.

General Health

The importance of good basic health may seem self evident, but often a busy practitioner may not go into it in sufficient detail. Factors such as smoking, hypertension, obesity, diabetes, thyroid condition, and liver disease can influence the outcome of the surgery. Small infections anywhere in the body should be eliminated in advance because they can contaminate the surgery site. Any drug use, including such common medications as aspirin, must be established. Aspirin decreases platelet agglutination and can lead to intraoperative and postoperative hemorrhage. Smoking increases the risk of skin necrosis following surgery. This is especially true in face lifts, and the patient should stop for a period prior to and just after the surgery.

For best results, preoperative counseling should be considered an integral part of the treatment and should include, when appropriate, the subjects of weight reduction, exercise, hair style and make-up. There are exceptions to any rule, of course, but it is generally absurd to perform a face lift on patients who are alcoholic, grossly overweight, or are three-pack-a-day smokers because their addictions will quickly reverse the benefits of the surgery. A potential candidate for aesthetic surgery may not be able to attain all of his desired goals through surgery, but those goals should be openly discussed. This total patient approach is the mark of a superior plastic surgeon.

?? aggregation

Psychological Factors

The chance of uncovering a personality disorder in a patient seeking aesthetic surgery is greater than that for the general population; however, 98 percent of these patients can be helped. This high rate of success baffles psychiatrists, but can perhaps be explained by the fact that seeking aesthetic surgery is in itself a positive sign because such patients are taking an active role in directing their lives.

The level of psychopathology found in seekers of aesthetic surgery has lessened in the last 20 years as aesthetic surgery has become more accepted. Nevertheless, thinking in terms of basic personality types helps to alert the plastic surgeon to potential problems and also prepares him for any postoperative personality changes. These postoperative changes are usually temporary, but they are found in a high percentage of patients undergoing this type of surgery. Usually they are represented by an "intensification" of the preoperative personality factors. The main personality types tending to seek aesthetic surgery follow (Fig. 8-1).

Passive-Dependent Type

Symbolically, passive-dependent type patients substitute others (in this case, the surgeon) for parents. They are compliant and want the surgeon to tell them what to do and to reassure and support them. Key words in the interview are, "You tell me, Doc. You are the expert." Ironically, these patients nevertheless often seek an opportunity to prove the "parent" (surgeon) wrong.

Obsessive-Compulsive Type

These patients like to discuss endless details and tend to intellectualize their problems. They have denial patterns and feelings of isolation. The best way to help these patients is to provide a written list of postoperative instructions. Endless questions and emphasis on tiny details should serve as a warning that the patient is probably of this type.

Hysterical Type

These patients also have endless questions, but their questions relate more to their postoperative appearance than to the substance of the operation. Such patients are fearful that their appearance is their only asset. Key words to listen for are, "What will I look like?" The best way to handle this type of patient is with reassurance. Once healed, these patients are often the most grateful and become the most enthusiastic referral sources.

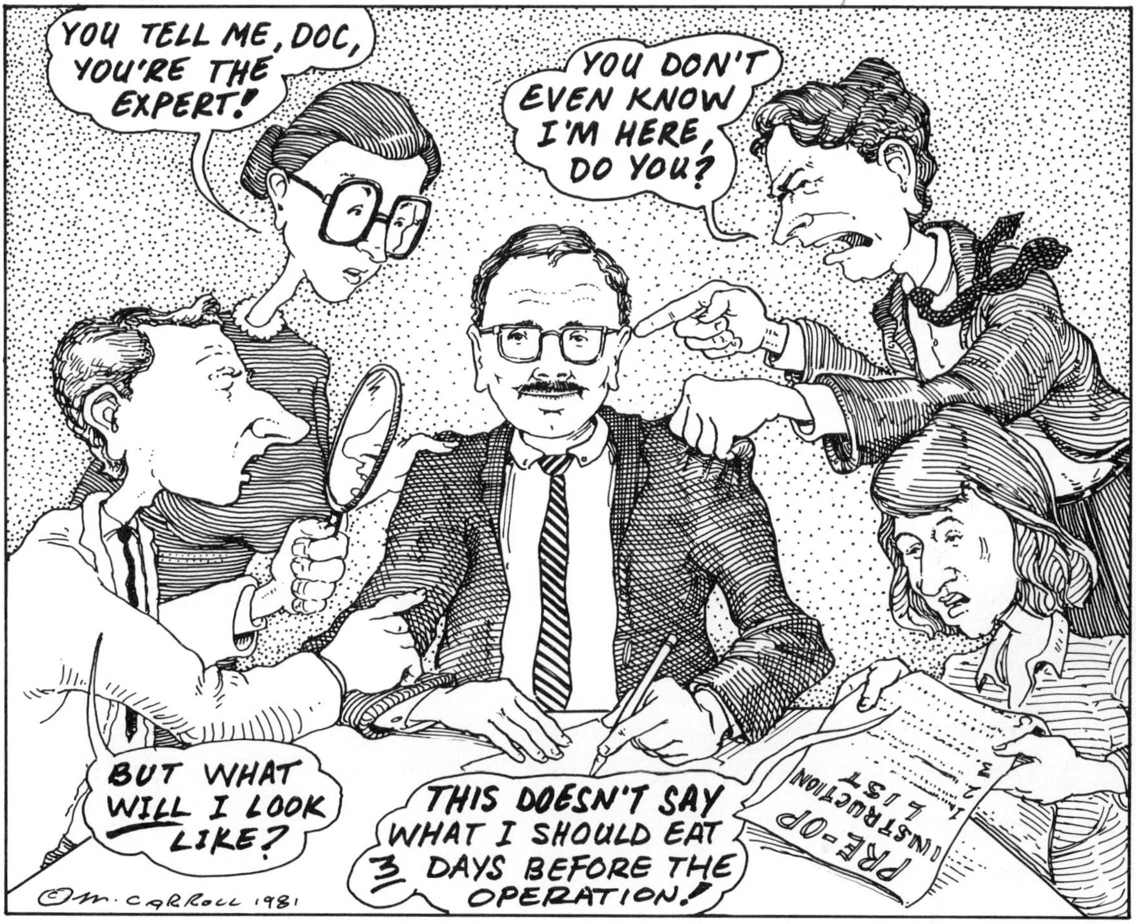
YOU TELL ME, DOC, YOU'RE THE EXPERT!
YOU DON'T EVEN KNOW I'M HERE, DO YOU?
BUT WHAT WILL I LOOK LIKE?
THIS DOESN'T SAY WHAT I SHOULD EAT 3 DAYS BEFORE THE OPERATION!
PRE-OP INSTRUCTION LIST
©M. CARROLL 1981

Figure 8-1. **Recognizing personality differences.** Recognizing different personality types and reacting to patients according to personality differences will aid the surgeon in helping the patient in the pre- and postoperative periods. Listening during the interview is a key factor in being able to make such an assessment.

Paranoid Type

The paranoid type patients feel useless and angry and are full of suspicion. It is important to recognize that their feelings of anger are attempts at self-preservation. Clues to a paranoid personality are accusations of neglect and lack of interest on the part of the surgeon.

Additional Psychological Factors

Generally speaking, a practitioner will be wise to handle a patient who has a seemingly minimal defect with a great deal of care. Wanting to eliminate a small defect may represent a patient's exaggeration of a minimal problem, but this is not always the case. A scar revision or dermabrasion, although revealing no significant change to the surgeon, may be of enormous importance to the patient. The surgery, in these cases, may represent the obliteration of a painful memory, as in the case of a divorced woman who has sustained a laceration from a drunken former husband. The surgeon should not be misled by a gross defect so obvious that he neglects to explore the patient's psychological goals in desiring its removal.

If a patient is vague, indecisive and skips from subject to subject, he is likely to be revealing unrealistic goals. Such a patient may not be satisfied with the postoperative results and is usually not a good candidate for surgery.

If the patient refuses to discuss goals and expectations or if the surgeon himself does not feel comfortable about the anticipated procedure, he should not operate. In such cases, if a problem develops following surgery, the surgeon's attitude is likely to be, "I never should have accepted this patient." The patient senses these feelings, and this usually leads to a psychologically unsatisfying conclusion for both parties.

Although plastic surgery for men is more accepted today, especially among business executives, a man feels more guilt than does a woman about what he regards as his narcissistic tendencies, and he also harbors fears about his sexual identity when he finds himself wanting to get "beautified." These fears will express themselves in various ways, but men are apt to be more difficult to manage because of it. This is especially true in rhinoplasty patients where there is a strong identification of the nose as a phallic symbol.

There is an additional question to be considered in the case of any patient who has had previous aesthetic surgery: Does the desire for a repetition merely represent reasonable attention to body maintenance, or does it represent a desperate desire to remain forever young?

Another question to be asked is, "Why does the patient request surgery now?" If the request comes in the middle of an emotional trauma or in an attempt to rekindle the flames of a lost romance, the ensuing disappointment may be profound. Asking this simple question may reveal a great deal and spare the patient much future disappointment.

Prepayment of surgical fees is an essential part of the treatment. It injects a needed note of reality into the relationship, and it permits the patient to concentrate on getting well rather than on finding fault with the surgery.

Three Guidelines

Psychopathology alone is not a contraindication to surgery. A physician's understanding of the patient's state of mind can prevent misunderstanding and can help sustain a supportive relationship which will carry the patient through this temporary psychological dislocation.

In assessing a patient for aesthetic surgery, the following should be considered:

- The patient's expectations. How realistic are they?
- The possibility, or even likelihood, of an imperfect result. Can the patient accept such an outcome?
- The psychological hazards of the postoperative healing period. Can the patient be brought successfully through the temporary postoperative psychological dislocation with the surgeon as a temporary psychotherapist?

With experience, the successful aesthetic surgeon will find himself developing certain criteria which will serve to alert him to potential problems of communication between himself and the patient.

Types of Surgery

Rhinoplasty, Septoplasty

To determine how early one can operate, preoperative evaluation of patients seeking rhinoplasty should detail the patient's growth history (including menses, height gain, etc.) and previous nose injury or surgery. Repeated operations and repeated trauma both affect healing because the increased amount of scar tissue cannot be completely removed and can eventually cause a change in vascularization. A nose that is twisted and asymmetrical to begin with may be improved, but it can never be completely straightened.

Evaluating preoperative nasal patency requires careful clinical judgment as there is no reliable laboratory test to measure this, and the patient's feelings of obstruction are subjective. The surgeon should note the condition of the mucous membranes. The septum can be straightened and the turbinates modified, if necessary, but the covering mucosa can still swell and block the airways in the presence of smoke, pollutants, hay fever, or other allergies.

Atopic rhinitis can cause dry crusting. Chronic use of nasal spray can lead to rhinitis medicamentosa and a dependency on the spray. Withdrawal may have to be accomplished by steroid injections to the turbinates. These conditions should be identified and treated medically prior to surgery.

Repeated rhinoplasty may lead to excision of too much cartilage in the internal valve area. This, in turn, may lead to inspiratory collapse of the nose as the osteocartilagenous support gives way because of the negative inspiratory pressure. Injury to the inferior turbinates may interfere with their role as the regulatory valve of the nose and an aggressive infracture may cause bony obstruction. These latter conditions can be treated surgically.

The quality of the overlying skin is important. The surgeon should realize that active sebaceous glands thicken the skin so that it does not drape well over the new framework. The skin should be treated preoperatively to reduce acne and oil, and the limits of correction should be explained to the patient. The ideal candidate would be a 16-year-old with thin, dry skin, no history of acne, and a straight nose with minimal deformity.

The operation is performed through the nostrils with an incision made internally between the upper and lower cartilages. The skin is elevated from the nasal dorsum. The lower alar cartilages are delivered into the operative field by a bipedicle incision and trimmed to reduce the bulb of the tip. The hump of nasal bone and cartilage (upper lateral and septum) is removed with a rasp or chisel. Finally, a lateral osteotomy narrows the vault, completing the alteration of the cartilagenous skeletal framework of the nose (Fig. 8-2).

Alterations to a deviated septum and turbinates may improve breathing. This is usually accomplished through a submucous resection of the deformed cartilage, taking care to leave enough cartilage to support the nose.

From a review of 407 consecutive rhinoplasties performed by the senior author and followed an average of several months, the most common complications of rhinoplasty include hemorrhage (2 percent), septal perforation (1 percent) and residual deformity (12 percent).

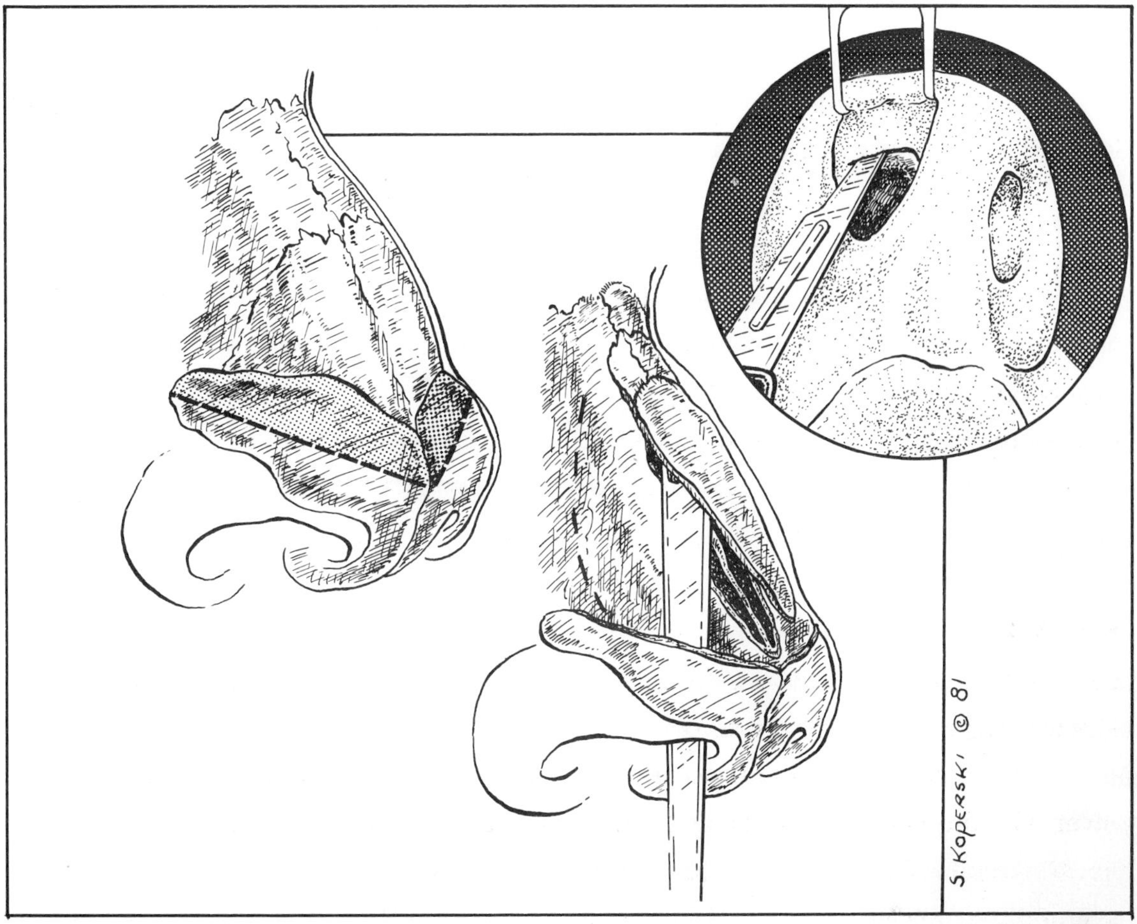

Figure 8-2. **Rhinoplasty.** Altering a nasal shape requires a surgical modification of the osseocartilaginous framework of the upper lateral cartilage and nasal bone and the lower lateral cartilages (left). The incision is intranasal, usually between the upper and lower lateral cartilages (circular inset). After the caudal aspect of the lower cartilages is modified, the hump (upper lateral cartilage and nasal bone) is removed, in this case by an osteotome (center). A fracture of the maxilla narrows the vault and completes the procedure (dotted lines in center illustration).

Residual external deformity that requires revision may arise from a technical flaw in the surgical procedure or from the healing process itself. Almost one-half of these problems are due to a residual bulbous tip and one-fifth are caused by irregular nasal bones requiring further rasping. Previous scars, from fracture or other injury, and preexisting asymmetry both contribute to the problem. Continued or worsened airway obstruction is normal for a month or more, owing to postoperative swelling. It may actually take over a year for the swelling to subside completely and for the final shape of the nose to emerge, especially in the thicker skin of the tip.

Hemorrhage may occur either at the time of surgery or 10 to 14 days later. Epistaxis should be treated by internal packing and application of an external splint to maintain the postoperative shape. Ligation of the maxillary artery is rarely necessary, although it has been reported.

Septal perforation may occur in those patients with friable membranes when a submucous resection is done. Symptoms may include whistling on nasal inspiration, crusting or intermittent hemorrhage. Intranasal examination reveals the fistula in the septum.

Postoperative care includes head elevation to reduce venous congestion and cold compresses to the eyes to reduce swelling. Direct pressure applied at the time of the nasal fracture does the most to reduce subcutaneous hematoma leading to "black eye." A nasal splint is applied in the operating room. Packs of soft rubber drains are employed overnight and removed in the morning. The splint is removed five to seven days later. The patient should avoid stress for two to four weeks. If the patient wears glasses, they must be taped to the forehead for a similar length of time to avoid pressure on the fractured nasal bones.

Mentoplasty

Frequently, patients who request a rhinoplasty also have a recessed chin. Chin augmentation often results in a better facial balance. An incision under the chin, or intraorally in the buccal sulcus, allows access to the mentum for placement of bone, cartilage or a silicone rubber implant. The silicone implant, in sizes of 4 to 8 mm, is the most frequently used material since it requires no donor site. Assessment of occlusion is important, and occasionally a cephalometrogram is required to assess the interrelationship of the facial bones. In cases of facial bone deformity, osteotomy of the maxilla or mandible may be the proper treatment for recessed chin (Fig. 8-3).

If silicone is selected, it is important to place the implant on the tip of the mandible overlying the cortical bones. Experimental studies have suggested that there is greater absorption of underlying bone if the implant is placed subperiostally, and clinical studies have shown that up to 50 percent of patients experience some bony absorption. It is important, therefore, that the implant not overlay the thin cortical bone covering the roots of the teeth.

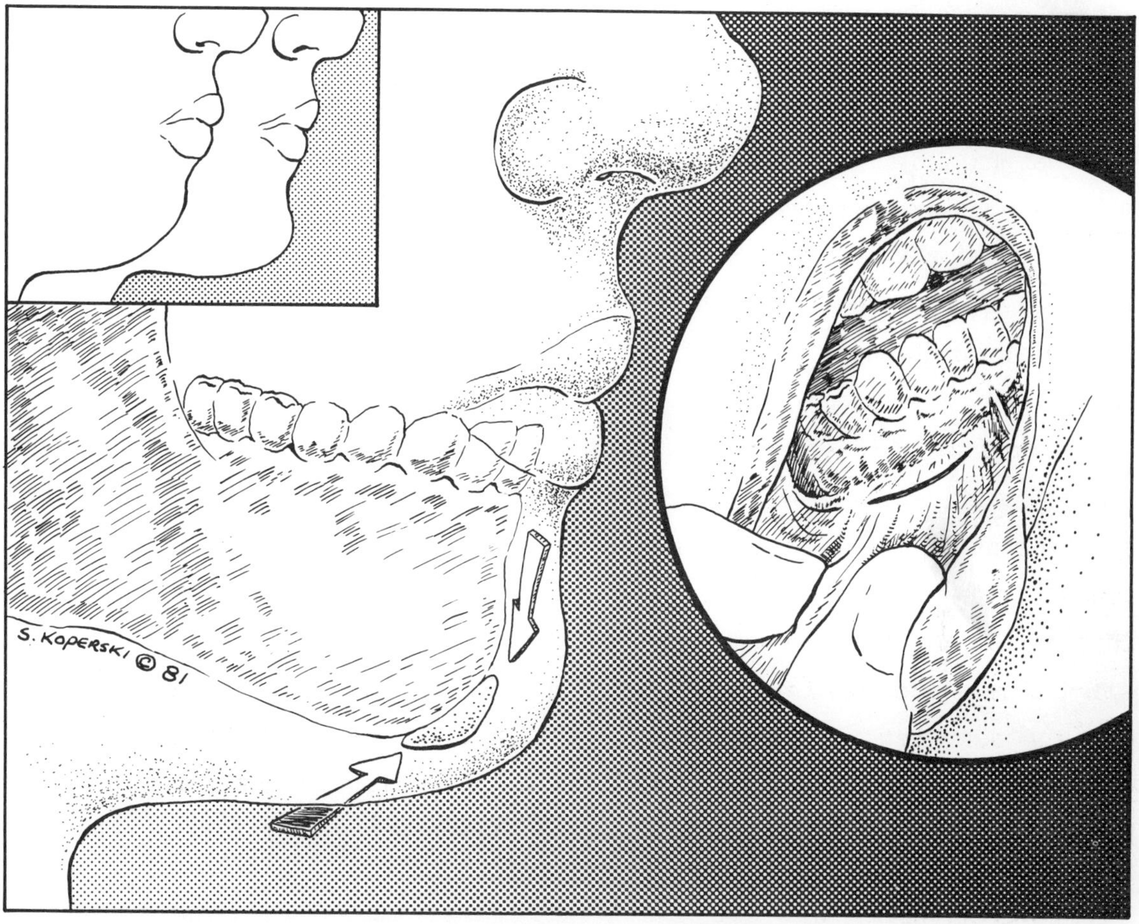

Figure 8-3. **Mentoplasty.** Augmentation of the chin may balance the profile (rectangular inset). The operation can be performed intraorally or through a submental incision as shown by arrows in center illustration. If it is performed intraorally, a 1.5 cm incision is made on the lip mucosa to one side of the frenulum (circular inset). Leaving the frenulum and the midline attachments of the lower lip may help to prevent cephalad migration of the implant if the intraoral route is used.

Postoperative care includes reducing motion of the face by prescribing a liquid diet. A pressure dressing helps hold the prosthesis in place.

Blepharoplasty

Blepharoplasty is designed to correct blepharochalazia (atonia of the eyelid skin), dermatochalazia (hypertrophy of the eyelid skin), and pseudoptosis (lower lid "bags"). Most commonly, the operation removes excess skin above the upper lids and bags under the lower lids. This involves excision of skin, muscle and fat from the upper lid and incision at the lower lid margin to remove fat and skin. "Malar puffs" are not eradicated. The surgeon must evaluate the position of the eyebrow; if it is severely ptotic, it must be raised (Fig. 8-4).

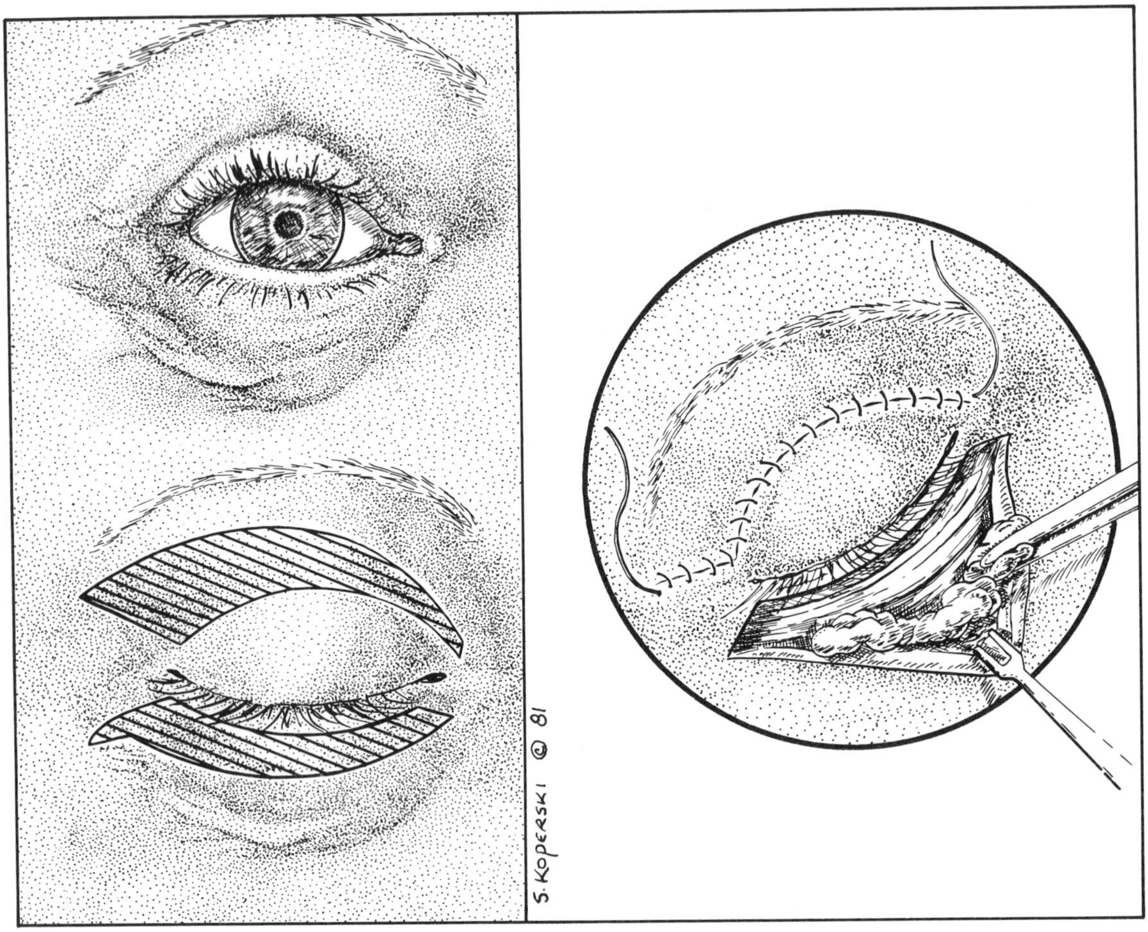

Figure 8-4. **Blepharoplasty.** In essence, eyelid plasty is most effective for redundant skin of the upper lid and for fat "bags" of the lower lid. The amount of skin usually resected is shown in the shaded areas (left). Note that the incision is made in the tarsal crease in the case of the upper lid and at the lash border in the case of the lower. Fat can be removed from either lid as desired. The upper lid incision is closed with a running suture. In this patient, a skin flap is used for the lower lid and the muscle opened in the area of the three pockets for access to the fat (circular inset). Many surgeons prefer a skin-muscle flap in order to have direct access to the fat.

The preoperative evaluation includes assessment of ocular movements, tear production and vision. It is also necessary to check for ptosis and for Bell's phenomenon (which would protect the cornea in the initial postoperative period). Tarsal plate tone should also be assessed. Problems in any of these areas must be pointed out to the patient as surgery may magnify existing defects. The appearance of the eyes, for example, may be affected by squinting due to poor refraction. This results in hypertrophy of the obicularis oculi and pretarsal muscles. If pigment is present in the lower lids, it may be intensified postoperatively.

Serious complications include ectropion, corneal abrasion and blindness. Ectropion occurred in 2 out of 600 patients in our series and therefore is rare, but it can be very difficult to treat. In older patients, tightening the tarsal plate and adding skin is the most effective treatment. The normal amount of skin removed is 10 to 15 mm from the upper lids and 3 to 8 mm from the lower lids. Blindness has been reported from infection, hematoma, spasm of the central retinal artery, and glaucoma, but it is extremely rare (0.04 percent of patients).

Corneal abrasion is not uncommon, especially with general anesthesia. For patients operated on under general anesthesia, it is necessary to protect the eyes with an ocular lubricant. The postoperative complaint of pain or "sand in the eyes" is the key to diagnosis. Treatment consists of patching the eyes and applying topical antibiotics for 24 hours.

General postoperative care includes rest, elevation of the head, and ice compresses for 24 hours, followed by warm compresses for several days. Balanced salt solution for irrigation of mucus alleviates discomfort. Sterile ophthalmic lubrication may be necessary at night.

Rhytidectomy

Rhytidectomy (face lift) is one of the most common aesthetic operations. Essentially, the procedure involves the advancement of flaps from the cheek and neck, using incisions hidden in the hairline and around the ears. The skin is elevated from the underlying subcutaneous tissue, care being taken to avoid the facial nerve and great auricular nerve. The skin is placed under slight tension and the excess trimmed away. The superficial musculoaponeurotic system (SMAS) may be sutured to further tighten the face. The SMAS is the investing fascia of the facial muscles and extends from the frontalis to the platysma. Occasionally, the incision goes across the top of the head for a "forehead lift" which helps to elevate the brows (Fig. 8-5).

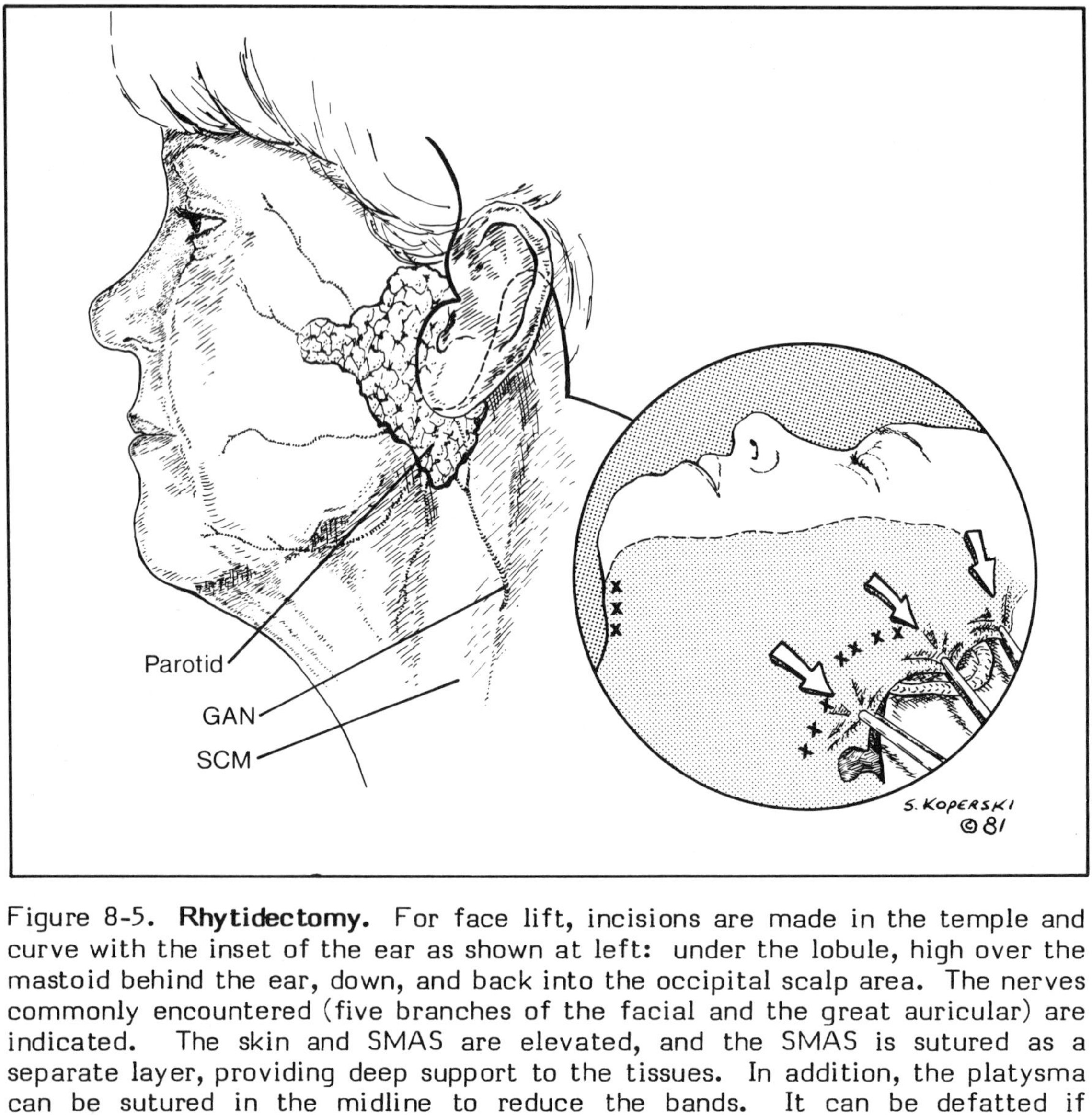

Figure 8-5. **Rhytidectomy.** For face lift, incisions are made in the temple and curve with the inset of the ear as shown at left: under the lobule, high over the mastoid behind the ear, down, and back into the occipital scalp area. The nerves commonly encountered (five branches of the facial and the great auricular) are indicated. The skin and SMAS are elevated, and the SMAS is sutured as a separate layer, providing deep support to the tissues. In addition, the platysma can be sutured in the midline to reduce the bands. It can be defatted if necessary. The skin is overlapped and trimmed. In the circular inset, the sutures in the SMAS are indicated by Xs and the direction of tightening by arrows.

Most patients seeking face lift (80 percent) have normal Minnesota multiphasic personality inventories. Adapting Edgerton's classification, patients requesting rhytidectomy fall into four groups:

- Those between the ages of 29 to 39 who are emotionally dependent. Members of this group often have highly unrealistic goals and are having difficulty making the transition into adulthood.
- Those between the ages of 40 to 50 who work for a living. Rhytidectomy is becoming more common among members of this group who

have to compete with younger individuals. The surgery may help, but, in itself, may not achieve the desired goal of promotion or job retention.

- Those, usually over the age of 50, who have suffered bereavement. Studies have shown that the operation may help to relieve women of the depression of being widowed.
- Men. Although this surgery is becoming more accepted for men, they still account only for roughly 10 percent of rhytidectomy patients and the psychology is different from that of women.

Preoperative preparations for rhytidectomy include performing the routine evaluation described earlier in this chapter under General Health and having the patient maintain normal diet and normal exercise. Specifically, the skin should be in good condition with no evidence of acne and no scalp infections. The patient should cease, or at least curtail, smoking because it constricts the blood vessels and increases the risk of postoperative flap loss. Evaluation must also include a neurological history and an examination to elicit any weakness of the seventh nerve. It is important to establish whether or not there is a history of Bell's palsy because it may recur under stress.

Postoperatively, control of the patient's blood pressure is extremely important because even a transient rise contributes to hematoma formation. Elevation of the head, sedation and rest all help keep the incidence of hematoma low. Also, the patient must recuperate in a setting where the personnel understand the particular needs of the plastic surgery patient.

Common complications of rhytidectomy include hematoma (5 percent of patients) and excessive postoperative sagging. More serious complications include nerve damage, the most common of which is to the great auricular nerve in the neck. Injury to the seventh nerve, with resultant paralysis of a muscle group, occurs in 0.5 to 2.5 percent of cases. Skin slough, most commonly in the postauricular region, occurs in 3 percent of cases.

Treatment of hematoma consists of evacuation. A hematoma will increase the chance of loss of skin flaps and will leave a wrinkled, woody appearance to the skin. Small hematomas may be evacuated by needle when they liquefy after 5 to 10 days; large ones require that the patient be returned to the operating room immediately.

Excessive postoperative sagging may occur because of the stretching of the collagen fibers, loss of resiliency of the elastic fibers, and compression of tissue fluid. Excessive preoperative sagging of the skin should alert the surgeon to this possibility, and the patient should be warned that a second lift may be necessary to obtain the best results.

Sensory nerve damage can be avoided by taking care to avoid the great auricular nerve. This nerve crosses the midpoint of the sternocleidomastoid (SCM) muscle 6.5 mm caudal to the bony exterior auditory canal.

The surgeon must also be familiar with the course of the seventh nerve in order to avoid injuring it, especially if a dissection of the SMAS is performed. The nerve emerges from the stylomastoid foramen and has five branches which become very superficial when they emerge from the parotid gland. The nerve is always beneath the SMAS. Awareness of how the parotid gland differs in size among individuals helps to avoid trouble; in some patients the parotid is very small and the dissection may reach the plane of the nerves very quickly (see Facial Fractures, Fig. 10-4).

Treatment of nerve laceration consists of approximating the ends, using magnification and fine sutures. Occasionally, weakness of the facial nerve may be temporary. In that case, it is caused by swelling, and function will return in two to three months.

Treatment for sloughed skin flaps includes debridement and application of saline dressings. Usually the wound will contract and epithelize. A subsequent rhytidectomy may excise a good portion of the scar.

Otoplasty

The ear forms from cartilagenous hillocks from the mandibular and hyoid arches. Prominent ears are usually caused by a lack of sufficient definition of the antihelical folds. The lop-eared appearance causes early psychological problems, beginning when the child enters school.

Correction requires an incision behind the ear. The spring of the abnormal cartilage is broken by cutting or abrading it to define the antihelical folds. This may be done as early as age five because 85 percent of ear growth has taken place by that time (Fig. 8-6).

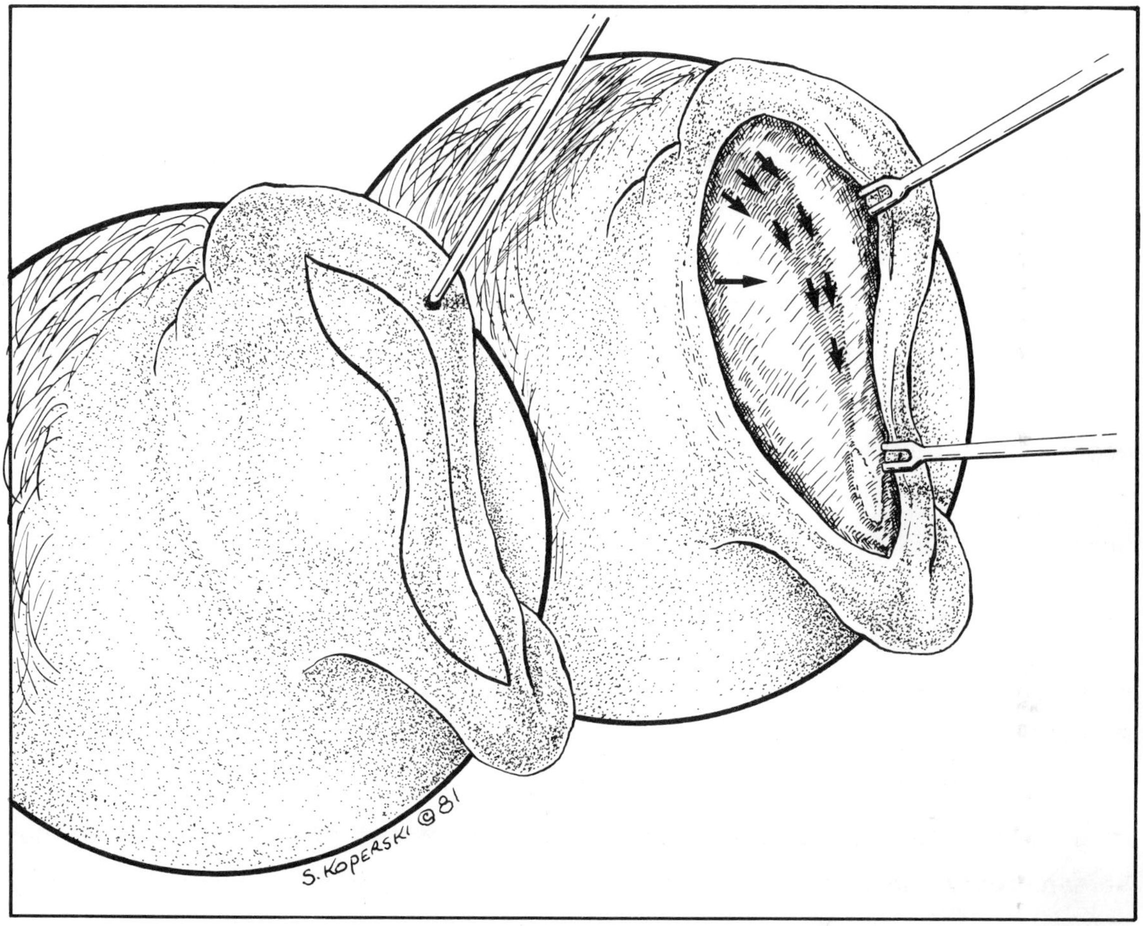

Figure 8-6. **Otoplasty.** To correct prominent ears, a posterior incision removing the dumbbell-shaped skin allows access to the cartilage of the helix (left). Abrading the cartilage in a funnel shape breaks the springs of this cartilage to create the superior and inferior crura which, along with the tail of the antihelix, can be held back to the mastoid fascia with sutures (arrows right). This places the rim of the helix about 15 mm from the mastoid.

Complications of this surgery may include telephone ear, where the middle portion is tighter than the top or the lobule, or sharp cartilage edges if the abrasions are made too deeply. Recurrence of the deformity is possible where there has been inadequate breaking of the cartilage spring. Chondritis is rare. This is fortunate because the resultant scar and deformity are severe. Hematoma is rare. The scar is rarely a problem as it is hidden behind the ear.

Postoperative care includes rest and an occlusive head dressing for five to seven days.

Chemical Peel

Chemical peel is used for smoothing very fine wrinkles in severely "weathered skin." In its most common form, chemical peel consists of an application of phenol to the defatted skin, causing a second-degree burn. It has been revealed in histological studies that this treatment increases the material that accepts elastic stain and makes the collagen more homogeneous. The results have been shown through biopsy studies to be effective for up to 13 years.

Phenol is absorbed through the lungs and skin and excreted by the kidneys. Dilute solutions are absorbed most freely. Stronger concentrations cause necrosis of the skin, blocking absorption. Absorption of phenol may produce toxicity, early manifestations of which are evidenced by changes in the electrocardiogram and a rise in blood pressure and pulse. After application of the agent, a frost occurs on the skin, followed by hyperemia. Taping the skin increases the depth of the burn and, hence, the effectiveness of the peel.

Complications may include hypertrophic scars, increased sensitivity to sunlight, and blotching of the skin. Phenol should never be applied to the neck or to undermined skin flaps.

Expected sequelae of chemical peel include a general reduction in pigmentation of the treated skin, since peeling decreases the number of melanophores in the basal layer of the epidermis. A prolonged erythema of the skin can result, and an alteration of existing skin lesions may occur. Frequently, telegectasias will be more pronounced, pores will increase in size, and nevi will darken.

Hair Transplantation

Hair transplant consists of grafting plugs of skin containing hair follicles to areas of alopecia from donor sites in the occipital region. The surgeon must take into consideration the progressive nature of baldness in order that the patient not end up with the donor site itself eventually uncovered. The best candidates for this surgery are men with late onset male pattern baldness. Shafts of thick hair which grow in a spiral pattern are the best donor type as these cover more area than does straight hair.

The punch grafts are usually 3 to 4 mm in diameter and must be cut on a bevel to correspond to the direction of the hair shafts. The donor site need not be closed primarily. The surgeon then cuts out a circle of scalp 1 mm less in diameter than the donor site. As the scalp retracts, it accommodates the larger donor plug. The shafts must be oriented in the proper direction to correspond to the rest of the hair pattern. All grafts lose their hair postoperatively, and regrowth takes up to six months.

Hair strips used as grafts and hair flaps have their uses, but they leave sharper demarcations than the staggered, more natural appearance obtained by plugs.

Breast

In our culture, the breast is a powerful psychosexual symbol which can profoundly affect an individual's self image. Problems may range from deformities such as small or asymmetrical breasts in women and gynecomastia in boys to breast reconstruction following mastectomy.

Augmentation Mammoplasty. This operation is usually performed by making an incision around the nipple and placing an implant of saline silicone or gel behind the breast and on top of, or sometimes beneath, the pectoralis major muscle. The incision may also be placed under the breast or in the armpit. Occasionally, the implant is placed under the pectoralis muscle (Fig. 8-7).

Preoperative evaluation includes a personal or family history of breast disease, previous biopsies and psychological motivation. The size of each breast and the position of the nipples should be noted as these features are often asymmetrical. Carcinoma of the breast has rarely been reported following this operation; the percentage is lower than that expected for the population generally (10 per 10,000 cases). Since breast tissue extends from the clavicle to the axilla to the waist and penetrates the pectoralis muscle, the implant may theoretically hinder early detection of a tumor. However, most of the tissue is in front of the implant and is, hence, accessible.

If the nipple is below the inframammary crease, a pexy or lift is indicated, otherwise the result will merely be a larger, droopier breast.

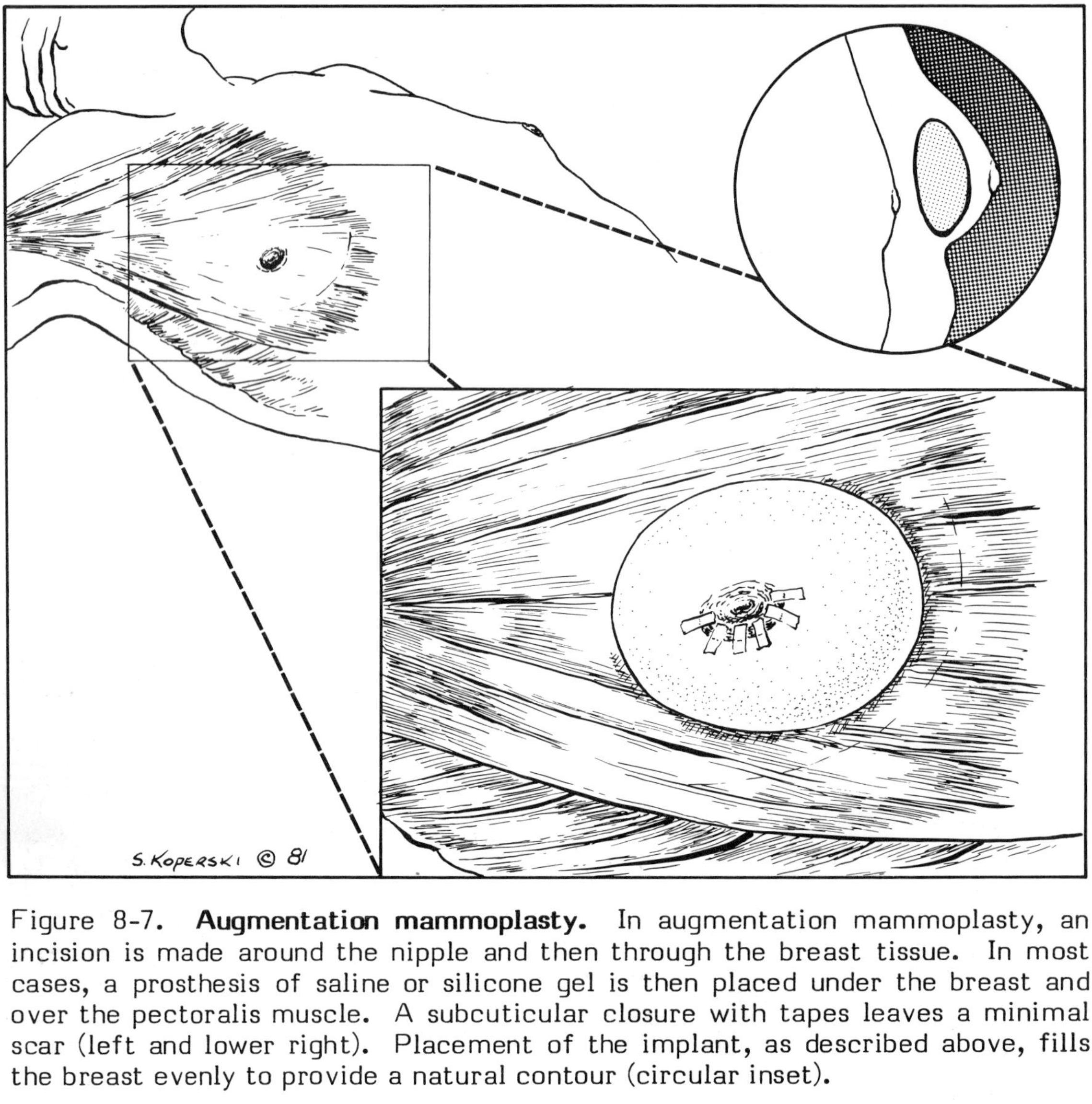

Figure 8-7. **Augmentation mammoplasty.** In augmentation mammoplasty, an incision is made around the nipple and then through the breast tissue. In most cases, a prosthesis of saline or silicone gel is then placed under the breast and over the pectoralis muscle. A subcuticular closure with tapes leaves a minimal scar (left and lower right). Placement of the implant, as described above, fills the breast evenly to provide a natural contour (circular inset).

Common complications include hardness from capsule formation (20 to 40 percent of patients), hematoma (3 percent), nipple numbness (4 to 7 percent), infection (2.5 percent), and malposition of the implant. Hardness results from excessive scar contracture in the pocket compressing the implant. The hardness varies; it can be mild or as hard as a tennis ball. The exact cause is unknown. Treatment is closed or open capsulotomy performed to reexpand the pocket. Continued pressure with an elastic bandage, massage and exercise are helpful. If severe and persistent capsules form, the implants may have to be removed, but this is rare.

Inflatable implants may leak (7 percent of patients) either from valve misfunction or fatigue of the implant. The resulting collapse requires reimplantation with a new prosthesis. Malposition may occur from scar contracture as well as from inaccurate placement at the time of surgery. Hematoma may be immediate or delayed. Evacuation is the required treatment.

The infection rate in this type of surgery is remarkably low. Prophylactic antibiotics are of unproven benefit. Infected implants may have to be removed and the infection treated. In such cases, the implants can be replaced in two to three months. Occasionally, an implant may be saved with intensive antibiotics. The periareolar incision, because of the thickness of coverage, seems to protect against extrusion of the implant more than does the inframammary incision.

Postoperative care includes reduced activity for 7 to 14 days. Drains are generally not used.

Gynecomastia. Gynecomastia is a normal occurrence at puberty; 70 percent of cases regress by the late teens. Late onset, however, may indicate tumor or endocrine disturbance. Gynecomastia can be psychologically crippling to a teenage boy. Operations performed through the areola remove the breast tissue and leave a small amount of tissue beneath the nipple so that the nipple does not "stick" to the chest wall. Drains are required because of the large flaps dissected.

The most common problems are technical. A "shelf effect" may be evident where the area of tissue removal abuts the normal tissue. Careful feathering of the junction will alleviate the problem.

Reduction Mammoplasty, Mastopexy. Hypertrophy of the breast in women can cause psychological problems as well as functional problems such as backache, kyphosis, shoulder pain and inability to participate in sports.

The operation consists of preservation of the nipple on a pedicle, amputation of the lower sections of the breast, and tailoring the skin envelope. An average of 400 g is removed per side in a hypertrophic breast (Fig. 8-8).

A ptotic breast is of normal size but the skin envelope is stretched, giving a drooping appearance. This may be the result of weight loss or, more commonly, pregnancy. In a mastopexy the nipple is lifted, but only the excess skin is removed. Occasionally, a mastopexy is combined with a small implant to increase the breast size and correct ptosis.

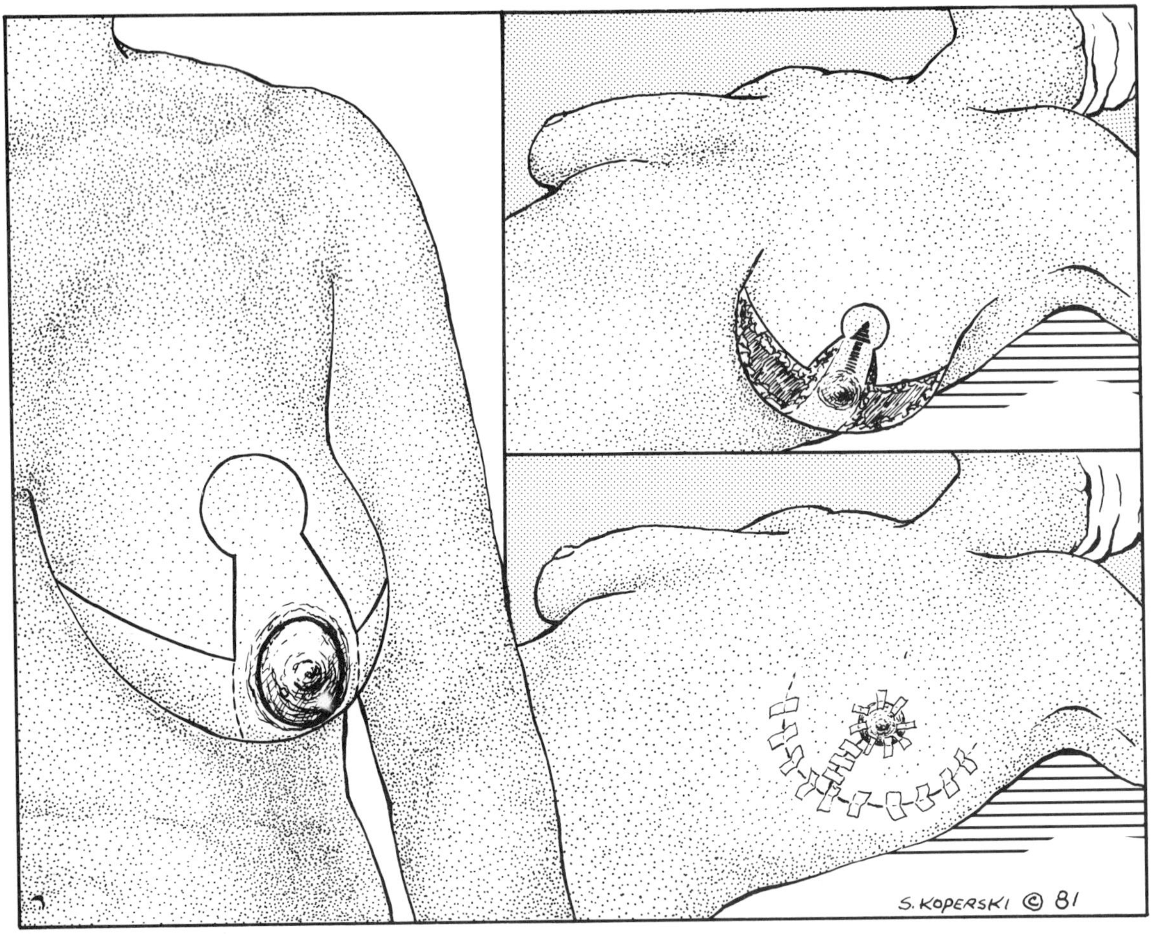

Figure 8-8. **Reduction mammoplasty.** In reduction mammoplasty, the usual markings (left) provide a keyhole for the nipple. Resection of the skin between the lines provides a skin "brassiere" to shape the breast. The nipple is preserved by deepithelizing a vertical dermal pedicle and resecting excess breast tissue beneath this as well as medially and laterally (right). A subcuticular suture and tapes complete the closure which forms an inverted "T" scar, most of which will be in the submammary fold (lower right).

Preoperative preparation includes weight loss, which causes more sagging of the breast. Patients must be warned that some postoperative sagging is to be expected owing to the nature of the tissue.

Common problems in breast reduction include hypertrophic scarring (1.8 percent of patients), numbness of nipple (70 percent), and postoperative sagging of the breast. This occurs in most patients because of the nature of the tissue preoperatively. Scarring is significant, and the patient must be willing to accept the scars in return for a better silhouette and a lighter chest.

The incisions run around the areola, down to the inframammary crease, and medially and laterally in the inframmary crease. It should be remembered that body scars are always larger than facial scars because of the increased tension on body skin and because of its relative thickness.

Change in nipple sensation will occur to some extent, and the further the nipple is shifted, the more likely this is to occur. Numbness may affect sensitivity or nursing ability as it is the stimulation of the nipple that signals the brain to release hormones to stimulate the breast for lactation. However, many patients with large breasts have decreased sensation of the nipple to begin with. When more than 500 g of tissue are excised, nursing ability is seriously affected.

Severe problems may include hematoma (5 percent of patients). Infection is extremely rare and must not be confused with fat necrosis. Nipple loss, fortunately, involves less than 1.0 percent of patients.

Subcutaneous Mastectomy. Subcutaneous mastectomy, with reconstruction with subcutaneous implants, may be indicated for those patients with a strong family history of breast carcinoma and multiple previous biopsies who are several years from menopause and have severe fibrocystic disease. All of the indications are usually necessary as the reconstructed breast is inferior to the original organ. Occasionally, a patient with cancer phobia, or one who has had previous breast cancer, can be helped by this procedure. The operation is similar to a gynecomastia procedure. It does not remove all of the breast tissue as the nipple remains and cancer can still develop. However, the incidence of breast cancer following subcutaneous mastectomy is much lower than would be expected (0.5 percent of patients), especially when one considers that it is reserved for high-risk individuals.

Abdominoplasty

Because of pregnancy or rapid weight gain, abdominal tissue may remain redundant after parturition or subsequent weight loss. This is caused by the rupture of the dermal collagen, resulting in "stretch mark" scars. Diastasis of the rectus muscle is another possible sequela.

The operation consists of a horizontal incision beginning below the anteriosuperior iliac spine and extending across the pubis to the other side. The skin is undermined at the level of the fascia, to the costal margins after circumscription of the umbilical stalk. The fascia is plicated horizontally and vertically and the excess skin drawn over and trimmed. The umbilicus is brought out on the skin of the abdomen. Usually, all tissue between the umbilicus and the pubis can be removed. This operation is not a substitute for weight loss. Complications of abdominoplasty include hematoma (2 percent of patients), infection (7 percent), skin loss (1 percent), dehiscense (5.4 percent), phlebitis (1 percent), emboli (0.8 percent), and gross scarring (3 percent) (Fig. 8-9).

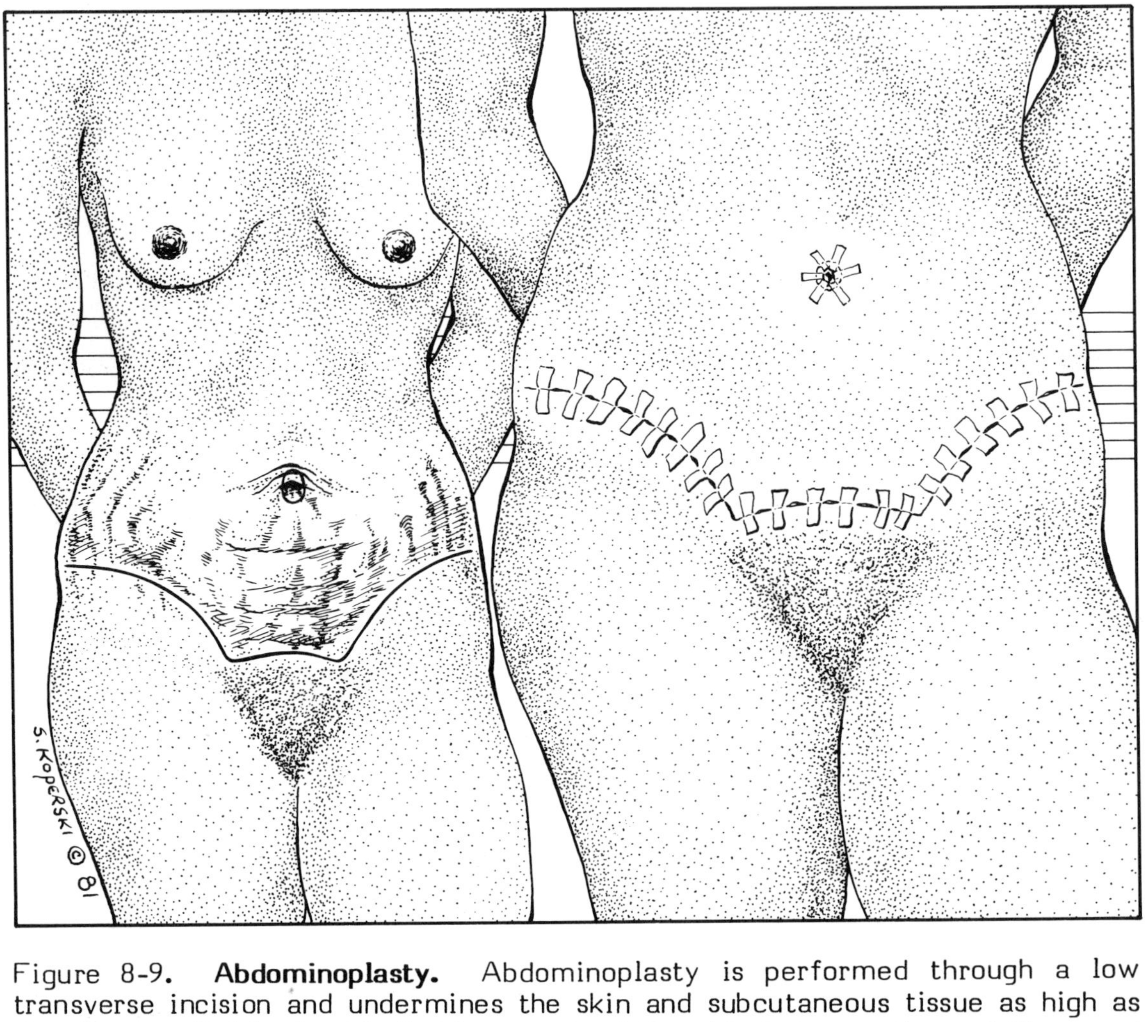

Figure 8-9. **Abdominoplasty.** Abdominoplasty is performed through a low transverse incision and undermines the skin and subcutaneous tissue as high as the rib cage (left). In this fashion, most of the skin between the umbilicus and the pubis can be resected. The umbilicus is circumscribed and sutured at the same level through the downward shifted abdominal flap (right). Note that not all stretch marks are removed but only those between the umbilicus and pubis.

Thigh Reduction

Thigh reduction is designed to remove skin and subcutaneous tissue over the greater trochanter to reduce the "jodhpur deformity." It does remove some tissue from the buttocks and medial thigh, but the best results are obtained in those patients who have fatty deposits over the greater trochanter. Poor results are achieved in those patients with complaints of drooping buttocks, fat legs or "large thighs."

The procedure involves an incision beginning below the anteriosuperior iliac spine and extending across the upper part of the greater trochanter to the gluteal fold around the perineum and part way up the groin crease. This surgery is not a substitute for weight loss, and the patient must be made to realize that the scars will be significant and will often drift downward with time rather than remaining hidden in the creases. Patients will look better in slacks and tight dresses, but dressed in shorts they may display a scar. In some instances, the newer technique of suction curettage of the involved fat may obviate the necessity of these large incisions for some patients (Fig. 8-10).

Complications include phlebitis, numbness, wide scar, double bulge deformity, hematoma and wound separation. Infection is rare in spite of proximity to the perineum. Numbness results when the lateral femoral cutaneous nerve is transected.

Postoperative care includes keeping the hips extended for two to four weeks because early flexion will cause dehiscence. Support hose and early ambulation reduce the risk of phlebitis.

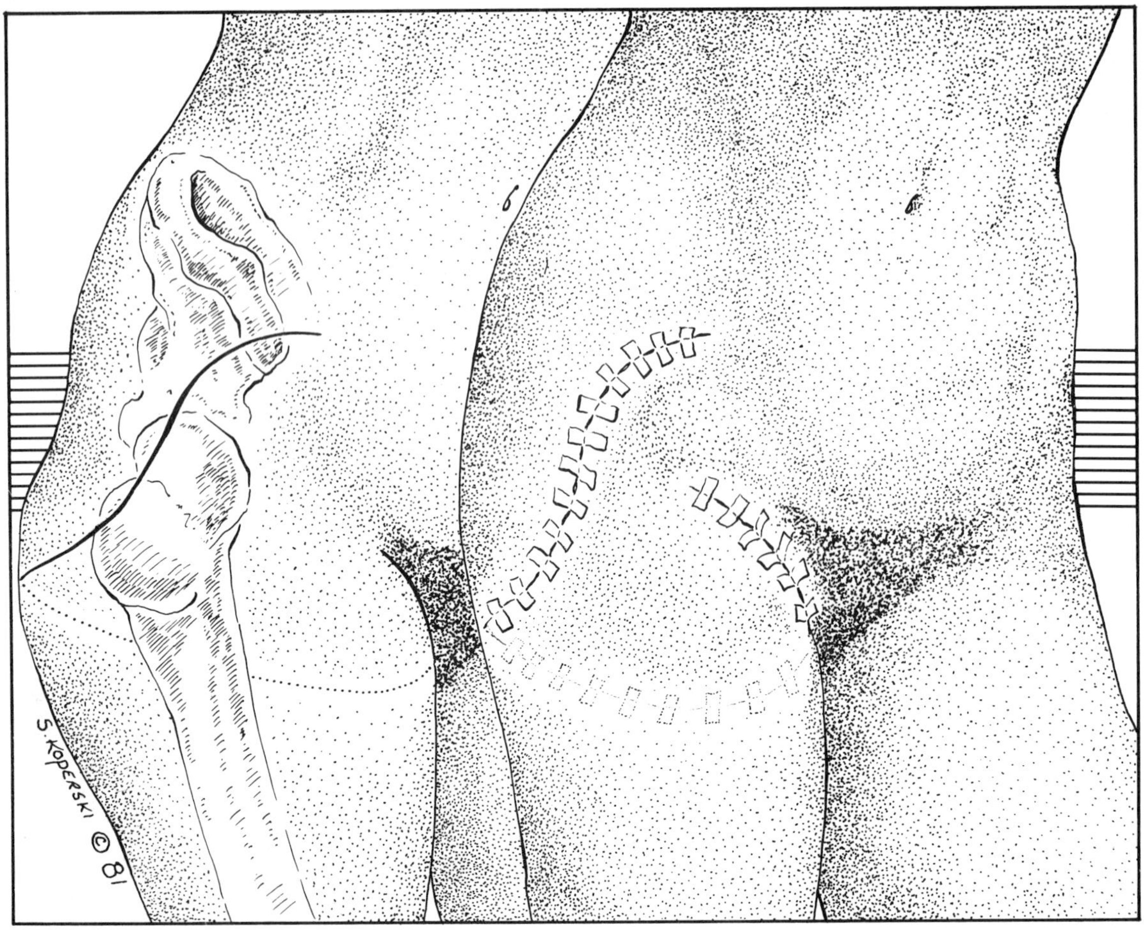

Figure 8-10. **Thigh reduction.** Thigh reduction removes skin and fat over the greater trochanter (left). The improved contour is shown at right. The scar, which is prominent as in the case of all body surgery, extends from the lateral hip to the gluteal fold and from there to the groin, thus almost girdling the leg.

Brachioplasty

Older patients, or patients who lose weight, often have redundant tissue over the triceps. This can be removed by an S-shaped incision from the axilla to the medial condyle. This produces a scar which is hidden when the arm is at the side. A prominent scar will show when the arm is raised. Occasionally, in very thin patients with minimal deformity, a transverse excision in the axilla will be sufficient and will produce a hidden scar. Damage to the thoracobrachial nerve is probable with resultant numbness of the inner aspect of the arm (Fig. 8-11).

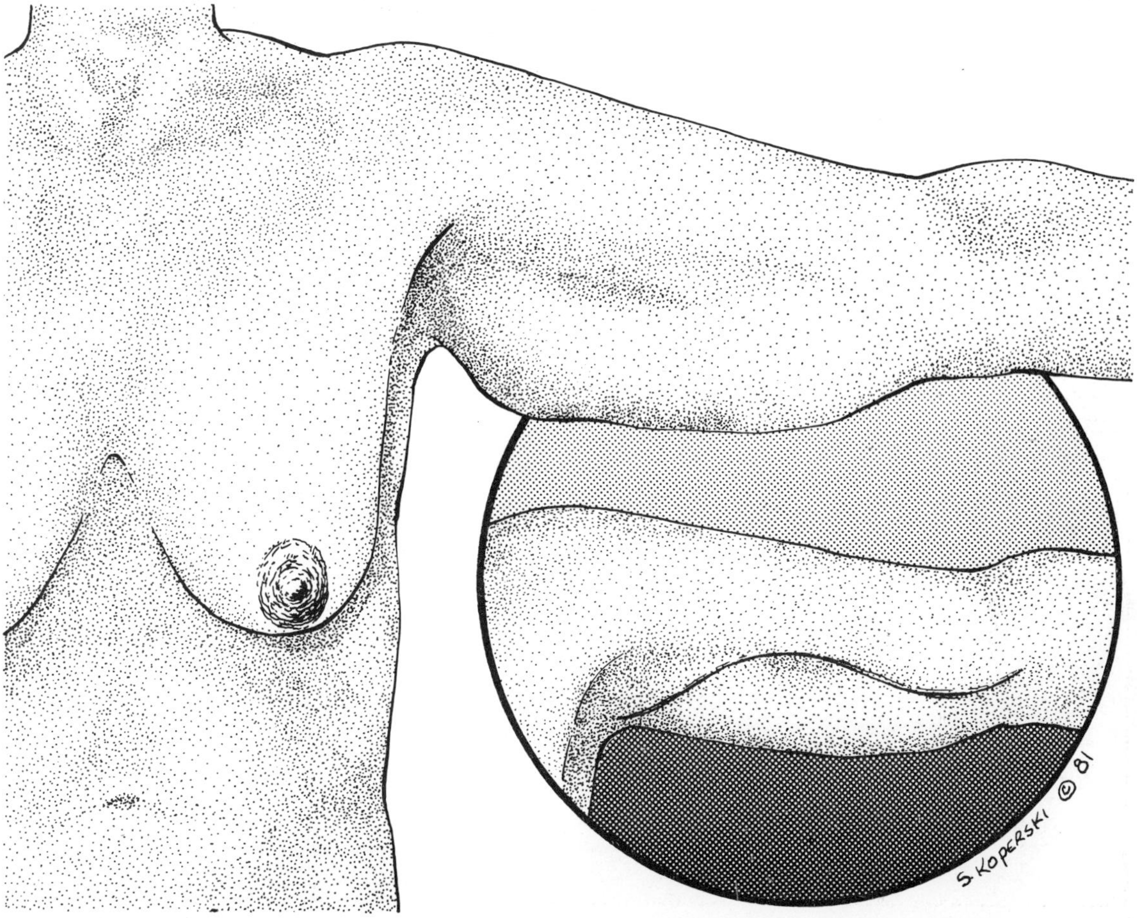

Figure 8-11. **Brachioplasty.** Brachioplasty removes the skin and subcutaneous tissue over the triceps which gives a bat-wing appearance to an older arm. The scar, which is prominent, is curved to reduce the likelihood of contracture and is kept on the inner aspect of the arm to make it less noticeable.

Summary

Aesthetic surgery combines the three principles of plastic surgery: elective incisions, wound care, and wound closure. Although standard procedures are used, the techniques are different and each operation requires individual variations according to these principles. In no other surgery is Q.S. (quantum sufficit) more appropriate.

The success of aesthetic surgery depends upon the expectations of the patient and the technical expertise of the surgeon. Despite the various psychological implications, the success rate for surgery is 90 percent and above. Physical complications are less than 1 to 2 percent of patients, but some can be quite serious, and patients should be apprised of their potential. Aesthetic surgery can be extremely satisfying to the surgeon, as these groups of patients are highly motivated to get well. Reduction of the incidence of the few adverse psychological reactions depends upon the surgeon's preoperative selection of patients which improves with experience.

CHAPTER 9

Breast Reconstruction

Loss or disfigurement of the female breast by mastectomy can cause the patient profound emotional and sexual disruption. Fortunately, earlier diagnosis of breast disease, recognition of the importance to the patient of her physical integrity, and improved reconstructive methods have liberalized medical opinion as to the advisability and feasibility of breast reconstruction.

The reconstructive surgeon who confronts a radical or modified radical mastectomy is faced with several problems. The most immediate is a shortage of skin and subcutaneous tissue. Complete reconstruction of the breast should include restoration of the nipple/areolar complex and the anterior axillary fold. The direction of the original scar is an important factor in the reconstruction process. Generally, a transverse incision is acceptable as it lies within the brassiere line, but it is often carried too far toward the sternum and restricts the types of clothing that can be worn. A slightly oblique incision is best, provided it permits sufficient access to the tumor, because it makes subsequent reconstruction easier.

Timing of Reconstruction

Some medical centers advocate breast reconstruction immediately following ablation of the tumor, but, in our opinion, the timing of the repair should be based upon the stage of the disease.

Patients with stage I disease should wait three to six months following surgery. This period allows for a proper histological examination to ascertain the extent of the disease, permits the scar tissue to soften, and gives the patient time to come to terms with her loss and to develop realistic expectations. A patient who expects a reconstructive operation to result in a normal breast will be disappointed. Reconstruction for patients with stage II or stage III disease should generally begin 6 to 12 months following completion of any subsequent chemo/radiotherapy.

Reconstruction for patients with stage IV disease is not entirely contra-indicated, but it must be undertaken with full realization of the very real possibility of further difficulty from the tumor. In the event that initial therapy is not curative, the disease is more likely to recur at a distant site rather than on the chest wall; therefore, we feel that reconstruction of the breast will not alter the final outcome of the disease.

The surgeon should discuss with the patient the possibility that a reconstruction could obscure the early detection of a chest wall recurrence and what this might mean in regard to further treatment. It is important to note that the presence of a prosthesis does not interfere with the administration of radiotherapy, if such should be needed at a future date.

Preoperative Evaluation

Adequate Skin Coverage

When anterior chest wall skin coverage is adequate, and if the pectoralis muscle remains completely intact, subcutaneous or submuscular pockets may be dissected to accommodate silicone mammary prostheses. For some patients this relatively simple operation is sufficient, and volume symmetry is achieved when wearing a brassiere. The nipple and areolar complex can be constructed at the same time or five to eight weeks after implantation of the prosthesis. If, however, the lateral border of the pectoralis is fibriotic following the modified radical mastectomy, this may render the submuscular pocket impractical (Fig. 9-1).

The most common problem following reconstruction is hardening of the breast, and this is more noticeable if the subcutaneous placement is utilized. The hardening occurs because the scar capsule around the implant contracts, compressing the prosthesis. The cause of this contracture is unknown, but leakage of silicone fluid, hematoma, or chronic infection are suspected causes. Some surgeons believe that muscle flaps appear to reduce the incidence of this problem.

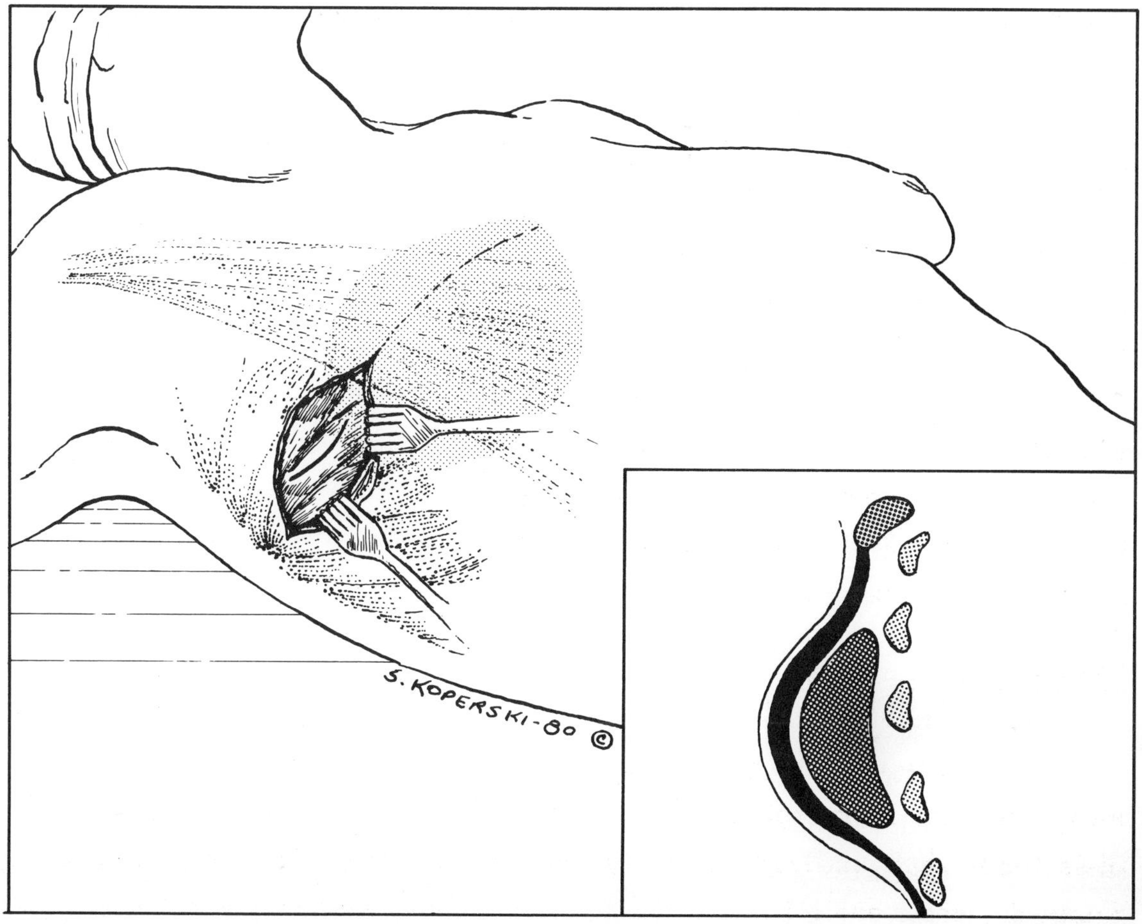

Figure 9-1. **Mammary prosthesis implantation.** For subcutaneous or submuscular implantation, the lateral aspect of the mastectomy scar is utilized. A pocket to receive the prosthesis is dissected in the area shaded. It is not necessary to make an additional cutaneous scar, such as a submammary incision. The inset shows the cross sectional relationship of the prosthesis in the subpectoral position.

Inadequate Skin Coverage

When there is inadequate skin coverage, either from radiation-induced changes or following wide resection of the original disease, skin and subcutaneous tissue must be added. This was originally accomplished by using local flaps. These procedures permit better padding over the prosthesis, adding both softness and protection. Also addition of tissue releases the tight skin envelope, presenting a more natural-appearing breast. In the past, these flaps required numerous stages, necessitating multiple hospital admissions over the course of months or years.

Recent developments in the understanding of flap physiology now permit the plastic surgeon to offer one-stage coverage with skin and subcutaneous tissue by way of an axial skin-muscle flap, utilizing the latissimus dorsi muscle. Isolating the neurovascular bundle permits transfer of the entire latissimus dorsi muscle with appropriate skin. The result is far preferable to that obtained by skin flaps alone.

The Latissimus Dorsi Muscle. The latissimus dorsi muscle takes its origin from the lower thoracic and lumbar vertebrae and from the iliac crest. This broad, fan-shaped muscle inserts into the intertubercular groove of the humerus. The blood supply from the thoracodorsal artery, a terminal branch of the subscapular artery, enters the deep aspect of the muscle in company with the thoracodorsal nerve. The vessel can reliably be found 10 cm from the insertion of the muscle. When possible, the vessel should be preserved during the extirpative surgery in order to facilitate any subsequent reconstruction. The muscle functions to extend, adduct and medially rotate the arm, and a switch of its origins to the chest wall poses little functional deficit (Fig. 9-2).

For breast reconstruction, the latissimus dorsi muscle is useful in three ways. First, if additional skin is required, a cutaneous island measuring as large as 12 by 20 cm can be transferred, yet the donor site can still be closed primarily. Further, the surgery can be designed so that most of the donor site scar can be concealed within the line of a brassiere. Second, where adequate skin coverage exists, the muscle alone can be used to provide subcutaneous padding. Third, the edge of the muscle can be used to simulate the anterior axillary fold in those patients who have lost the pectoralis major muscle.

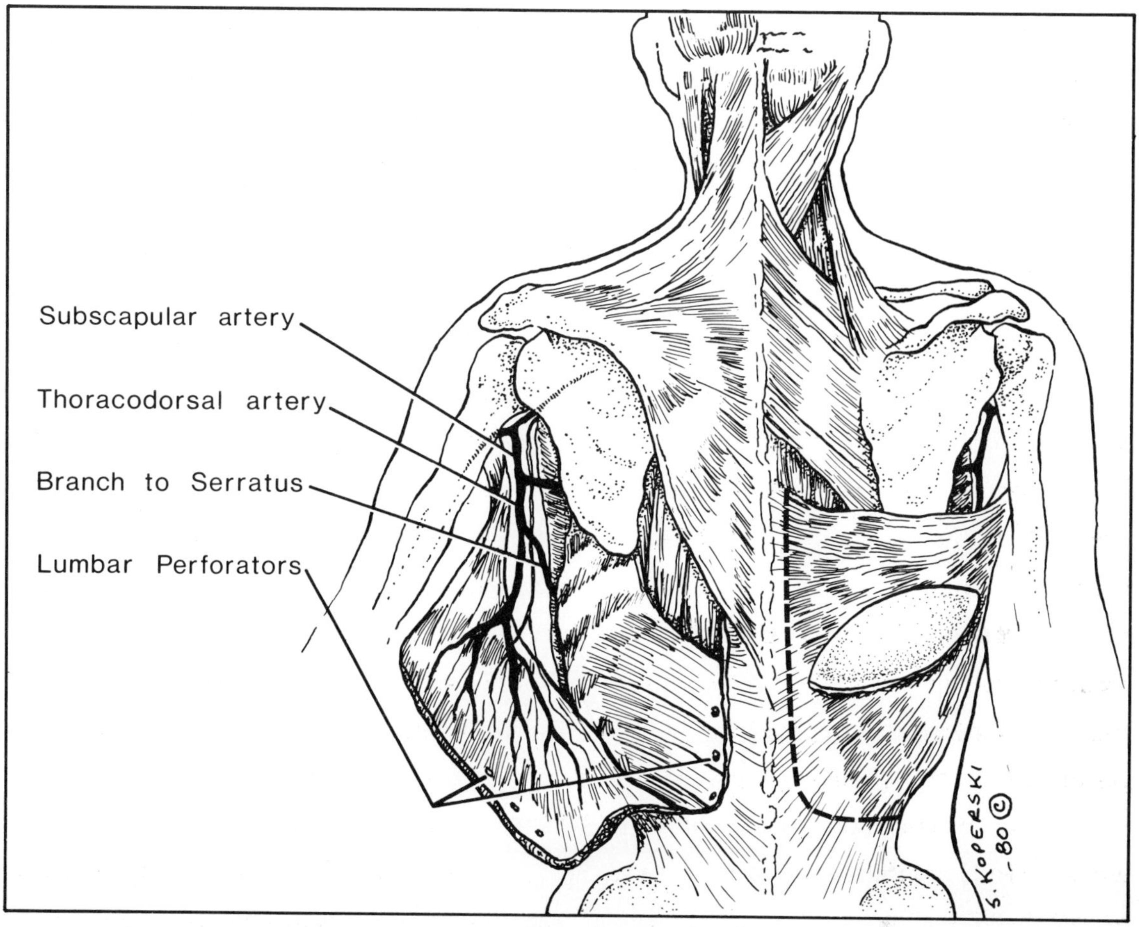

Figure 9-2. **Latissimus dorsi in original position.** The vascular anatomy of the latissimus dorsi muscle is demonstrated on the left. Note the origin of the thoracodorsal artery and nerve which accompanies it. If possible, these should be preserved at the time of the mastectomy. The right-hand side of the illustration shows the position of the skin island on the muscle before elevation. For clarity of demonstration, the rest of the skin has been removed.

Technique of Reconstruction

The vascular pedicle is isolated, with the aid of a Doppler probe, if necessary, through an incision that can be incorporated into the creation of the elliptical skin island. Using preoperative markings, the surgeon determines the size of the chest wall defect, then isolates an island of skin of appropriate dimension, retaining its muscular attachment. The latissimus muscle is separated from its origins. This flap of muscle and skin is then tunneled through the axilla to the chest wall and sutured to the sternum, the clavicle, and the edge of the deltoid muscle. The segment of skin fits into the incised breast scar. At the same time, a silicone prosthesis is placed beneath the flap to simulate the breast mound. The cutaneous island, if needed, is designed on the muscle in such a way as to fit into either a transverse or an oblique mastectomy scar (Fig. 9-3).

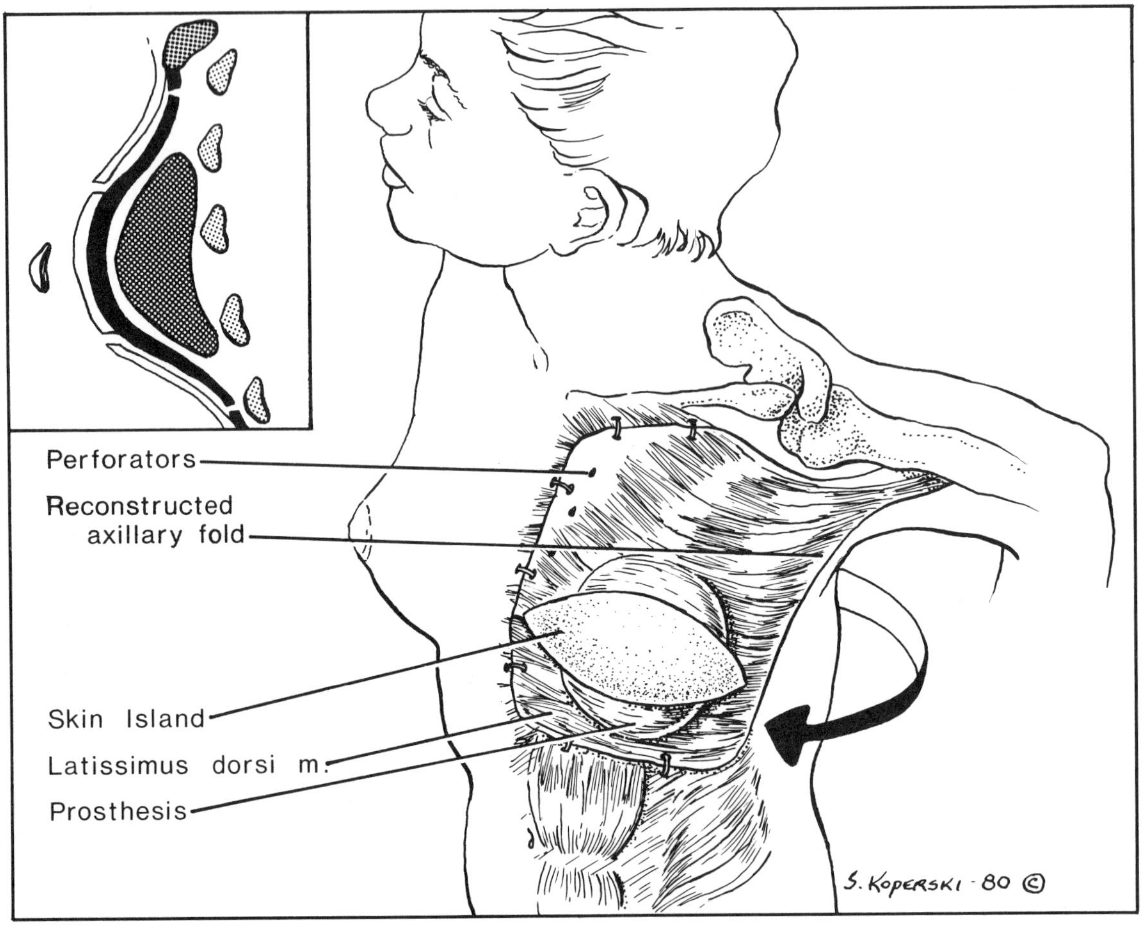

Figure 9-3. **Latissimus dorsi rotated.** Note the position of the prosthesis beneath the transposed flap. The inset shows the cross-sectional relationship of the prosthesis to the chest wall and the flap. There may be some pectoralis major muscle between the chest wall and the prosthesis in those patients who have had a modified radical mastectomy.

It is possible to reconstruct the nipple and areolar complex at the time of the initial procedure, but we believe it is advisable to do this at a later time because scar contracture may result in displacement of the nipple.

Ligation of the thoracodorsal artery at the time of resection of the tumor does not prevent use later of the latissimus flap since it may survive on the collaterals at its insertion. It is best, however, to preserve this artery during the ablation whenever possible. If ligation has occurred, one must wait six weeks for these collaterals to be effective.

The Contralateral Breast

Whether to treat the other breast is a matter of controversy. We believe that management of the opposite breast depends upon the age of the patient, the family history, and the patient's wishes. Current data support the concept of performing a subcutaneous mastectomy on the remaining breast. This seems to lower the risk of carcinoma, especially in patients in a high-risk category. This includes patients with multiple prior biopsies, a family history of carcinoma, or interductal hyperplasia with atypia. There is general agreement that the contralateral breast in a patient with prior carcinoma has a greater chance of developing a carcinoma of its own. Not all surgeons agree that prophylactic treatment is indicated. Some claim that the cure rate is just as high with early detection of the growth.

A subcutaneous mastectomy removes varying degrees of tissue, depending upon the technique used and the thinness of the flaps. The nipple and associated ducts are left, and some tissue remains at the periphery. The procedure does reduce the amount of tissue by 95 percent, and hence, it would seem, also reduces the chance of subsequent disease.

Some ablative surgeons advocate simple mastectomy on the opposite breast on the theory that a subcutaneous mastectomy removes insufficient amounts of tissue. It must be kept in mind that a simple mastectomy, and in some cases even a modified radical, does not necessarily remove all of the breast tissue. There is the possibility of breast tissue remaining within the pectoralis muscle as well as at the periphery of the resection.

In lower-risk individuals, if the opposite breast needs aesthetic treatment, a reduction mammoplasty or, if only ptosis is the problem, a pexy can be performed. This makes the contralateral breast, if ptotic, a better match with the reconstructed one. The argument has been advanced that the scar tissue left by the surgery may hide detection of a subsequent carcinoma. Other ablative surgeons feel that pexy and/or reduction will not interfere with their examination of that breast.

Mammography is a valuable follow-up technique, although recently controversy has developed as to the safety of its frequent use. The presence of a prosthesis will not interfere with this procedure.

Until recently, reconstruction following subcutaneous mastectomy has led to disappointment owing to a high complication rate. Infection, slough of skin or nipple, extrusion of the implant, and hardening due to spherical scar contraction around the implant have been commonplace. With the use of dermal flaps and muscle flaps to pad the implant and to provide subcutaneous tissues, these complications have been reduced considerably.

The use of latissimus or pectoralis muscle flaps offers a better reconstruction than the subcutaneous placement of the prosthesis. The subpectoral implant hides less tissue from examination. Frequently, however, the prosthesis is deformed by flexion of the pectoralis muscle. The latissimus flap requires considerably more surgery and can hide potential disease, but it gives an excellent reconstruction.

The real question is not whether subcutaneous mastectomy removes enough breast tissue, but rather whether the subsequent reconstruction hides treatable disease. That is a question that can only be answered at some future date.

Summary

Reconstruction of the female breast following a major extirpative operation has significantly improved. The latissimus dorsi flap provides the plastic surgeon with a reliable technique that permits a rapid reconstruction with better results than the earlier multistaged procedures. Preoperative planning prior to the extirpative surgery will further improve these results. Ablative surgery an be performed, therefore, without compromising the reconstruction. Subcutaneous mastectomy of the contralateral breast should be considered for high-risk individuals.

CHAPTER 10

Facial Injuries

Plastic surgeons are frequently called upon to treat victims of trauma to the face and skull. The etiological factors are many and varied, but the automobile is most often the cause of complex injuries. Victims of automobile accidents sustain injury to the head and facial region in 71 percent of cases requiring hospitalization.

Patients with facial fractures who sustain high velocity injuries have a life-threatening associated injury in 30 percent of cases and major nonlife-threatening injuries in another 30 percent. Low velocity injuries are caused by falls or by being struck by a fist or blunt object. Life-threatening associated injuries are present in 4 percent of patients sustaining low velocity injuries. Patients who have fractured strong facial bones, such as the supraorbital ridge or mandible, have major associated injuries 50 percent of the time.

The most significant priority in treating the patient with a facial injury is finding or ruling out life-threatening associated injuries. Often these associated injuries, especially of the abdomen or cervical spine, are not as striking as the severely disfiguring facial injury. When treating patients involved in significant trauma, all sites of injury should be thoroughly examined with a high index of suspicion. Treatment of multiple systemic injuries should take precedence over the management of facial wounds.

Even though treatment of other injuries may be more urgent, facial lacerations can be closed with a few strategically placed sutures and left to await definitive care when the patient's condition is more stable. If large soft tissue avulsions have occurred, sterile moist dressings are employed for coverage until reconstructive procedures can be completed. Few facial fractures require immediate attention. In most cases, it is best to wait several days, until the post-traumatic edema has subsided, before attempting reduction.

Establishment and maintenance of an airway is always the cardinal rule for management of an acutely injured patient. A physician who treats facial trauma must be deft in dealing with airway problems. Frequently, objects such as teeth, dentures or foreign bodies obstruct the airway of an injured or unconscious patient. These must be removed with dispatch. In certain types of mandible fractures, the structural stabilization of the mandibular arch is lost and the patient's tongue can be displaced posteriorly, obstructing the airway. It is possible to manage such situations by protruding the tongue with a suture or forceps, or by placing the patient in the prone position.

When the measures cited above are inadequate to restore a clear airway, endotracheal intubation or emergency tracheotomy may be necessary. When there is no time for an elective low tracheotomy, an emergency airway must be established by incising the skin and conic ligament between the thyroid and the cricoid cartilages. The airway can be maintained with a cannula or catheter until a more permanent airway is established.

When time permits, it is advisable to take the patient to an operating area and perform a standard low tracheostomy through the third or fourth endotracheal ring. This is particularly important for the patient whose airway will be compromised by progressive soft tissue edema following the initial trauma, or the patient with central nervous system depression who will require long-term intubation and positive pressure ventilation.

Examination

The general physical examination of a patient with facial injuries should be conducted in an unhurried, thorough manner in a well-lit room equipped with suction, nasal speculum, tongue blades and examination gloves. The wound should be cleansed to aid examination. Large particles of necrotic debris and foreign bodies can be debrided by gentle irrigation so that the wound can be thoroughly explored and evaluated.

When examining facial lacerations, the physician should be alert to the possibility of injury to the specialized soft tissues beneath the skin. Loss of facial animation or loss of sensation in the cheeks, gums and mouth are danger signs. Once the neurological status of the motor and sensory nerves has been established, the physician may infiltrate local anesthesia into the wound to facilitate further cleansing, debridement and repair.

If there is a laceration of the cheek or near the orbit, the surgeon should consider the possibility of lacerations of the parotid or lachrymal duct. Evaluation of vision and range of eye motion are essential parts of the examination. Diplopia may be a sign of an orbital wall fracture. Injury to the globe or impairment of visual acuity calls for an ophthalmological evaluation. The nasal cavity should be suctioned clear of debris and should be examined with a speculum to rule out a septal fracture or hematoma. Blood in the ear canal or behind the tympanic membrane may indicate a basilar skull fracture.

Careful observation will reveal considerable information regarding the bony structures of the face. Ecchymosis or contusion of the periorbital area or malar eminence or unequal level of the pupils on forward gaze should alert the surgeon to the possibility of a zygomatic fracture. Increased distance between the medial canthal ligaments may indicate a complex nasal fracture. Deviation of the jaw to one side may signify a mandibular fracture. Fracture of the nasal bones may be obvious initially. Later, however, it may be difficult to diagnose a nasal fracture owing to distortion of the nasal framework by edema.

Palpation of bony ridges, such as the zygomatic arch, nasal bridge, orbital rim and edge of the mandible, often reveals evidence of fracture. The maxillary teeth should be grasped between the thumb and forefinger and evaluated for tenderness and mobility. An unstable midfacial fracture or craniofacial separation can be diagnosed in this manner. To evaluate for mandibular fractures, the anterior portion of the mandible should be gently rocked while grasped by the thumbs and fingertips. Abnormal bite relationship of the teeth, called malocclusion, indicates a disruption of one of the dental arches. Since what is a "normal" dental occlusion varies from patient to patient, the patient should be asked to indicate how his teeth normally meet when he bites.

Diagnosis

Consideration of the mechanism of injury can help diagnose facial fractures. Direct impact to the chin which disrupts the normal bite relationship may lead the surgeon to suspect a fracture of the mandibular condyle. This is particularly true in the case of children where minor blows to the chin can cause fractures of the condyle. Direct blows over the nose or cheek may cause zygomatic or nasal bone fractures. When the eye is struct by a large blunt object, the force of impact can drive the orbital contents through the thin medial and inferior walls of the orbit (Fig. 10-1).

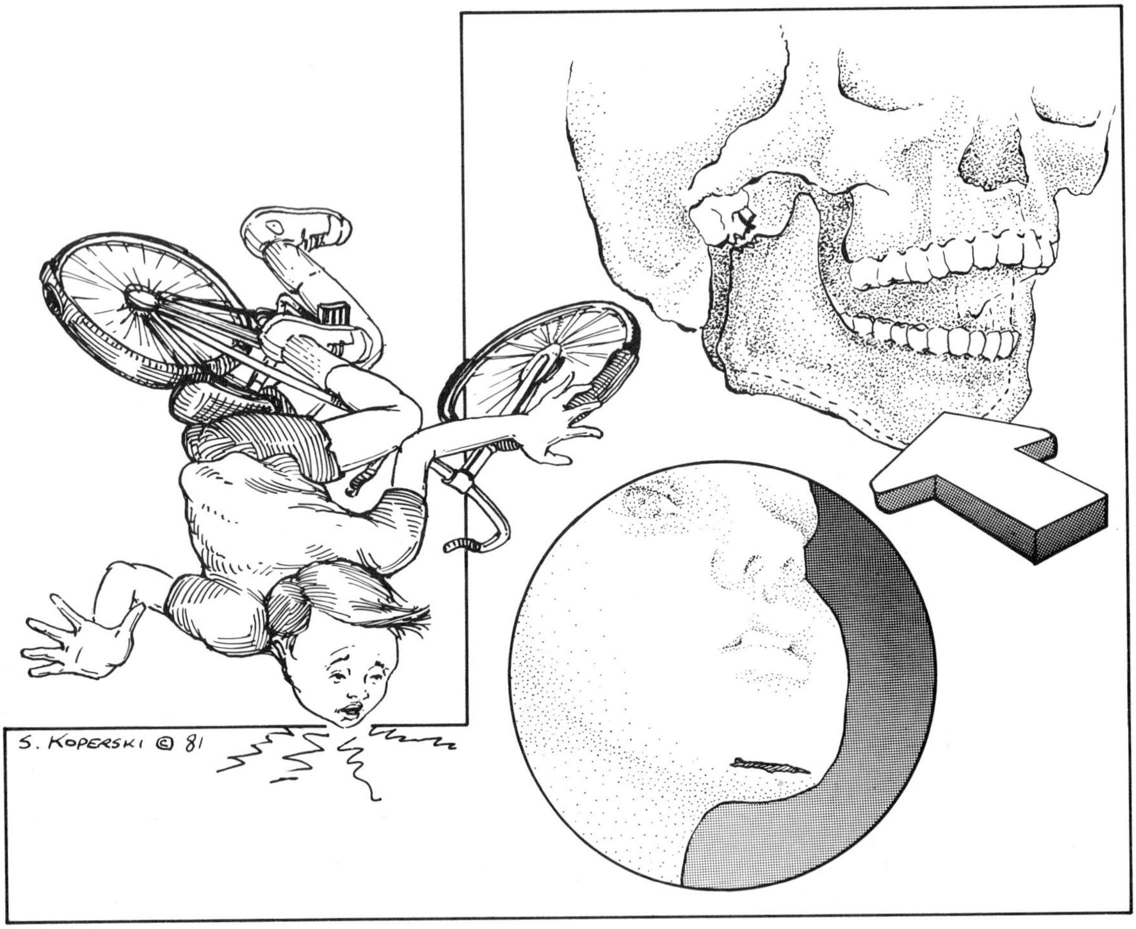

Figure 10-1. **Mandibular condyle fracture.** A submental laceration (circular inset) resulting from a fall, especially in a child, may fracture the condyles due to a backward thrust of the mandible (arrow). Such a fracture may be overlooked, but the laceration should evoke suspicion.

Additional studies, intelligently employed, often confirm suspicions aroused by the clinical examination and knowledge of the mechanism of injury. X-rays often provide additional information, even in the case of obvious fractures. Skull and cervical spine x-rays should always be considered because of the frequent association of facial injuries with skull fractures and cervical spine dislocations.

The most valuable and commonly employed x-ray views used in the diagnosis of facial fractures are the anterior-posterior and lateral of the skull and facial bones, including the Waters' view. The Waters' view is the single most useful examination of the facial bones, often revealing fractures of the orbit, zygoma, frontal bone, nasal bones and maxillary sinus. The reversed Waters' view can be used effectively when the patient cannot be placed in the prone position for examination (Fig. 10-2).

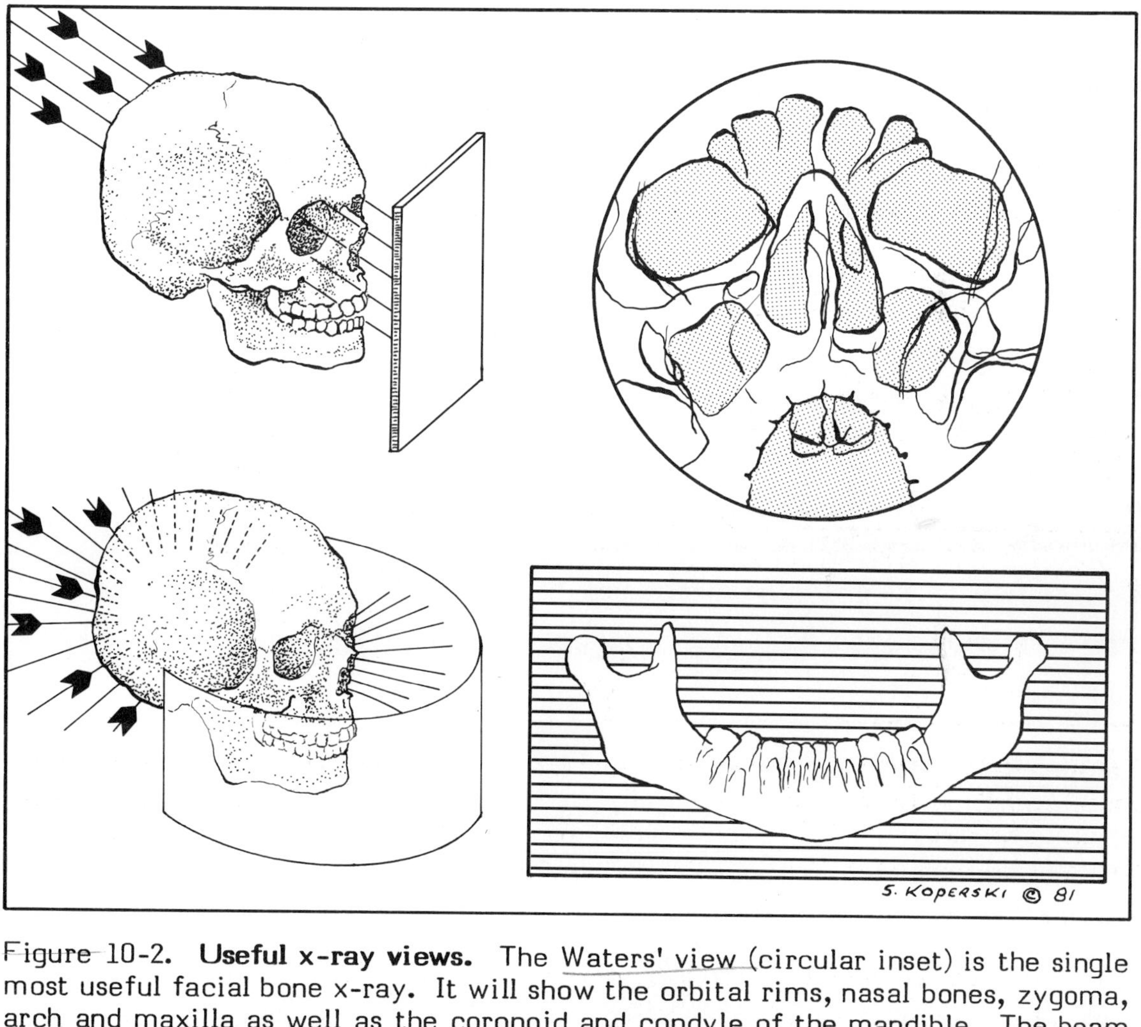

Figure 10-2. **Useful x-ray views.** The Waters' view (circular inset) is the single most useful facial bone x-ray. It will show the orbital rims, nasal bones, zygoma, arch and maxilla as well as the coronoid and condyle of the mandible. The beam is projected from back to front (top left). The panorex (bottom left) is the single most useful view for the mandible. The beam is projected from front to back but rotates with the plate to give a "mercator" projection of the mandible (rectangular inset).

Pantomogram

After the facial series survey has been completed, the surgeon can obtain more precise information by specialized roentgenograms. The clinical signs may indicate a zygomatic or orbital floor fracture, and a Waters' view may confirm this by showing blood in the maxillary antrum. In such cases, the full extent of the injury can be demonstrated by tomograms of the orbit. The lateral anterior projection, or "bucket handle view," dramatically reveals fractures of the zygomatic arch. X-rays of the nasal bones are often useless, since repair must be based upon the clinical examination rather than on the radiographic findings.

Posterior, anterior and lateral oblique views of the mandible can be employed to reveal the point of fracture of the ramus and body. Because it is difficult to view the condylar angle and the subcondylar areas, however, panoramic radiograms should be obtained when mandibular fractures are suspected. One should remember that old fracture lines may show on a radiograph years after the injury, due to the fact that facial bone healing is by fibrous union with little callous formation.

It is essential to maintain adequate records when performing plastic surgery, particularly in cases prone to litigation or those involving insurance judgments. Most patients with facial trauma enter these categories. It is important that the surgeon obtain accurate, high quality photographs before and immediately after giving primary care to a patient with facial injuries. No verbal description can adequately replace a photographic record of a patient's injury and progress.

Treatment of Soft Tissue Trauma

All facial lacerations must be regarded as potentially contaminated wounds, and tetanus prophylaxis should be administered. Patients who are certain they have been immunized within the previous five years need receive no toxoid. When the booster has been given more than 5 but less than 10 years prior, 0.5 cc of absorbed tetanus toxoid should be given intramuscularly. If a patient has not been immunized previously or has not had a booster shot within 10 years, 250 mg of hypertet (human tetanus antitoxin) and 0.5 cc of absorbed tetanus toxoid should be given.

Many lacerations and minor soft tissue injuries can be treated effectively in the emergency room setting. If fractures are exposed through the soft tissues, or if underlying structures such as the parotid duct, facial nerve or eyelid are injured, primary treatment should be given in the formal operating room where conditions for successful repair are optimal.

Infiltration of local anesthetic or regional nerve blocks achieve excellent anesthesia for repair of most minor facial lacerations. If depression of the central nervous system is not in question, premedication can also be administered. Xylocaine, 5 to 7 mg per kilogram of body weight per hour with 1:200,000 epinephrine, can be given without significant risk of central nervous system toxicity.

Local infiltration through the wound margins with 30 gauge needles provides satisfactory anesthesia and reduces bleeding. However, this technique has the disadvantage of distorting the tissues to some degree. Regional blocks of the major sensory branches of the trigeminal nerve provide excellent analgesia but provide no local hemostasis. A combination of regional block with minimal local infiltration of anesthetic and vasopressor will usually provide an excellent analgesia with good hemostasis and minimal distortion of the tissues.

While many cleansing agents have been advocated, few offer significant advantages over copious irrigation of the wound with saline solution. Many soaps and cleansing solutions have been shown to be associated with local tissue damage to already traumatized soft tissue. Canine and human bites should be particularly well irrigated since the necrotizing enzymes present in saliva contribute to wound morbidity. A brush or scalpel blade will remove embedded foreign bodies such as metal, dust, cinders, gravel and glass. If dirt tattooed into the skin is not removed, it may result in permanent pigmentation.

Contused lacerations with devitalized tissue at the edges should be conservatively debrided using techniques described in Chapter 4 under Mechanical Factors. Most clean facial wounds can be safely closed up to 48 hours after injury. The surgeon must use his best clinical judgment in the case of dirty or contaminated wounds.

It is best not to undertake major reconstruction of the wound at the time of original care because elaborate reconstruction might jeopardize the main objective which is primary wound healing. If there has been extensive soft tissue loss, it is better to do a skin graft, or to suture the skin to oral mucosa, rather than to attempt to reconstruct the defect with a rotation flap, Z-plasty or advancement flap employing traumatized or contused soft tissue. Once primary wound healing has been achieved, cosmetic aspects can be improved.

Generally speaking, each tissue plane violated should be closed carefully following the precepts given in Chapter 5. Each such area should be repaired separately. Wound closure should begin with the careful orientation of strategic landmarks, such as the skin of the vermilion border, eyelid margins and eyebrows, before proceeding to less critical areas.

A through-and-through lip laceration, for example, should be closed in three layers. Absorbable catgut sutures can be used to close the oral mucosa after the vermilion border has been precisely aligned. Following this, absorbable sutures should be used to repair the oral musculature. In cases where the integrity of the oral, or other facial, muscle has not been restored, a noticeable soft tissue defect, which may require later revision, can develop. Finally, the skin must be closed under no tension, with the vermilion border and white roll of the lip precisely aligned.

Scalp and Forehead

As with most injuries over a bony prominence, minor degrees of trauma can cause a laceration to the depth of the periosteum. Inspection of the bone through the wound will reveal small linear fractures more readily than will radiographs. Skin edges are frequently crushed and require debridement. Large full thickness sutures can be used in hair-bearing areas to promote hemostasis. The frontalis muscle must be repaired as a separate layer in forehead lacerations. Scalp hair should rarely be shaved; the eyebrow should never be shaved as regrowth may result in coarser, thicker hairs.

Eyelids

The delicate structure of the eyelids requires careful handling and meticulous closure of all three tissue layers. Prior to repairing a lacerated eyelid, the surgeon should conduct a careful examination to evaluate damage to associated structures such as the cornea, lachrymal gland or lachrymal cannicula.

The tarsal plate and conjunctiva can be closed with 6-0 absorbable sutures. Care must be taken to protect the cornea by tying the knots on the muscle side. The key skin suture at the grey line must then be placed. The muscle and skin edges should be closed separately and the eye dressed with a soft ocular patch which should be left in place for at least 24 hours (Fig. 10-3).

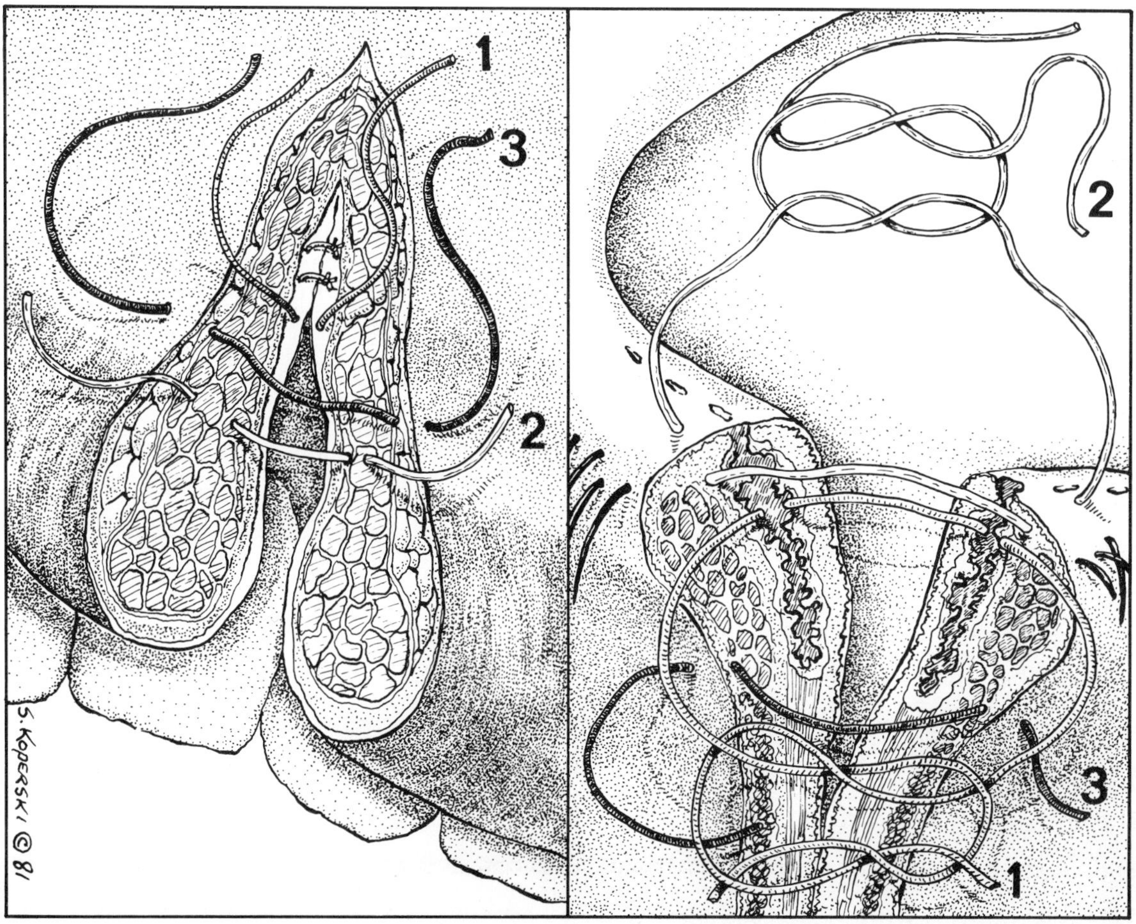

Figure 10-3. **Closure of lip and eyelid lacerations.** Anatomical realignment is important in full thickness lacerations. Such a laceration of the lip (left) may require three separate layers for best approximation: suture in the musoca (1); sutures in the muscle (2); and sutures in the skin (3), the first of which should be at the white roll to help with the alignment. For such a laceration of the eyelid (right), the first suture is in the tarsal plate (1), since the conjunctiva does not need to be closed as a separate layer. The second suture is at the grey line (2) and left long for taping down to the skin so that the cut edges do not irritate the globe. Skin sutures complete the closure (3). As the skin and muscle are an integral unit, they need not be closed separately.

Lacerations of the medial aspect of the eyelid may involve the canthal ligament or the lachrymal duct. Injuries to these structures usually require hospitalization and repair in the operating room. During this procedure, the surgeon explores the lachrymal duct with a probe, then places a fine polyurethane tube through the duct to splint the repair.

Disruptions of the medial canthus are frequently associated with complex nasal bone fractures. Repair can be effected only by the creation of a new bony insertion for the ligament. The surgeon passes a wire suture through the ligament and fastens it to the bone by tying it over a button or bolster on the opposite side of the nose. The wire is kept in position for several weeks while the canthal ligament develops a new bony insertion.

Ears

The ear is frequently injured in fights or automobile accidents. Injuries may range from simple lacerations through skin and cartilage to complete avulsion of the auricle. Because of the rich blood supply to the ear, an incompletely severed auricle usually survives when it is carefully reattached.

If a completely severed ear is recovered, the epidermis can be removed using a dermabrader. The dermis-cartilage unit is banked under the skin of the mastoid area or of the abdominal wall, to be employed in later reconstruction. Through-and-through lacerations of cartilage should be repaired with several fine absorbable sutures. If necessary, the cartilage should be trimmed so that the skin will be sutured without tension and all the remaining cartilage will be covered with skin. Skin avulsions can be replaced with a full thickness skin graft from the contralateral postauricular area.

Contusions of the ear can result in a hematoma between the cartilage and perichondrium. This must be aspirated to prevent deformities of the cartilage, such as the "cauliflower ear." After evacuating a hematoma, the surgeon makes a compression dressing of cotton soaked in saline solution and mineral oil and molds it to the contour of the ear. This is done to prevent recurrence of the hematoma. Because cartilage is an avascular structure and its resistance to infection is low, the administration of antibiotics is indicated.

Parotid Duct

The course of the parotid duct follows the line from the tragus of the ear to just above the corner of the mouth. When the patient has sustained deep lacerations in this area, parotid duct laceration should be suspected. To evaluate the duct, the surgeon introduces a small Silastic tube into the opening of Stenson's duct, which is opposite the second upper molar. If the tube can be advanced into the wound, the duct is lacerated. In that case, the tube is then placed in the proximal portion of the duct, which is located by milking saliva distally. It is then advanced, and the lacerated areas are approximated with several sutures. The Silastic tube is left as a splint for the duct repair and is secured to the oral mucosa with an absorbable suture. It should be left in place for one week. Failure to identify this injury can result in a parotid fistula.

Facial Nerve

The buccal branch of the facial nerve parallels the duct, and its laceration must be presumed when the parotid duct is transected. When major branches of the facial nerve are lacerated proximal to a line dropped from the lateral canthus, they must be repaired in the operating room under magnification. (The technique of microscopic repair of small nerves will be discussed in Chapter 16.) The small terminal branches of the facial nerve usually regenerate, and function is restored without approximation (Fig. 10-4).

Function will return to the buccal and ocular branches of the facial nerve because of numerous interconnections with other branches. However, the frontal and marginal branches do not communicate with other branches and these must be repaired, even in the case of distal lacerations. Temporary tarsorrhaphy may be required in order to protect the cornea until the orbicularis muscle function has returned. The loss of the cervical branch to the platysma has few clinical sequelae.

When optimal conditions exist, nerve repair is best undertaken at the time of wound closure. Primary repair, however, is not an emergency and can be undertaken within 72 hours of injury. Up to this time, the distal nerve ends can be identified with the aid of a nerve stimulator. However, repair subsequent to that time is extremely difficult and, if repair must be delayed, the nerve ends should be marked with sutures for later identification. Our experience has shown that the distal branches of the nerve are extremely difficult to find on later exploration because they are embedded in scar tissue.

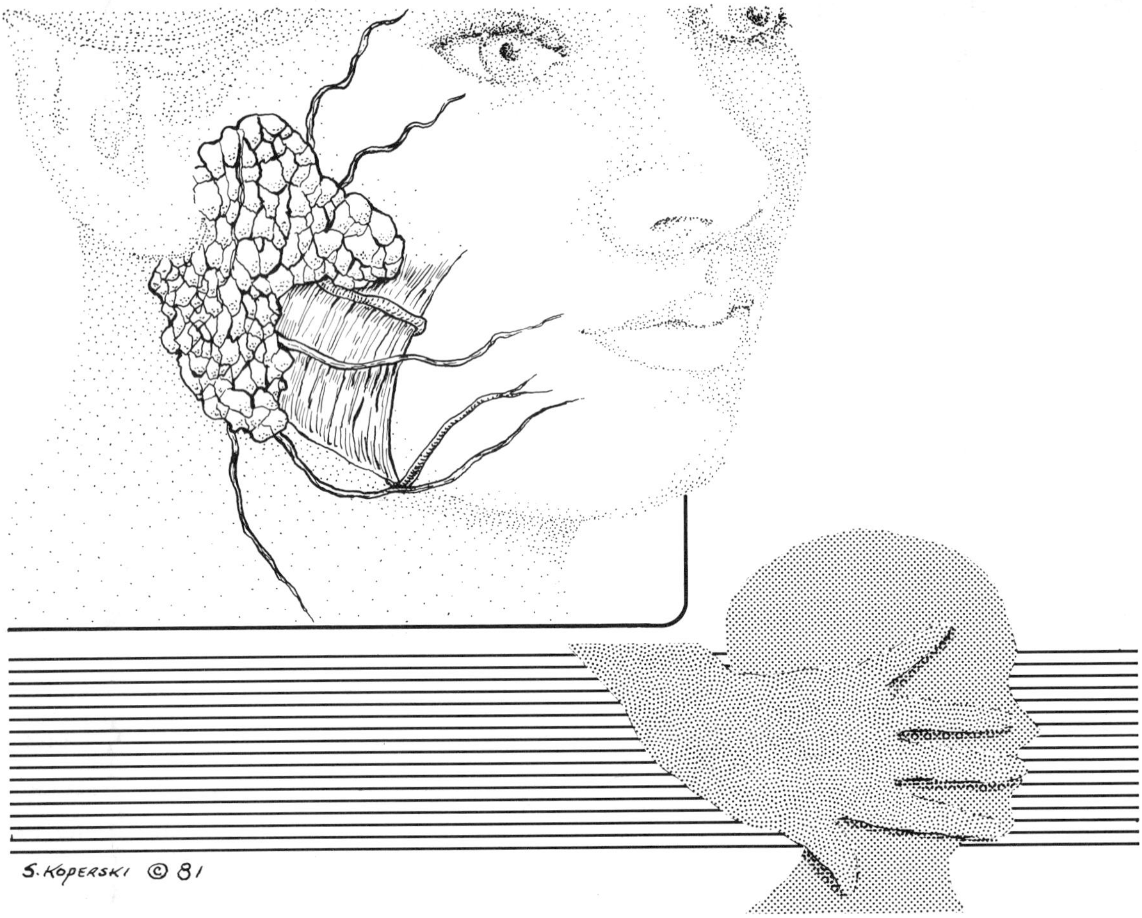

Figure 10-4. **Seventh nerve branches.** The seventh nerve is motor to the muscles of facial expression. It has five branches. If the left hand is placed on the right face (lower right), the thumb corresponds to the cervical branch, the index to the marginal mandibular, the long to the buccal, the ring to the zygomatic, and the little finger to the temporal branch. In the top illustration, the skin and SMAS have been removed to reveal the nerve's relationship to the parotid (within) and the masseter muscle (above). The parotid duct can be seen crossing the masseter. Note the relationship of the marginal branch to the mandible: dorsal to the facial artery it loops below the mandible; ventral to the facial artery it is always above the rim of the mandible.

Treatment of Facial Fractures

Two goals guide the repair of facial fractures: proper functioning and pleasing appearance.

Facial fractures, like fractures elsewhere in the body, must be anatomically reduced and properly immobilized. Some fracture sites can be exposed directly and the fracture immobilized with stainless steel wire. Other fractures must be reduced and wired indirectly. Fractures of the jaw are reduced by using the teeth as a guide to reduction. The unstable fragments are immobilized by attaching them firmly to the more stable segments.

Proper anatomical reduction of fractures of the jaws and face requires an understanding of the principles of occlusion. Occlusion refers to the meshing together of the working surfaces of the teeth. Mandibular and maxillary first molars are used as reference points for normal, or median, occlusion.

These teeth have two grinding surfaces: the mesial, or proximal, cusp and the distal cusp. These names are based on their proximity to the examiner with the mesial cusp being anterior and the distal posterior. The surface closest to the tongue is called the lingual surface and the surface abutting the cheeks is called the buccal surface. The lower arch is smaller than the upper arch, and the mandibular teeth fit inside the maxillary teeth.

Neutroclusion is defined as the fitting of the mesiobuccal cusp of the first maxillary molar into the mesiobuccal groove of the first mandibular molar. This relationship serves as a guide to the normal bite. It is important to remember, however, that many patients do not have a normal bite. When the preinjury bite relationship has been disrupted by mandibular or maxillary fractures, its restoration is the key to anatomical reduction of the fracture. The surgeon usually establishes this relationship by inspection and verifies his finding by asking the patient how his teeth fit together normally (Fig. 10-5).

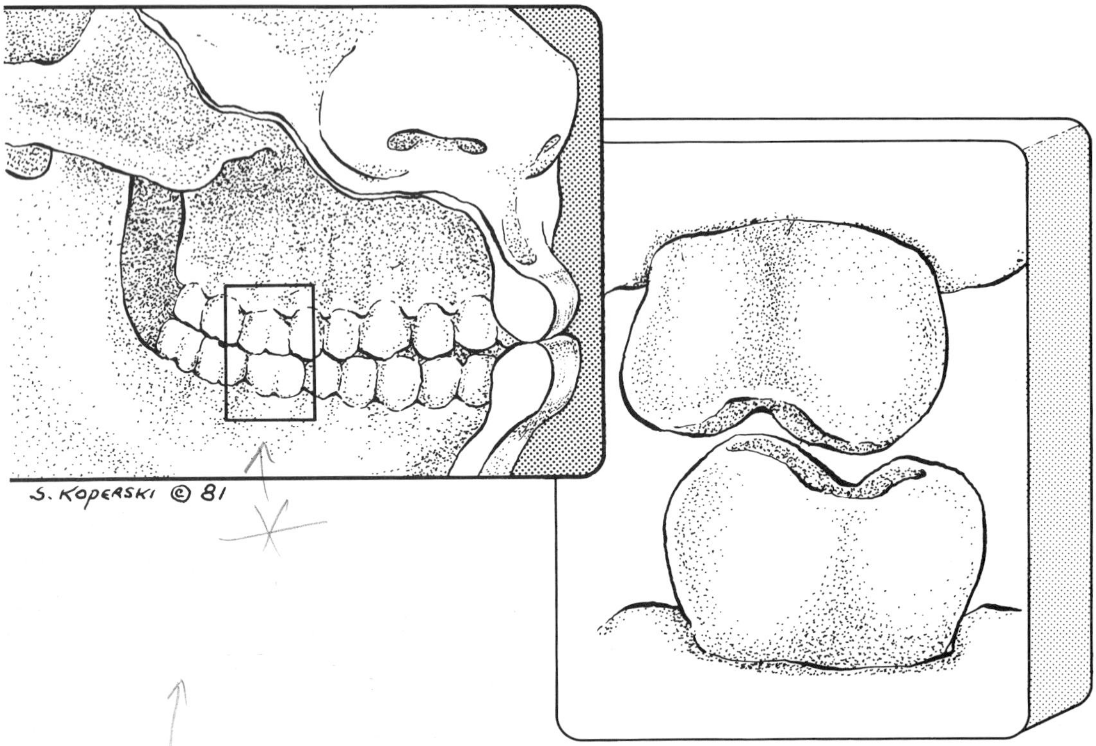

Figure 10-5. **Neutroclusion.** The proper occlusal relationship is measured from the first molar (inset left). Right: the maxillary first molar mesiobuccal cusp interdigitates with the mesiobuccal groove of the mandibular first molar (neutroclusion).

Once the fracture has been anatomically reduced, the surgeon must immobilize the fracture site until solid bony union is complete. While many methods exist for holding the surfaces of the teeth in solid contact, the most commonly employed method involves the use of prefabricated metal arch bars and elastic bands. The arch bars are ligated to the necks of the available teeth with wire loops, and the jaws are held together by the elastic bands, hooked into prefabricated tabs on the arch bars (Fig. 10-6).

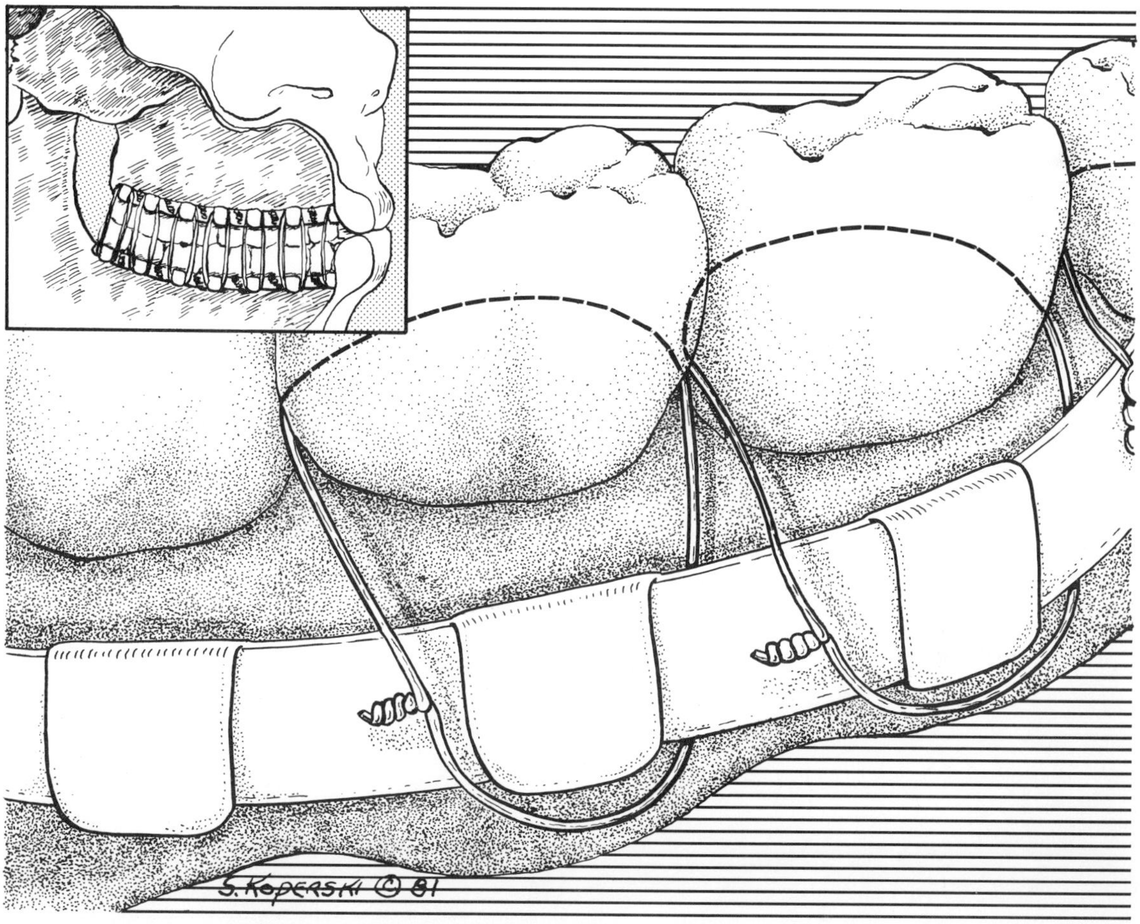

Figure 10-6. **Immobilizing the fracture site.** Arch bars are wired around the neck of the stable teeth. Elastic bands applied to the hooks of the arch bars hold the teeth in fixation until the adjacent bone heals. If the wire loops around the root of the tooth, it may cause distraction. If placed around the crown of the tooth, it may slip off.

If an insufficient number of teeth is available for attachment of the arch bars, dental splints, resembling dentures, can be wired to the mandible or maxilla to act as a guide for reduction of the fracture. Such fixation is generally maintained for from four to six weeks, by which time the fracture has become stable. Meanwhile, the patient is able to take liquid and eat blenderized meals. Oral hygiene is maintained with the aid of an irrigating appliance (Fig. 10-7).

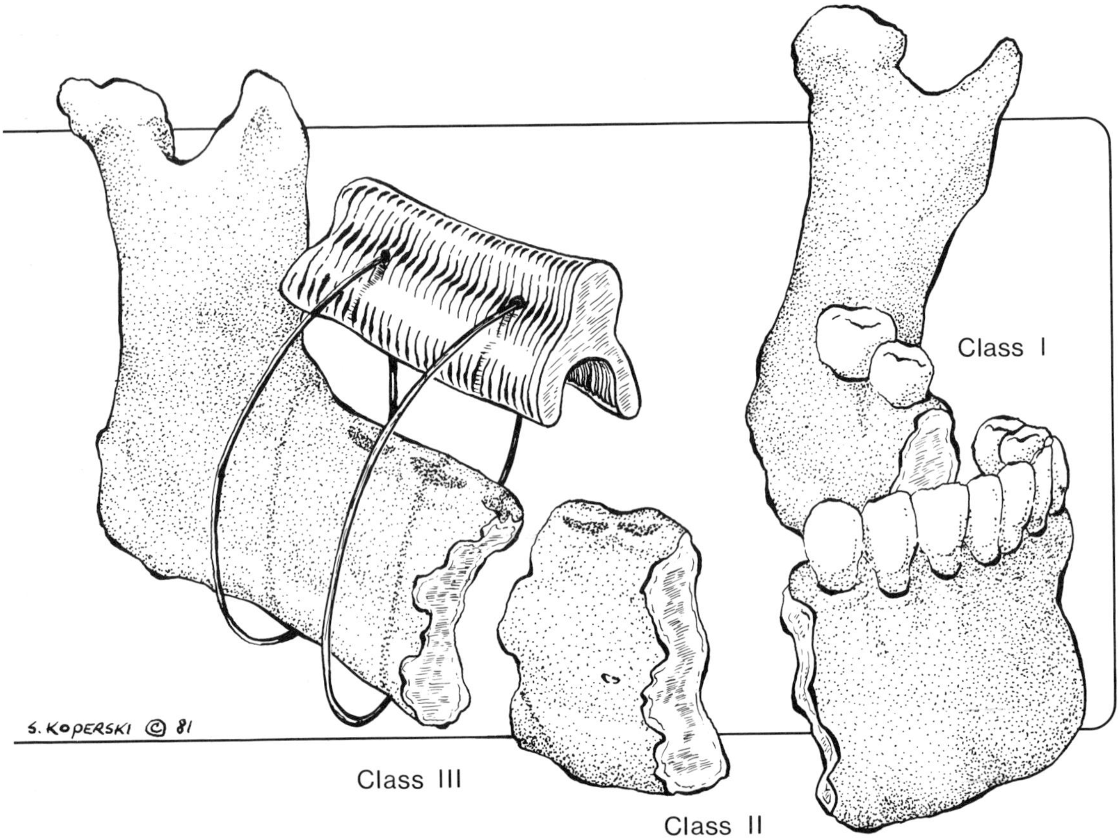

Figure 10-7. **Dental splint.** If the mandible is edentulous, a splint can be wired to the jaw to provide the stability and space that would normally be maintained by the teeth. Class I, II, and III fractures are shown.

Healing of the fracture is verified clinically rather than by x-rays. The surgeon simply removes the arch bars and evaluates the area for pain and tenderness by applying stress to the fracture site. Once the intermaxillary fixation is removed, the jaws are stiff and require weeks of exercise before the normal excursion is regained.

Mandible

Mandibular fractures illustrate many of the principles employed in the treatment of facial fractures. Mandibular fractures are described according to the anatomical region of fracture. Classification is based on the location of the fracture in relation to the teeth present on the mandible.

In class I fractures there are teeth on both sides of the fracture site which can be used for attachment of arch bars. In class II fractures there are teeth present on only one side of the fracture. In such cases, fabrication of a dental splint is often required. In class III fractures there are no mandibular teeth on either side of the fracture. In these cases, splints must be attached to the mandible by circummandibular wires (see Fig. 10-7).

Often direct wiring of the fracture site is necessary to maintain immobilization of a facial fracture. Certain mandibular fractures are rendered unstable because of the disruptive force of the muscles of mastication attached to the mandible. The angle of pull of these muscles tends to distract the fracture site.

An example of this is a fracture angled through the body of the mandible so that the pterygoid and temporalis muscles pull the posterior fragment upward while the digastric and geniohyoid muscles distract the anterior fragment downward. Such a fracture cannot be adequately stabilized by intermaxillary fixation alone. Direct wiring of the fracture site is required (Fig. 10-8).

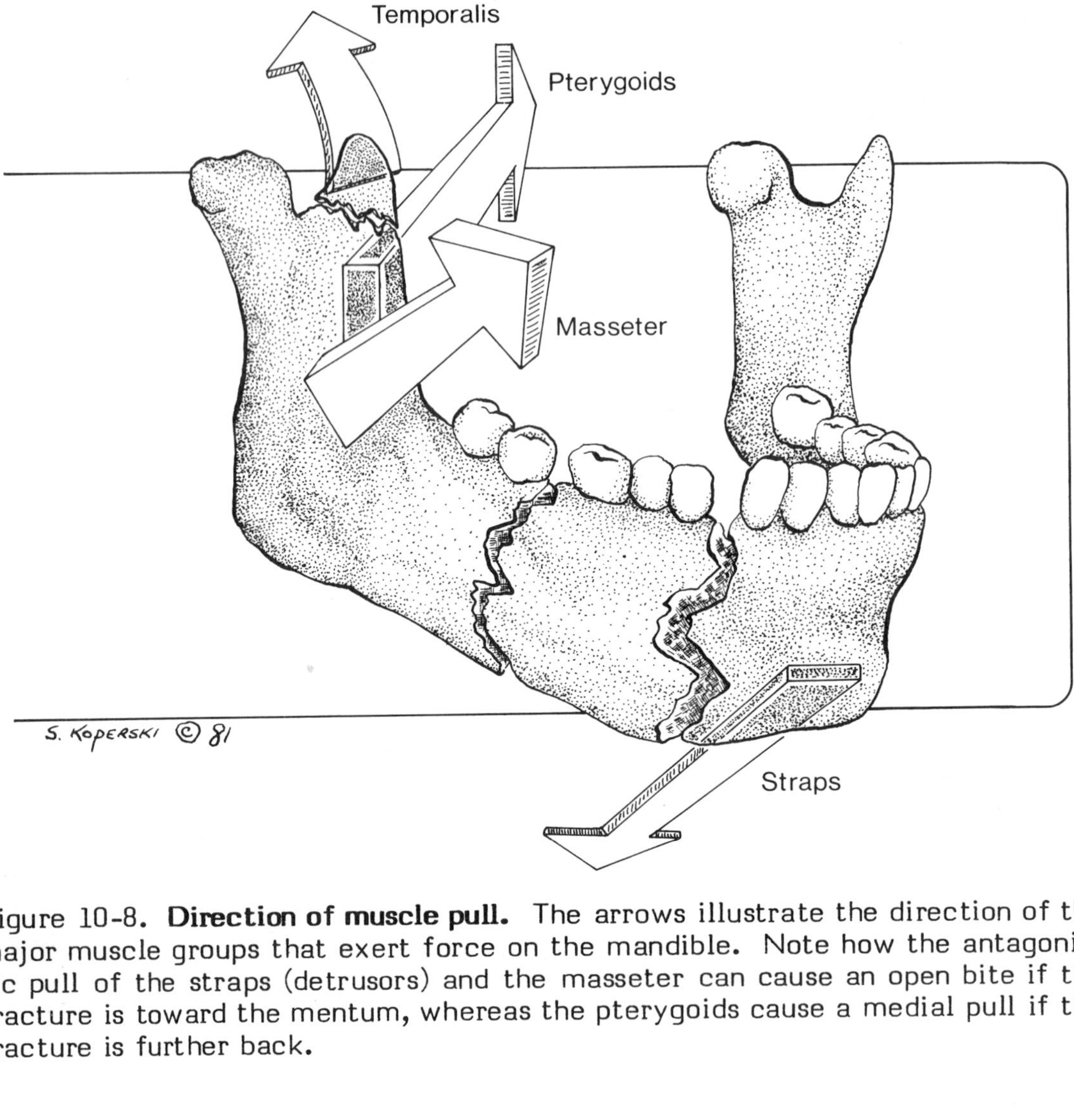

Figure 10-8. **Direction of muscle pull.** The arrows illustrate the direction of the major muscle groups that exert force on the mandible. Note how the antagonistic pull of the straps (detrusors) and the masseter can cause an open bite if the fracture is toward the mentum, whereas the pterygoids cause a medial pull if the fracture is further back.

For an open reduction, the inferior surface of the mandible is exposed through an incision beneath the mandible and over the fracture site. Care must be taken to avoid the marginal mandibular branch of the facial nerve. The periosteum must be stripped from the mandible, and all soft tissue and necrotic bone fragments that would interfere with healing must be removed from the fracture site. Using an air-driven drill, the surgeon makes two holes in the mandible. A 24 gauge stainless steel wire is passed through the holes and the ends of the wire are twisted together. This direct wiring, combined with intermaxillary fixation, holds the fracture site stable while healing takes place (Fig. 10-9).

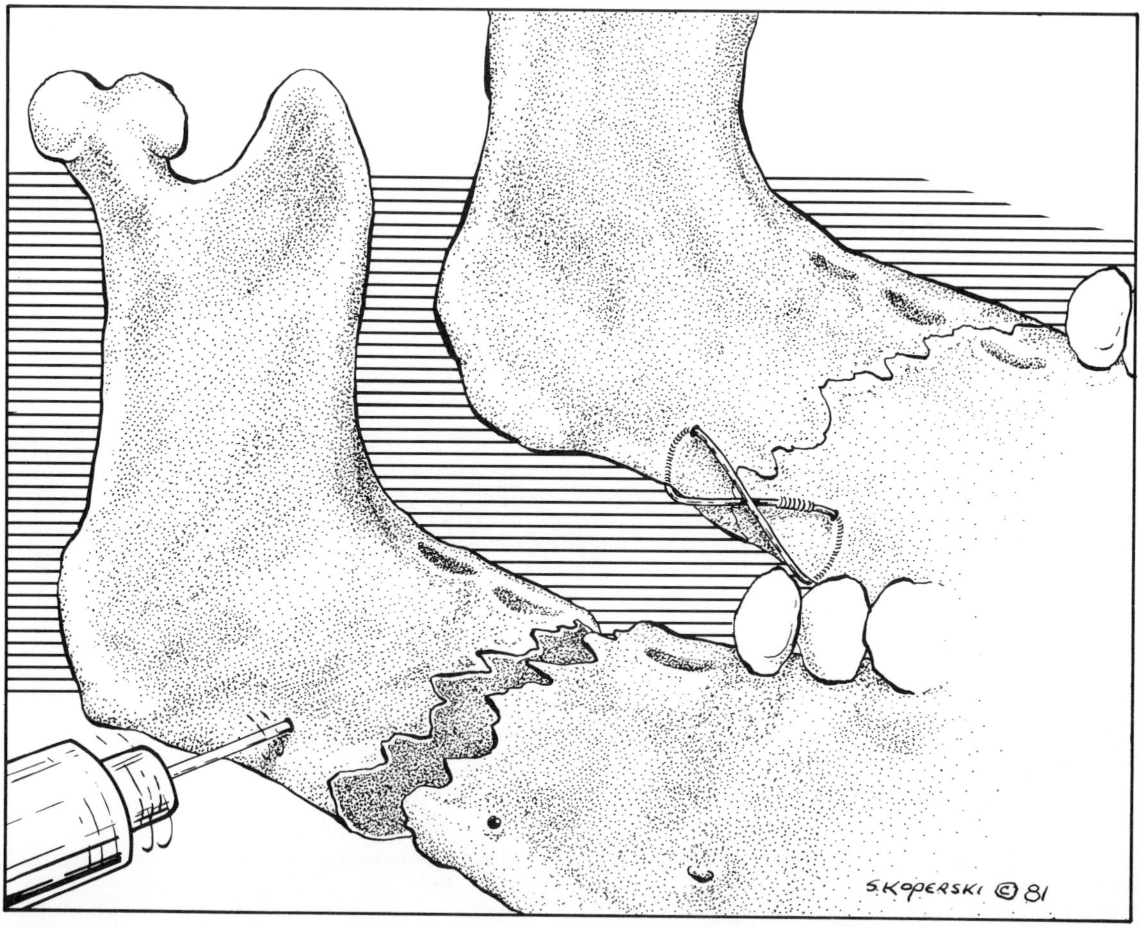

Figure 10-9. **Figure-8 wires.** A figure-8 wire may be all that is required for an edentulous mandible as any change in occlusion may be adjusted by the dentures. Two holes are drilled through the mandible (bottom left). A wire is passed through these holes and tightened in a crossed position. This configuration stabilizes the fracture in both the horizontal and vertical planes.

Maxilla

Fractures of the upper jaw are not uncommon following automobile accidents in which the face is smashed against the steering wheel or dashboard. Maxillary fractures follow certain predictable patterns which were described in 1900 by Le Fort. From his experimental work, classification of fractures of the maxilla evolved.

The simplest maxillary fracture, called the Le Fort I Guérin fracture, runs horizontally through the maxilla above the level of the teeth. The Le Fort II, or pyramidal, fracture traverses the nasal bones and inferior rims of the orbit and passes near, or through, the zygomaticomaxillary suture. In the most serious maxillary fracture, Le Fort III, the facial bones are separated from their cranial attachments (Fig. 10-10).

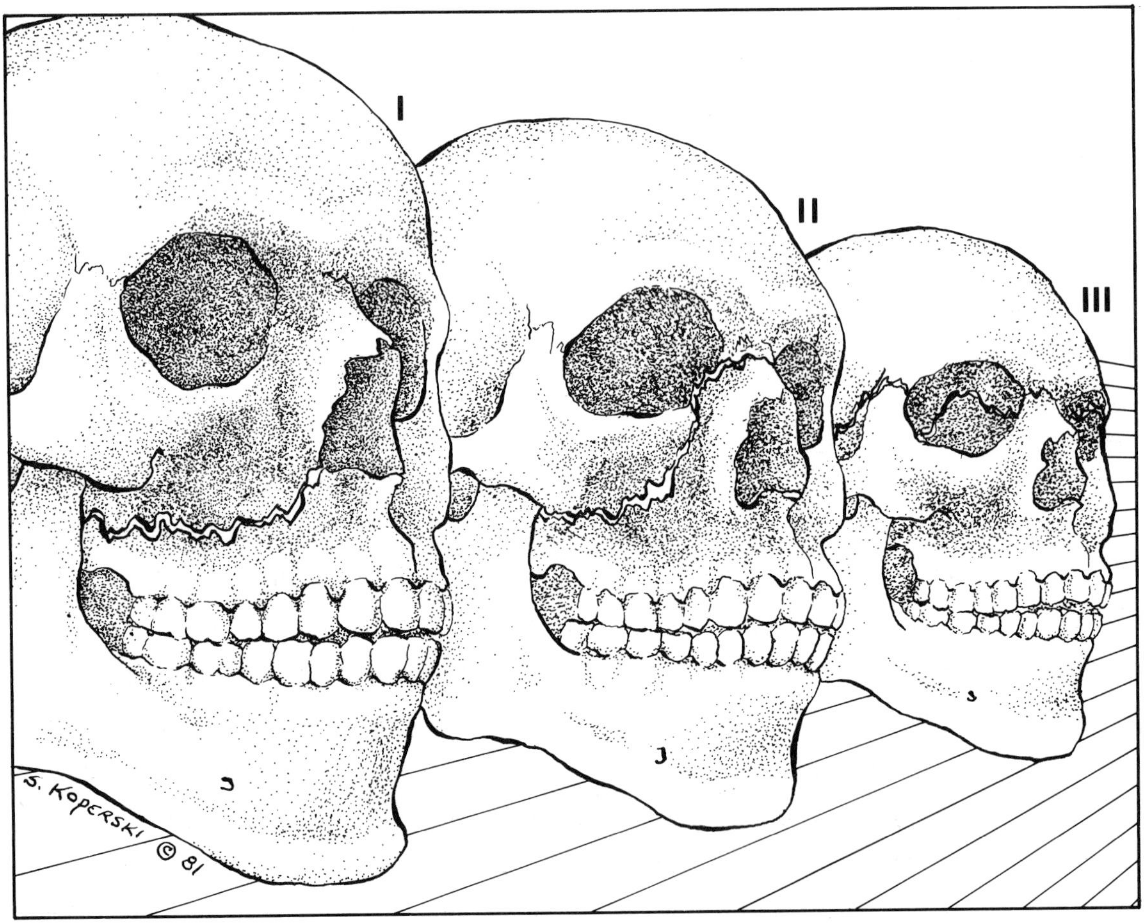

Figure 10-10. **Classifying facial fractures.** The Le Fort classification provides a guide to the expected stability of a facial fracture. A complete craniofacial disjunction, as in a Le Fort III, requires fixation to the cranial vault, whereas Le Forts I and II can be immobilized by fixation to the remaining facial bones. All three types of fracture may require interdental fixation.

The surgeon diagnoses maxillary fractures by grasping the alveolar ridge between thumb and forefinger and checking for mobility. With a Le Fort III fracture, the entire middle third of the face can be seen to move. These fractures are very likely to obstruct the airway. Fractures of the midface may be complicated by disruption of the cribriform plate with ensuing cerebrospinal fluid rhinorrhea. Malocclusion is invariably present. Untreated midface fractures result in an elongated and retruded maxilla, or "dish face."

As in mandibular fractures, the surgeon ensures anatomical reduction by establishing the pretrauma occlusion. The occlusive relationship is maintained by intermaxillary fixation to the mandible. Because opening the mouth would tend to cause the mandible to distract the fracture, the surgeon maintains fracture site stability by wiring the fracture segment to an adjacent stable bony area. Le Fort I fractures can be suspended from the infraorbital ridge with wires attached to the mandibular arch bar. Pyramidal and Le Fort III fractures are wired to the zygomatic arch or supraorbital ridge to maintain fixation.

Complex fractures of the midface may require a combination of fixation strategies. Smaller unstable fractures are wired to more stable segments. Some fractures are sustained with such force that the maxilla is impacted into the adjacent structures. A disimpaction forceps is required to reposition the segment anteriorly prior to fixation.

Zygoma

Fractures of the zygoma most frequently result from impact with a fist or blunt object. Before the effects of edema complicate the examination, a depression of the cheek is often visible. Owing to disturbance of the infraorbital nerve as it runs through the roof of the maxillary sinus, the patient may experience numbness of the cheek and lip. Pressure on the coronoid process of the mandible by the displaced zygomatic complex produces pain when the mouth is moved, a condition known as trismus. Palpation of the infraorbital rim may reveal a step-off deformity signifying disruption of the zygomatic maxillary suture. Occasionally the arch alone is fractured. In such a case, the arch can impinge on the coronoid process and cause trismus.

There are several excellent methods of reducing zygomatic fractures. Two of the most useful methods bear the names of famous plastic surgeons. Both involve placing incisions in unobtrusive sites and reducing the fracture by applying leverage force to the underside of the zygomatic complex. The zygoma is then wired into position to prevent a relapse.

The Gillies approach is made through the temporalis fascia. The incision is hidden in the temporal scalp. The temporalis fascia is incised, and an elevator is passed between the fascia and the temporalis muscle to the undersurface of the zygoma. Because of the powerful leverage force generated by this approach, it is particularly suitable for fractures of the arch and zygoma when treatment has been delayed and partial malunion has occurred (Fig. 10-11).

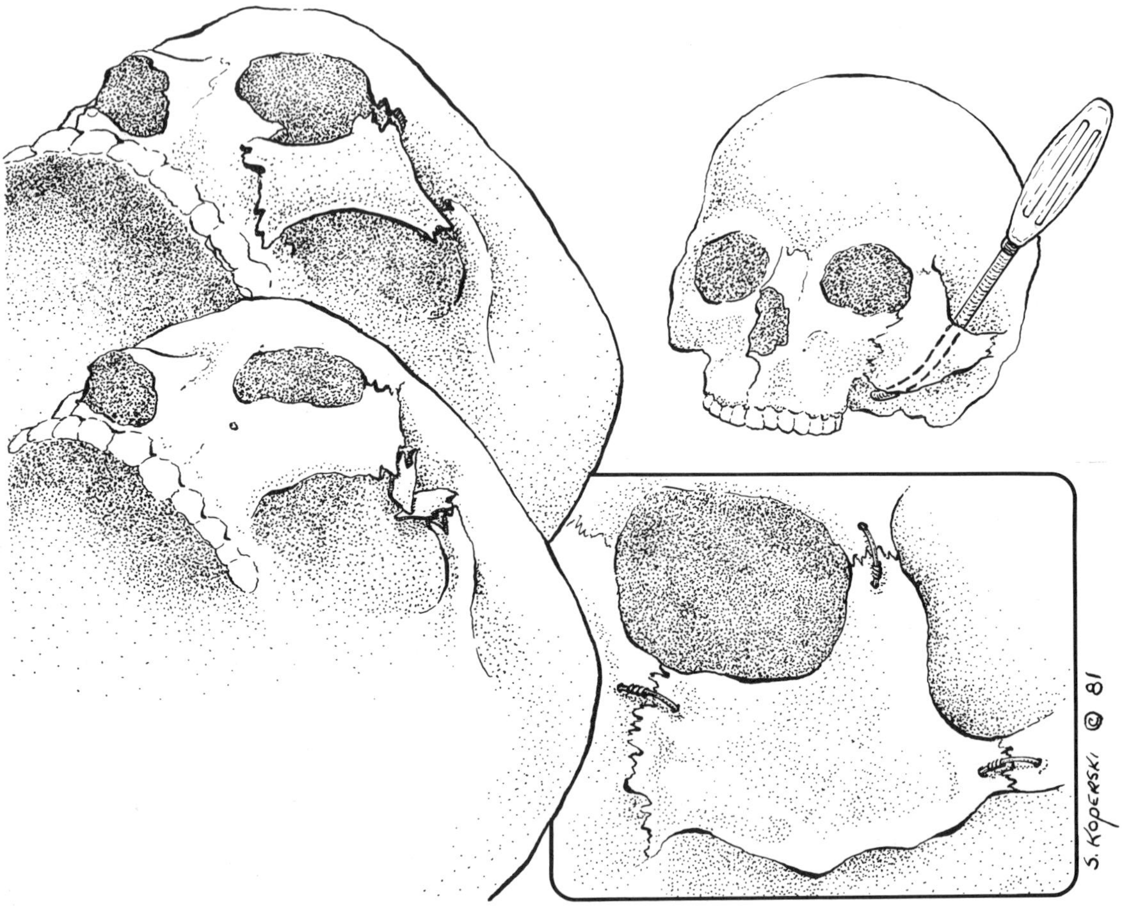

Figure 10-11. **Reducing zygomatic fractures.** Zygomatic fractures may involve the lateral wall of the orbit in one piece ("tripod") (top left), or they may be an M-shaped fracture of the arch (bottom left). The top right illustration shows the Gillies approach to the reduction. It is illustrated here for the tripod type but is useful also for the arch fractures. If the tripod is unstable, direct wiring or pins will be required (inset). The arch fractures are usually stable after reduction.

The Dingman approach utilizes an incision placed in the lateral eyebrow for reduction of the zygomatic complex. The zygomaticofrontal suture is exposed through this incision and it can be wired directly if the zygomatic complex fails to hold its reduced position. If necessary, the surgeon can expose the infraorbital rim through an incision in the lower eyelid and can wire the zygomaticomaxillary separation directly. A well-reduced fracture should restore normal cheek contour. In most cases the traumatized infraorbital nerve regains function.

Orbital Floor

Fractures of the orbital floor may be found in association with zygomatic fractures or encountered separately. The characteristic mechanism of injury is a sudden traumatic force applied against the orbital contents. A ball, fist or other object larger than the orbital opening (greater than 5 cm) compresses the orbital contents into the confined orbital cavity. The force is transmitted to the thin bones of the orbital floor and medial wall and, if great enough, can fracture and herniate the orbital contents.

The most frequently herniated structures are periorbital fat and the inferior rectus muscle. This muscle can become entrapped by the bony fragments of the orbital floor, giving rise to diplopia and limitation of upward eye movement. The discontinuity of the orbital floor and herniation of the orbital contents result in enophthalmos, although the early post-traumatic edema usually masks this finding. Disruption of the orbital floor with accompanying injury to the infraorbital nerve commonly results in anesthesia of the cheek (Fig. 10-12).

The red lens test is an excellent screening device for identifying patients with diplopia. The patient is asked to follow a flashing light with his eyes while one eye is covered with a red lens. In areas of diplopia, the patient will see two lights, one red and one white. Results can be charted for the nine cardinal ocular positions by noting the results on a grid chart.

The extent of orbital floor damage must be confirmed by tomographic studies. Ophthalmological evaluation of the status of the globe and extraocular muscles is an essential part of the examination. When the inferior rectus musculature is not released and the continuity of the orbital floor is not restored, diplopia and enophthalmos are long-term results. Even following correct reduction of the orbital floor, enophthalmos may persist because of destruction and resorption of periorbital fat.

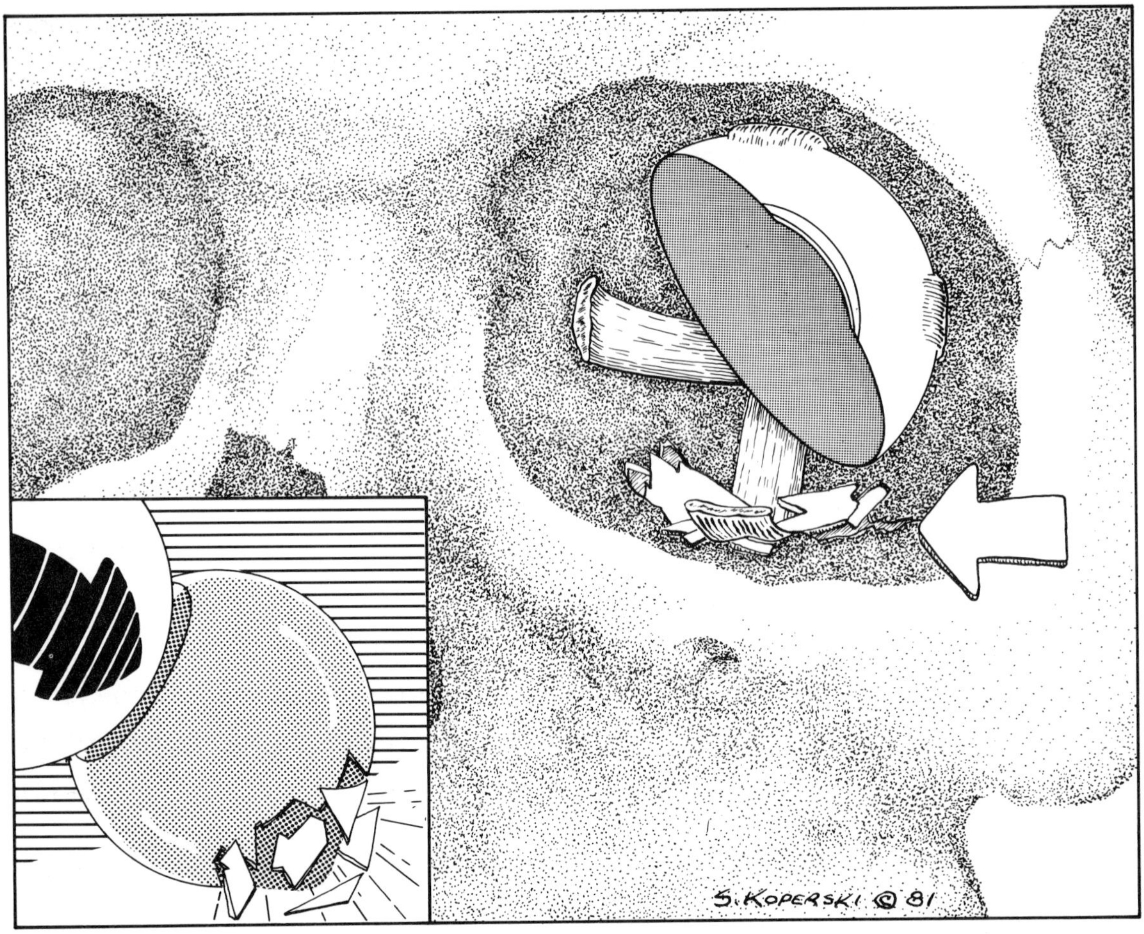

Figure 10-12. **Orbital fracture.** A "blow out" fracture of the orbital bones results from a direct blow on the globe which expands smartly against the thin orbital bones medially or inferiorly (arrow, inset). In the large illustration, the globe is partially cut away to demonstrate the possible entrapment of the orbital contents (fat or inferior rectus muscle), located by the arrow.

The surgeon explores the orbital floor through an incision in the lower eyelid. Periosteum is stripped from the floor of the orbit, and the herniated fat and musculature are restored to the orbital cavity. The defect in the orbital floor is reconstructed using either a synthetic implant or autogenous material such as nasal septal cartilage. Autogenous material is generally preferred. The correction is most effective when it is performed before scarring and fibrosis of the entrapped musculature have begun.

Nasal Bones

The nasal bones and cartilages are delicate structures that are easily damaged by even moderate force. Fractures may involve only the nasal bones and septum. In more severe injuries, the entire nasofrontal complex may be shattered and impacted into the orbital region.

Simple fractures of the nasal bones and septum can be treated in the emergency room. If the fracture is discovered prior to development of soft tissue edema, it can be reduced immediately. The nose can be packed with 5 percent cocaine solution to obtain anesthesia and an Asche or Walshom forceps introduced through the nares to precisely realign the fragments. The septal cartilage should always be checked for a hematoma. If a hematoma is present, it should be drained. Septal alignment should be corrected at the time of nasal fracture reduction.

If the surgeon discovers a fracture after considerable soft tissue edema has developed, the definitive correction is best postponed for five to seven days, at which time the edema will have subsided, the nasal bones and cartilages are still mobile and they can be maneuvered into position without difficulty. A dorsal splint made of plaster or molded metal is placed over the dorsum of the nose to protect the bones during the first week to 10 days of healing (Fig. 10-13).

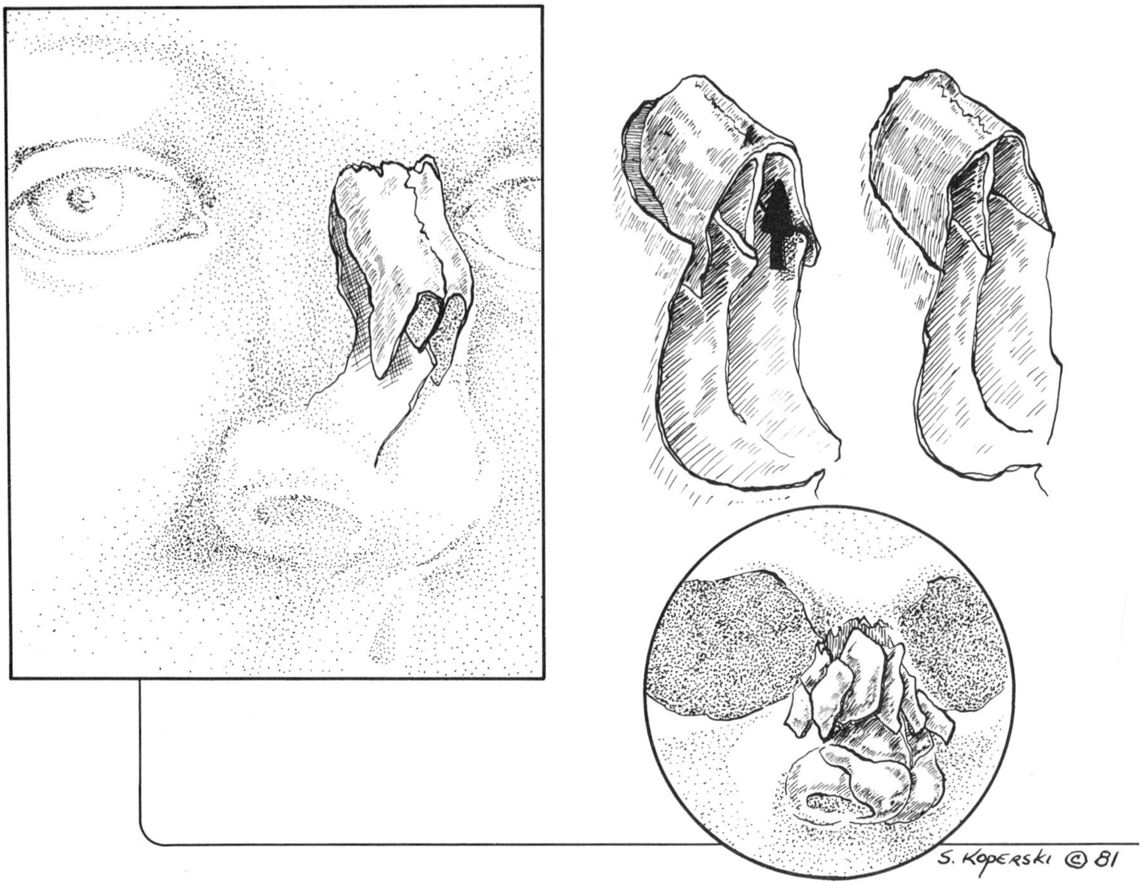

Figure 10-13. **Nasal fractures.** A sidewise blow to the nasal complex frequently shifts the nasal bones in a unit formed like the letter M (rectangular inset). The treatment is to elevate the M-shaped unit and shift it appropriately (top right). A blow straight on, with no sidewise deflection, may result in shattering of the nasal bones (circular inset). After elevation, this type of injury may require molding with internal packs.

More complicated nasofrontal fractures require direct exposure and wiring of the many fragments. These fractures can be exposed through the coronal incision used for craniofacial surgery. In such cases, the lacrimal apparatus is usually damaged and requires reconstruction. New bony insertions can be created for the disrupted canthal ligaments. Often the surgeon faces the task of molding small shattered fragments of bone together and holding them in place with a dorsal metal splint. Complex nasal fractures frequently require subsequent revision.

CHAPTER 11

Thermal Injuries

Burns, with an estimated 2 million a year in the United States alone, are common injuries. Of this total, over half are so minor that ambulatory outpatient care is all that is required. However, some 75,000 burn victims require hospitalization, and 12,000 of these succumb to their injuries. The mortality rate for severe burns is approximately 20 percent. Seventy-five percent of all thermal injuries are flame or flash burns, and most of these are sustained at home. Approximately 10 percent of burns are scald burns, with electrical and chemical burns being far less frequent.

During resuscitation of the severely burned patient, the basic principles of emergency care should be observed. The patient's general state of health should be evaluated and tetanus prophylaxis administered as indicated. As with any severely injured patient, control and maintenance of a patent airway is imperative. This is particularly true where smoke inhalation or burns of the oral or nasal mucosa may have occurred.

The edema associated with burns of the face and neck may also serve to severely compromise the airway, making subsequent intubation all the more difficult. It is better to employ an indwelling nasotracheal tube until the edema subsides rather than to perform tracheostomy through the burned neck.

The initial evaluation of the patient can be carried out in the burn unit or the emergency room. Minor burns can be dressed and the patients discharged. Generally, burns in children; second-degree burns covering more than 15 percent of the body surface in adults; third-degree burns; and burns of the face, hands or genitalia require hospital admission and care.

A patient with severe burns should be treated in a specialized facility where intensive care is available. These patients require massive fluid resuscitation through large-bore intravenous lines. They require an indwelling urinary catheter to follow fluid output and careful cardiovascular-pulmonary monitoring. Arterial line monitoring to obtain blood bases is useful in patients who have sustained severe smoke inhalation and respiratory burns.

Initial Evaluation

The most serious immediate problem for a patient who has sustained a thermal injury is the loss of fluid and electrolytes. Following a burn, there is increased capillary permeability in the area of the injury and massive amounts of plasma, electrolytes and proteins are lost by seepage into the burn wound. This fluid extravasation is at a maximum within the first 12 to 18 hours but continues for 24 to 48 hours following injury. In severe injuries, profound hypovolemia and hemoconcentration can result.

The immediate task confronting the physician treating a seriously burned patient is rapid restoration of fluid volume. There are several formulas that can aid fluid replacement, but to use them correctly the physician must accurately determine the surface area and depth of the burn.

The "rule of nines" is a helpful guide to ascertaining the burn surface area in adults but special charts are necessary for evaluating surface area in children because of the relatively greater surface area of the head and relatively smaller surface area of the extremities. In the adult, 9 percent of the body surface is allowed for the head and neck, 18 percent for the anterior thorax and abdomen, and 18 percent for the posterior portion of that area. Each upper extremity represents 9 percent of the body surface and each lower extremity represents 18 percent. The most accurate way to determine the extent of a burn is by reproducing the burned area on a standardized body surface chart (Fig. 11-1).

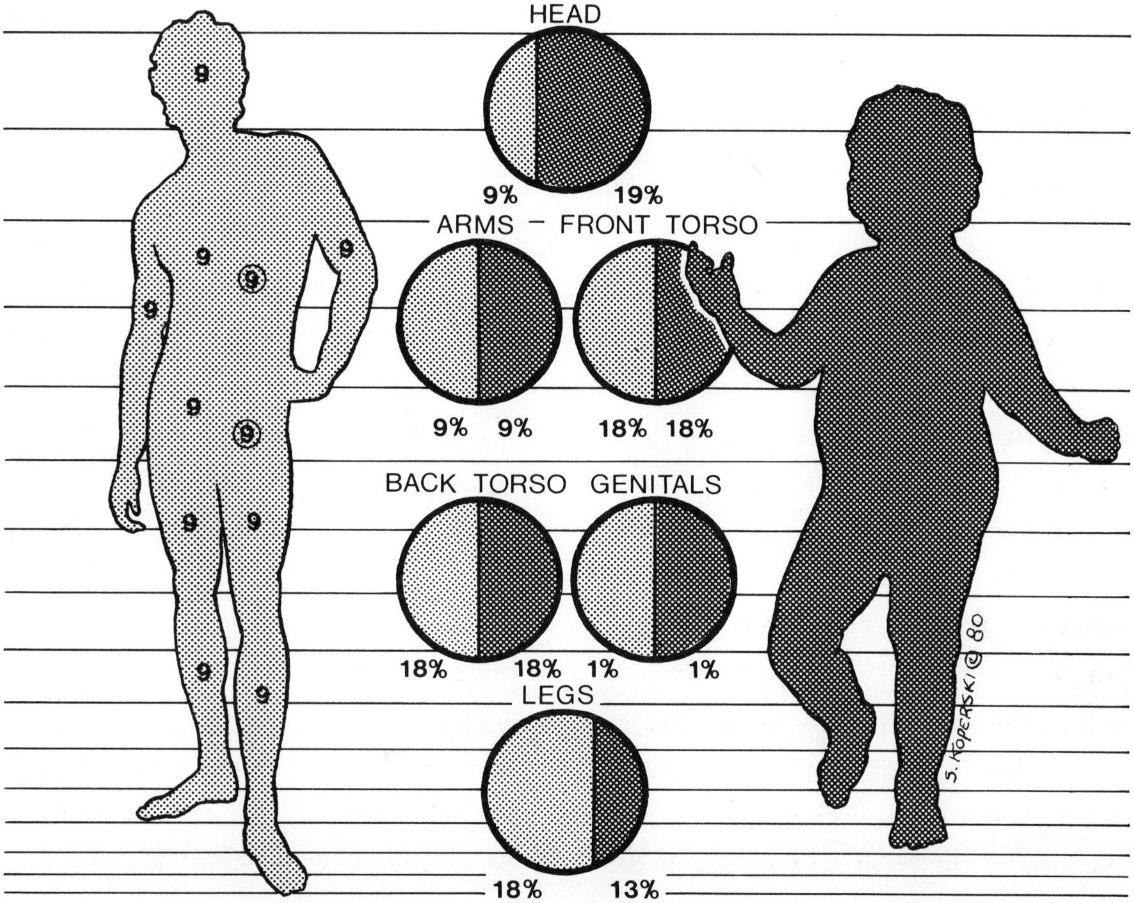

Figure 11-1. **"Rule of nines."** In judging burn surface area, the adult body can be divided into 11 regions of 9 percent each (left figure). In the child, however, the head represents a proportionately greater area while the lower extremities represent a smaller percentage (right figure). Center of illustration gives comparative percentages for adults (light shading) and children (dark shading).

The depth of a burn is a function of the agent of injury and the duration of contact. First-degree burns injure only the epidermis. In a second-degree burn, the level of injury reaches into the dermis, but the skin appendages remain intact and serve as a source of epithelization that will resurface most burn wounds spontaneously within two to four weeks. Some second-degree burns are so deep that few appendages survive, and grafting, as in third-degree burns, will not only hasten healing but provide a better quality of skin. Third-degree burns destroy all the skin appendages and can only heal, therefore, from the edges. If large in area, they will require grafts of skin for repair (Fig. 11-2).

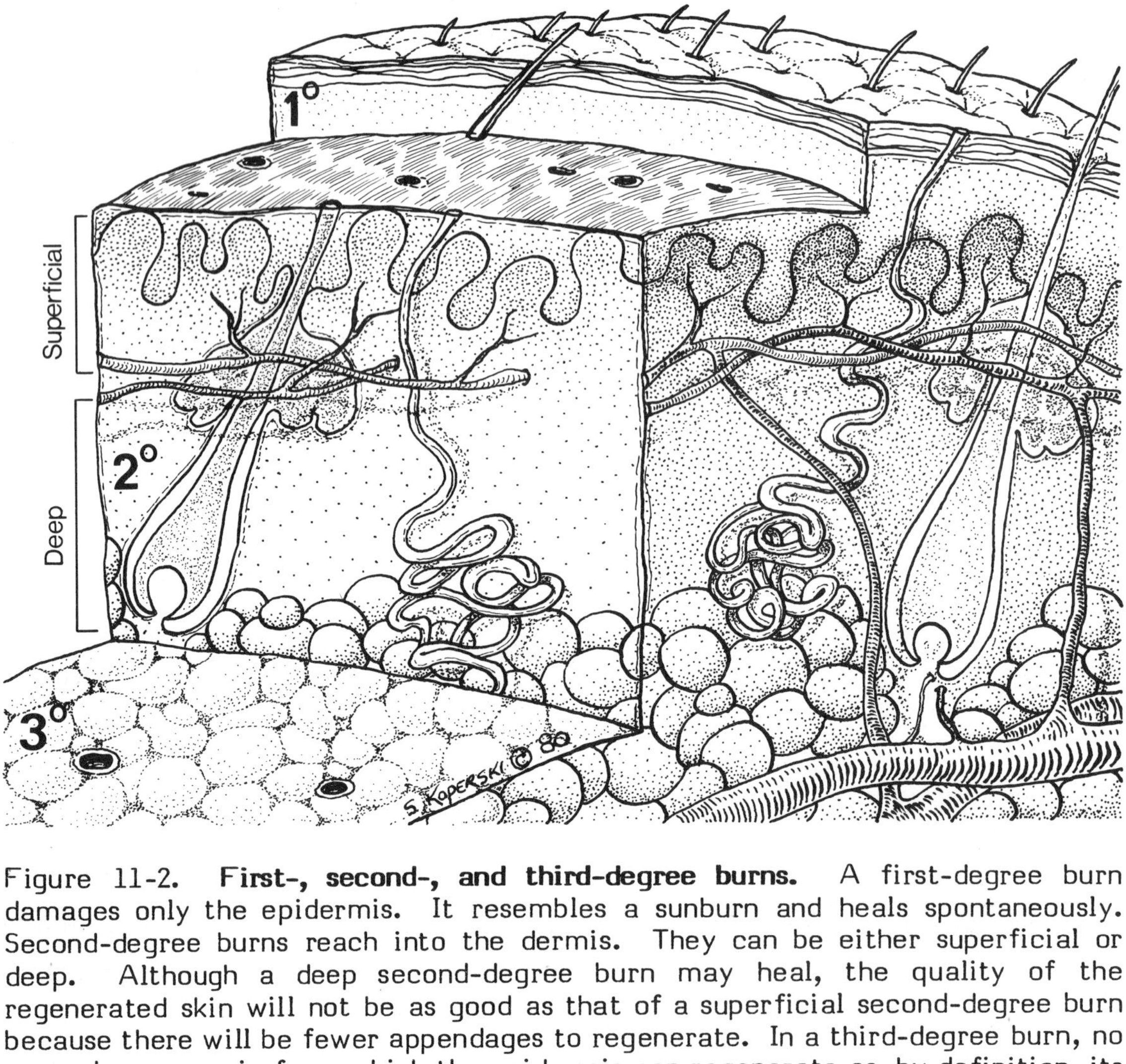

Figure 11-2. **First-, second-, and third-degree burns.** A first-degree burn damages only the epidermis. It resembles a sunburn and heals spontaneously. Second-degree burns reach into the dermis. They can be either superficial or deep. Although a deep second-degree burn may heal, the quality of the regenerated skin will not be as good as that of a superficial second-degree burn because there will be fewer appendages to regenerate. In a third-degree burn, no appendages remain from which the epidermis can regenerate as, by definition, its damage extends below the level of hair and sweat follicles.

The depth of the injury must be determined at the time of initial clinical examination and is based on the appearance of the wound (Table 11-1). First-degree burns are erythematous and painful. The presence of blisters and a weeping surface indicate a second-degree burn. Third-degree burns have a leathery brown or pale appearance and contain coagulated blood vessels. A sensation of pain in a burn wound tested with a pin suggests that the nerve endings are intact and, hence, that the burn is no greater than second degree. In third-degree burns, no nerve endings exist, and no pain to testing is elicited.

Table 11-1. Clinical Determination of Burn Depth

Criterion	First-Degree	Second-Degree	Third-Degree
Color	Erythema	More intense erythema	White, brown or charred
Blister	Absent	Present, with a weeping surface if blisters are broken	Absent
Sensation to pin prick	Present	Present	Absent
Wound surface	At level of unburned skin	Frequently elevated above normal skin	Frequently depressed below surrounding unburned skin
Healing tendency	Epithelizes	Epithelizes	Produces granulating wounds

Electrical Burns

Accurate assessment of the extent of an electrical burn is important but is extremely difficult to ascertain. In such burns, the extent of injury is usually significantly underestimated because of the innocuous appearance of the wound at the entrance and exit sites of the electrical current.

The heat generated as current passes through a solid conductor results in coagulation necrosis when that solid conductor is the human body. The amount of heat generated depends on the local tissue resistance, the path of the current, the type of current, and the duration of contact. The skin's resistance tends to concentrate the heat at the sites of entrance and exit.

After the skin is penetrated, the current tends to follow the path of least resistance. Tissues have various degrees of electrical resistance. Bone and fat have high resistance to electricity while muscle, blood vessels and nerves have lower resistance.

Alternating current, especially at low voltages, causes the most dangerous electrical injuries. This is because the muscle spasm produced immobilizes the patient, prolonging the contact with the electrical source and the duration of the injury. In the case of high voltage direct current, the massive reflex spasm produced tends to release the patient from contact with the electrical source.

Sudden death can occur from electrical injuries through ventricular fibrillation or ventilatory paralysis. Cardiac conduction is most significantly affected by low voltage injuries. High tension line injuries more commonly cause ventilatory paralysis.

Because of the massive destruction of muscle that can result from electrical injuries, myohemoglobinuria can be a significant problem. This renal damage is aggravated if the patient becomes hypovolemic. Therapy includes hydration and diuretics. The tissue necrosis results in systemic acidosis which must be reversed with sodium bicarbonate.

The high heat generated by the resistance of the tissues as the current passes through them results in extensive coagulation necrosis. This may not be evident until tissue edema develops. In these cases, fluid resuscitation must be continued until urine volumes and central venous pressure measurement indicate successful reversal of burn shock. These patients require extensive debridement of the necrotic tissue when they become clinically stable.

Pulmonary Injury

Smoke injury is sustained through prolonged exposure to hot gases in a confined space. Such a patient may arrive unconscious. Upper airway mucosal burns are sustained upon exposure to a flame or flash explosion. Lower airway injuries to the alveoli are not due to heat, but rather they are the result of prolonged exposure to chemical fumes and smoke particles. Burn patients with severe pulmonary injury carry a significant morbidity and must be treated aggressively.

Diagnosis of smoke inhalation is made through physical examination. There may be obvious burns and blistering of the oral mucosa. The nasal hairs may be singed and smoke particles may coat the tongue. Wheezing and coughing indicate lower airway injury. Blood levels of carbon monoxide should be measured. Arterial blood gases should be monitored regularly if pulmonary injury is suspected.

Injury to the airway from smoke and toxic chemicals can result in a massive slough of the pulmonary lining. This results in an obstruction of ventilation with shunting and hypoxia. Severe pulmonary infections follow loss of pulmonary mucosa.

In mild injuries physical therapy, postural drainage and oxygen therapy may be adequate. In more severe cases repeated bronchoscopy, prolonged intubation, high concentration oxygen therapy and positive pressure ventilation may be necessary. The role of steroids in treating airway injury associated with burns remains controversial. In most centers steroids are believed to be contraindicated. Systemic antibiotics are necessary to control pulmonary infections.

Fluid Replacement

Following the preliminary evaluation and the estimation of the extent of burn damage, fluid resuscitation should begin. There are several formulas to guide fluid replacement (Table 11-2). All of them relate the amount of fluid given to the weight of the patient and the percentage of body surface covered by the burn. It should be remembered that the amount of fluid loss is closely related to the extent of the burn up to an area of 50 percent of the body surface. After that, fluid loss cannot be calculated as a function of burn area; therefore, 50 percent is the maximum entered into the formulas for fluid replacement.

Table 11-2. Representative Types of Replacement Fluid Formulas

Formula	Colloid	Electrolyte Solution	H_2O (ml)
Brooke	0.5 ml/kg/%	1.5 mlg/%	2000
Evans	1 ml/kg/%	1 ml/kg/%	2000
MGH	125 ml plasma/%	15 ml/%	2000
Parkland Hospital	--	4 ml/kg/%	--

The formula serves as a guide to the total fluid requirement for the first 24 hours. One-half the total volume should be given in the first eight hours to compensate for the increased fluid extravasation during that period. The remaining one-half should be given over the rest of the 24-hour period. The fluid given over the second 24 hours should be about one-half that of the first 24-hour period.

Controversy exists regarding the best choice of fluid for resuscitation. Some authorities advocate the use of a colloid solution (plasma, dextran, albumen) on the theory that it prevents some of the fluid loss at the burn site by increasing colloid pressure. This results in administration of a lower total volume of fluid administered and may have advantages for the elderly patient.

It has been conclusively shown that adequate resuscitation can be achieved with electrolyte solutions alone, using 4 ml of solution per kg per percent of body surface burned. The best choice of resuscitation fluid for any patient in shock is lactated Ringer's solution.

Formulas are only rough guides to fluid administration. Replacement should ultimately be judged by the clinical condition of the patient. Renal perfusion is a sensitive index of hydration for a patient in shock. A urine output of 30 to 50 cc an hour is a sign that adequate hydration has been attained. For the infant or for the elderly patient, monitoring of the central venous pressure and pulmonary wedge pressure is a useful adjunct to fluid management. Weight should be monitored daily.

The administration of prophylactic antibiotics at the time of hospital admission represents another controversial area in burn care. Infection and burn sepsis are uncommon for 72 hours except by beta-hemolytic streptococcus. Burn wounds infected with this organism can rapidly prove fatal. For this reason, penicillin (500,000 units three times a day) has been administered prophylactically to burn patients by some centers. With the advent of improved topical agents, the necessity for penicillin prophylaxis has become debatable.

Third-Degree Burns

Burn Eschar

In the immediate post-burn period, third-degree burns are recognizable as thick, pale, leathery patches called eschars. They are often depressed below the level of surrounding, unburned skin. These thick, unyielding areas may be present on the thorax, neck or, circumferentially, on an extremity. The soft tissue burn edema cannot expand against the rigid eschar. This can result in compromised circulation to an extremity, or impaired ventilation if the eschar is on the chest or neck.

These tight, constricting bands should be treated immediately by incising completely through the eschar. Escharotomy should be carried out in a sterile fashion. Because of the insensitivity of third-degree burns, the escharotomy can be performed in the burn unit without a general anesthetic (Fig. 11-3).

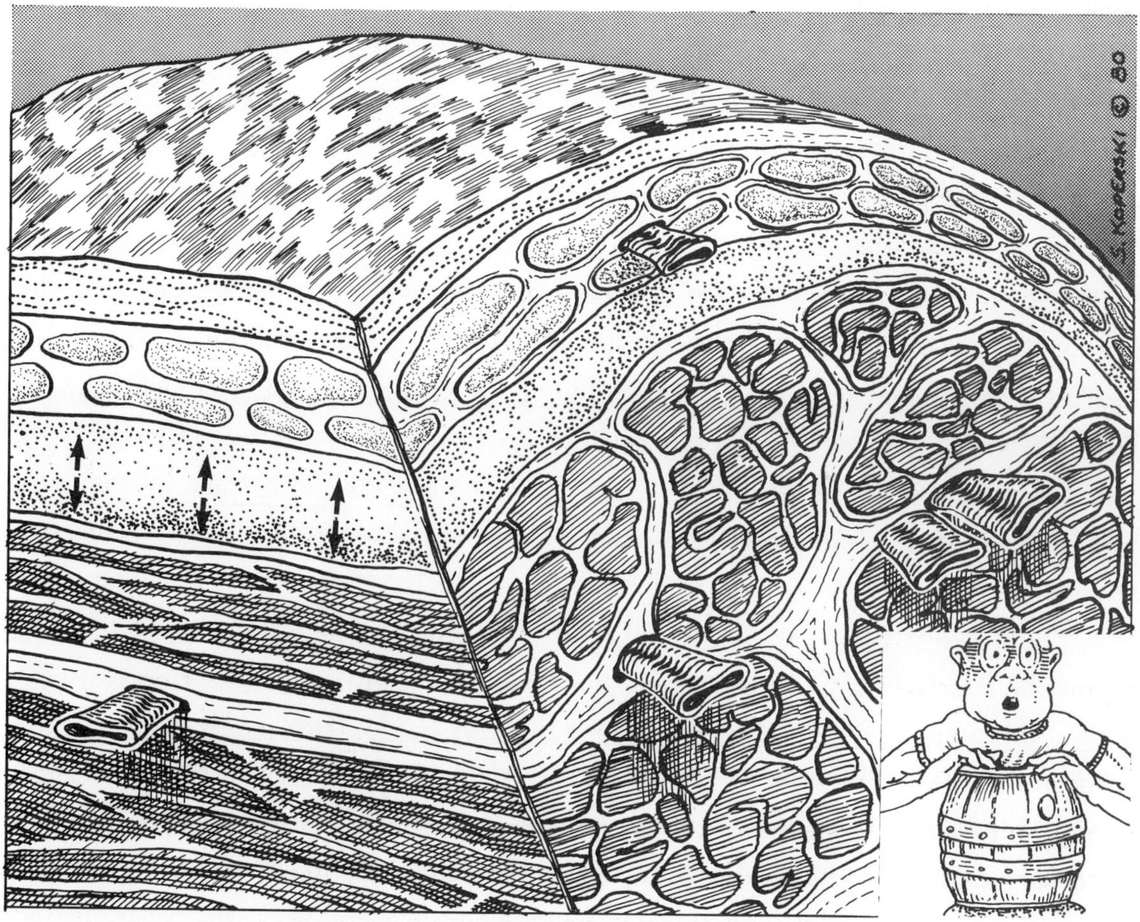

Figure 11-3. **Burn eschar.** A burn eschar results from coagulation of the dermis. If circumferential, this can compress the underlying vessels and nerves, especially when the tissue edema causes tissue expansion (arrows). If located in the thorax, an eschar may impair respiration (inset).

Preparation for Grafting

Following initial stabilization and care, the patient with deep burns must be prepared for wound closure by grafting skin. A diet including 50 to 80 calories per kilogram of body weight and 2 to 5 g of protein per kilogram must be maintained. While most patients tolerate this nutritional load orally, some patients, especially children, require supplementation of the diet. High calorie food supplements can be given through a nasogastric tube. Because of the risk of sepsis, intravenous hyperalimentation should be avoided.

Multiple gastric ulcerations with major gastrointestinal bleeding, called Curling's ulcers, can occur in the first weeks after a burn. A major hemorrhage at this time can be catastrophic. Patients should be treated prophylactically with frequent feedings and antacids. Cimetadine can be given to selected patients who exhibit symptoms or who have a history of ulcer diathasis.

The burn wound should be inspected and redressed daily. This is best carried out with the aid of a large Hubbard tank where the patient is fully immersed and the dressings are soaked off. The eschar can be examined and debrided as necessary with the patient in the tank. Topical agents can be applied when the patient leaves the tank and can be held in place with light gauze dressings.

It is important, especially when the hands and neck are burned, to institute active physical therapy to prevent wound contracture. The hands can be placed in splints which maintain the position of function. Several times a day active and passive therapy should be applied to all joints. Full neck extension should be maintained with splints.

The most serious problem for the burn patient during the three to six weeks prior to grafting, while the thick eschar is separating from the underlying tissue, is burn wound sepsis. Vigorous debridement and topical antimicrobials are the major means of preventing an overwhelming infection in the burn eschar.

The most popular antimicrobial agent at present is silver sulfadiazine (Silvadine). A thin paste of the cream is applied to the surface of the burned area daily. Silvadine penetrates the eschar, controlling proliferation of bacteria. Silvadine is painless and relatively easy for the nursing staff to apply.

Another common topical antimicrobial, Sulfamylon, has been used frequently in the past. However, this agent is a carbonic anhydrase inhibitor and can lead to significant metabolic derangement. In addition, Sulfamylon is very painful when applied.

Two to six weeks are required for complete separation of the eschar and for a healthy recipient site to be ready for skin grafting. The loose burn eschar is removed daily after soaking in a Hubbard tank. The process of eschar separation may be promoted by a grid escharotomy. This consists of cross-cutting the eschar down to normal tissue, creating 2 to 4 cm squares. Escharotomy increases the total surface area of the burn available for debridement during dressing changes.

In patients who have an area ready for grafting that exceeds the size of the potential donor site, temporary coverage of the wound is possible. Allografts and porcine (pig) skin have been used as well as synthetics, and amniotic membranes. This temporary cover seals the wound and minimizes loss of fluid, electrolyte and protein through the burn wound. The allografts usually survive at least two weeks before they are rejected.

The Grafting Procedure

In small, well demarcated third-degree burns, complete surgical excision of the eschar can be accomplished, followed by immediate skin grafting. Tangential excision, as it is called, eliminates the time necessary for eschar separation. This is especially useful for burns of the dorsum of the hand where early coverage is important in order to avoid scar contracture and joint stiffness.

After the eschar separates or is debrided away, granulation tissue develops on the surface of the burn. It is best to perform the skin grafting before the granulation tissue becomes thick and exuberant. Aesthetically important areas, such as the face and trunk; and functional areas, such as the hand and joint surfaces, should be grafted first. Large sheets of uniform thickness taken with a drum dermatone are best for these areas.

Frequently, skin graft placement and donor site choice must be planned in advance by bearing in mind the patient's resting position during the period of recuperation. Such procedures may have to be carried out in several stages. In some cases, the extremities can be suspended from an orthopedic bed frame with skeletal traction to avoid disruption of the skin graft in the postoperative period, as well as to facilitate dressing changes. Skin grafts can often be harvested from normal skin on the side of the body that is to receive the graft so that the patient is not compelled to lie on painful donor areas.

In cases where the donor sites are limited, consideration should be given to expanding the graft in a 6:1 or 3:1 ratio. While the resultant mesh-grafted area is not as cosmetically acceptable as a sheet graft, it allows the surgeon to maximize the donor site areas and to provide early coverage. Following healing and wound closure, the meshed areas can be excised and covered with sheet grafts.

The skin grafts are easily spread out on the granulation surface. Several sutures are needed to hold the grafts in place. A light dressing of saline or Neomycin-soaked gauze is placed over the grafts to provide stability and protection. When possible, it is best to splint joints in a position that will minimize scar contracture.

Post-Graft Care

The dressings should be changed daily for several days and the grafts inspected and debrided as necessary. The gauze dressing should be moistened as it is removed to prevent adherence and disruption of the graft. Thereafter, daily dressing changes are continued for five to seven days as necessary until the graft has taken. Treatments in the Hubbard tank can begin again when the graft is stable.

Once grafting is completed, care must be taken to prevent wound contracture deformities caused by scarring in the split thickness graft. Orthopedic splints must be applied and an active physical therapy program employed for at least six months to maintain full extension of the neck and extremities. If an active physical therapy program is not instituted, subsequent procedures may be necessary to release and skin graft the burn scar contractures.

Hypertrophic scarring of the grafted areas, and occasionally of the donor site itself, is sometimes a problem following burn reconstruction. The affected area becomes red, raised and uncomfortable. Employing a custom-made elastic garment to apply continuous pressure on the scar is the best method of preventing hypertrophic burn scars. A clear plastic mask, made from a facial moulage, can be used to apply pressure to the face and neck. The pressure should be applied immediately after wound closure and maintained for six to eight months or until the scars are white, flat, soft and no longer symptomatic (Fig. 11-4).

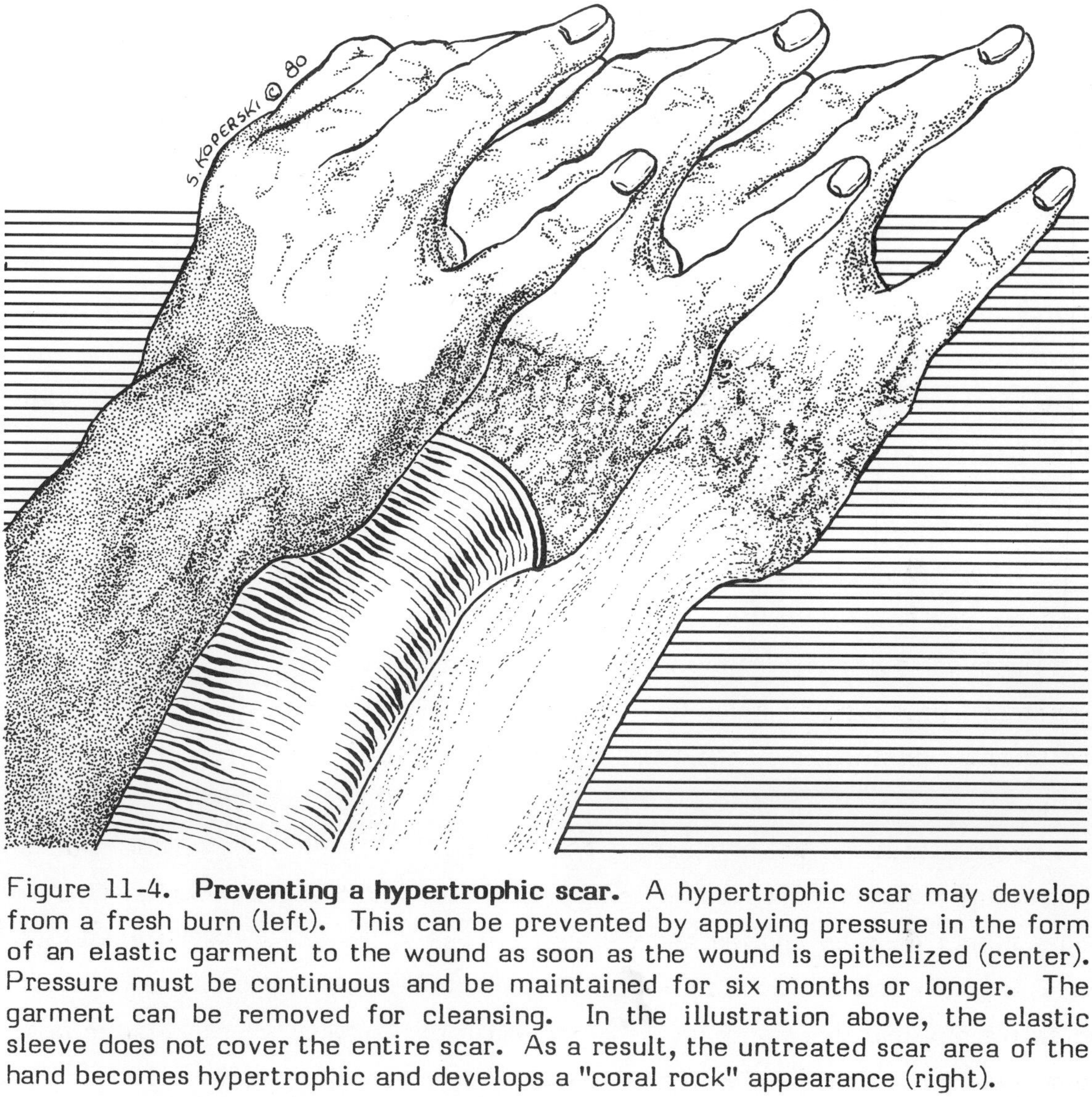

Figure 11-4. **Preventing a hypertrophic scar.** A hypertrophic scar may develop from a fresh burn (left). This can be prevented by applying pressure in the form of an elastic garment to the wound as soon as the wound is epithelized (center). Pressure must be continuous and be maintained for six months or longer. The garment can be removed for cleansing. In the illustration above, the elastic sleeve does not cover the entire scar. As a result, the untreated scar area of the hand becomes hypertrophic and develops a "coral rock" appearance (right).

The skin of healed donor sites is initially very fragile. Such areas are easily traumatized, may blister, and tend to be dry because of diminished sebaceous gland secretion. These areas should be protected from trauma. Lubrication of the skin with lanolin oil is helpful and often alleviates dryness and itching.

CHAPTER 12

Skin Tumors

One of the most common reasons for a patient seeking medical consultation is a skin lesion. A basic familiarity with frequently encountered benign and malignant lesions is essential for all plastic surgeons.

Benign Lesions

Nevus-Cell Nevus

Pigmented lesions comprise the majority of benign skin lesions evaluated by the clinician. The threat of malignant disease is a real concern to the patient seeking advice. Nevus-cell nevus is the most common pigmented lesion. The nevus cell is thought to arise from the neural crest. The location of nevus cell activity in the lesion is the basis for classification of the three histological types as either intradermal, junctional or compound.

Intradermal nevi are the predominant type seen in adults. These may be flat or elevated and may contain hair. Nevus cell activity in this lesion is found in the dermis. Junctional nevi are more common in childhood and adolescence. The lesions are usually flat, and the nevus cells are seen at the junction of the dermis and the epidermis. In a compound nevus, the cells are found in both the dermis and the epidermis.

Consideration should be given to excision of nevi, especially when junctional elements are present, because these are thought to be more prone to transformation into malignant melanoma than are other nevus types. While most nevi do not require excision, those that are subject to repeated irritation, those located on the palm, sole or genitalia and those which undergo a change in appearance or color, should be removed (Fig. 12-1).

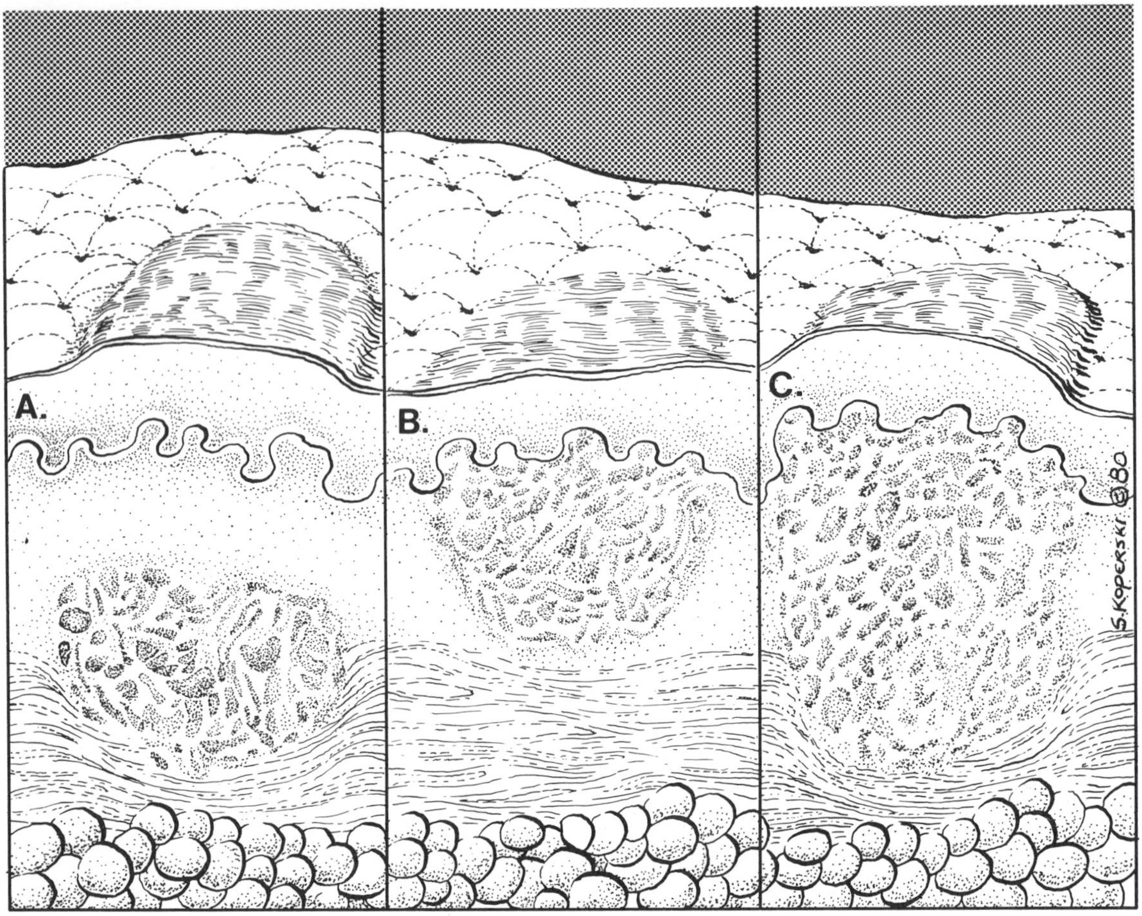

Figure 12-1. **Nevi are classified according to location in the dermis.** Intradermal nevi have the nevus cells deep in the dermis (A). Junctional nevi are in the upper dermis at the dermal epidermal junction (B). Compound nevi are found in both locations (C). Generally, the older the patient the less junctional activity should be present.

Congenital Pigmented Nevus

One percent of children are born with congenital pigmented nevus. The giant hairy type of nevus is always congenital. These lesions are different biochemically and histologically from the nevi that appear later in life. There is evidence to suggest that the congenital nevi are more metabolically active than acquired nevi.

The congenital nevus has been known to turn into malignant melanoma. Estimates of the rate of change from benign to malignant in giant congenital nevi range from 2 to 40 percent. Once transformation has occurred, however, the disease is rapidly fatal. It is because of the danger of malignant change that many authorities recommend early complete excision of congenital pigmented nevi. The lesion may be removed and closed or skin-grafted primarily. Subsequent scar revisions are performed on the grafted area as the child grows older (Fig. 12-2).

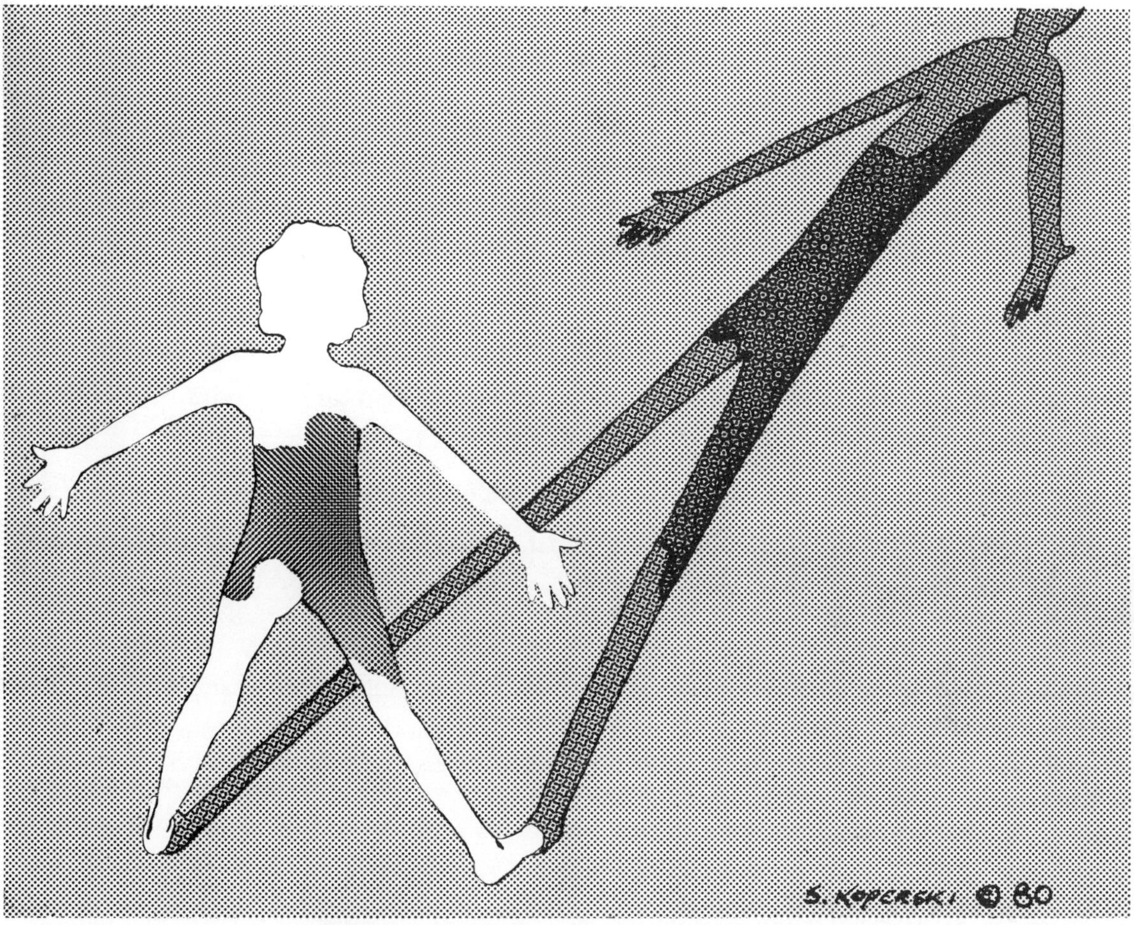

Figure 12-2. **Giant hairy nevi.** Giant hairy nevi are congenital lesions that have a higher rate of malignant potential than nevi that appear later in life. This patient has such a lesion, and because of its location it has attracted the additional sobriquet of a "bathing trunk nevus."

Hemangioma

The proliferation of vascular tissue of mesodermal origin represents the most common benign tumor of infancy, present in 10 percent of children. The lesions are seen at birth or appear in the first year of life. These hemangiomas are classified pathologically as capillary, cavernous or mixed.

The capillary hemangioma, or port wine stain, is flat and is usually present at birth. This lesion is discretely outlined and consists of capillaries with mature vascular endothelium. The lesions are most common on the face and neck and are often found in the distribution of one or more branches of the trigeminal nerve. These hemangiomas may develop purplish excrescences later, but otherwise change little during the individual's lifetime and always occupy the same relative area on the face as a child grows. It is important to remember that a few capillary hemangiomas may be associated with serious anomalies of the central nervous tract, such as the Sturge-Weber syndrome.

Numerous therapeutic modalities, including surgical excision, radiotherapy, tattooing, cryosurgery and, recently, laser beam surgery, have been employed to treat capillary hemangiomas. In the past, staged surgical excision, followed by reconstruction with skin grafts or local flaps, represented the best therapy. Lesions located deep in the dermis may be amenable to multiple tattooing procedures in which skin-colored pigment is placed superficial to the hemangioma.

Recent work with the argon laser has added a promising new dimension to treatment of capillary hemangioma. Several series have been reported in which the laser produced a desirable result without significant scarring. More experience is needed before widespread employment of this new modality becomes practical. In many cases, the use of an opaque cosmetic remains the best treatment.

The cavernous hemangioma or "strawberry" hemangioma comprises 90 percent of the hemangiomas of infancy. The lesions are often seen at birth but can appear within the first year of life. The capillaries are composed of immature or embryonal type endothelium, which explains why 80 to 90 percent spontaneously involute by the fifth year of life. The lesions may increase very rapidly in the first six to eight months. They can be of varying size. They may involve just the skin and subcutaneous tissue, or they may ramify deep into the tissue affecting the underlying muscle and bone.

Treatment involves repeated observation and often requires continued reassurance of the parents until the child reaches the age of five, at which time the decision regarding surgical excision of the lesion can best be made. Pressure dressings, particularly on an extremity, may speed the involution of the lesion. Corticosteroids have been of benefit in controlling rapidly expanding lesions, particularly those encroaching on vital structures. Oral prednisone (20 to 30 mg) is given every other day for four weeks, and then the dose is tapered. Response may be immediate and dramatic.

Hemangiomas that are difficult to manage because of increasing size, bleeding, development of a coagulopathy, or placement that threatens an important anatomical structure, such as the eye or mouth, should be treated without waiting. Lesions that appear after the age of two years and that increase in size are not likely to involute. These hemangiomas should be treated early.

Surgical excision, with reconstruction employing regional flaps or skin grafts, is the best treatment for cavernous hemangiomas. Occasionally, ligation of the major feeding vessels may induce involution. Recently lesions have been treated by intra-arterial embolization. Under fluoroscopic control, muscle or other materials are injected to induce thrombosis in the lesion. This method has had limited success. Irradiation should be avoided because of the high incidence of radiation-related late complications.

Lipoma

Lipomas are tumors composed of fat cells. They can be found anywhere in the body but are most frequently seen as painless subcutaneous nodules. The size of a lipoma may vary from 2 to 4 cm. They are soft, freely mobile and not attached to the overlying skin. Treatment consists of surgical excision. Multiple lesions need not be excised because malignant change is extremely rare. Liposarcomas are probably not related to benign subcutaneous lipomas.

Epidemoid and Sebaceous Cyst

These common lesions arise from epidermal elements located within the dermis. They may present as painless subcutaneous nodules or as a painful inflamed mass. They are usually freely mobile but are attached at some point to the overlying skin. The lesions are found most frequently in adults or late adolescents. They are most common on the face, over the malar eminence, or in the scalp. The differentiation of sebaceous and epidemoid cysts cannot be made clinically. Treatment consists of complete removal of the contents of the cyst as well as the cyst wall itself. The cysts should not be excised during active inflammation. A standard excision may be performed or, in some cases, the sac may be removed through a small incision after the contents have been expressed.

Malignant Lesions

The most frequently encountered malignancies of the skin are basal cell carcinoma, squamous cell carcinoma and malignant melanoma. Skin cancer is by far the most common type of malignancy in the human body. Skin cancers are probably related to damage to the skin by ultraviolet radiation from the sun. Ninety-six percent of these lesions occur in areas exposed to the sun. People with blonde or red hair and ruddy, Anglo-Saxon complexions are more prone to skin cancers than those with darker complexions. Negroes are rarely affected.

Other suspected causes are x-irradiation and direct contact with arsenic and paraffin compounds. Certain genetic diseases, such as xerodema pigmentosum, are associated with an increased incidence of skin malignancies. Patients who are immunologically suppressed following renal or cardiac transplantation have an increased risk of cutaneous malignancy. In contrast, pigmented races appear to be protected from skin cancer because their stratum corneum contains many active melanophores.

Basal Cell Carcinoma

Basal cell cancer is the most common skin cancer in Caucasians. The lesion arises from the pluri-potential cells of the epidermis or hair follicles. There are basically two clinical types of basal cell epithelioma: the isolated, nodular type and the more infiltrating type with vague borders.

The nodular type usually presents itself as a single, discrete, nodular lesion with a central ulcer and rolled or heaped-up pearly edges. They occur most frequently on exposed areas such as the face and the anterior chest. The ulcer is caused by necrosis in the lesion. Such lesions enlarge slowly along the skin plane and occasionally extend into the underlying subcutaneous tissue or cartilage. Histologically, the borders of this type of lesion show sharp demarcation on microscopic section.

The infiltrating type, which includes morpheic and sclerosing basal cell lesions, tends to extend beneath the skin like the roots of a tree. This is confirmed by the microscope view which shows tumor nests scattered throughout the entire field. These lesions are much more likely to invade underlying structures (Fig. 12-3).

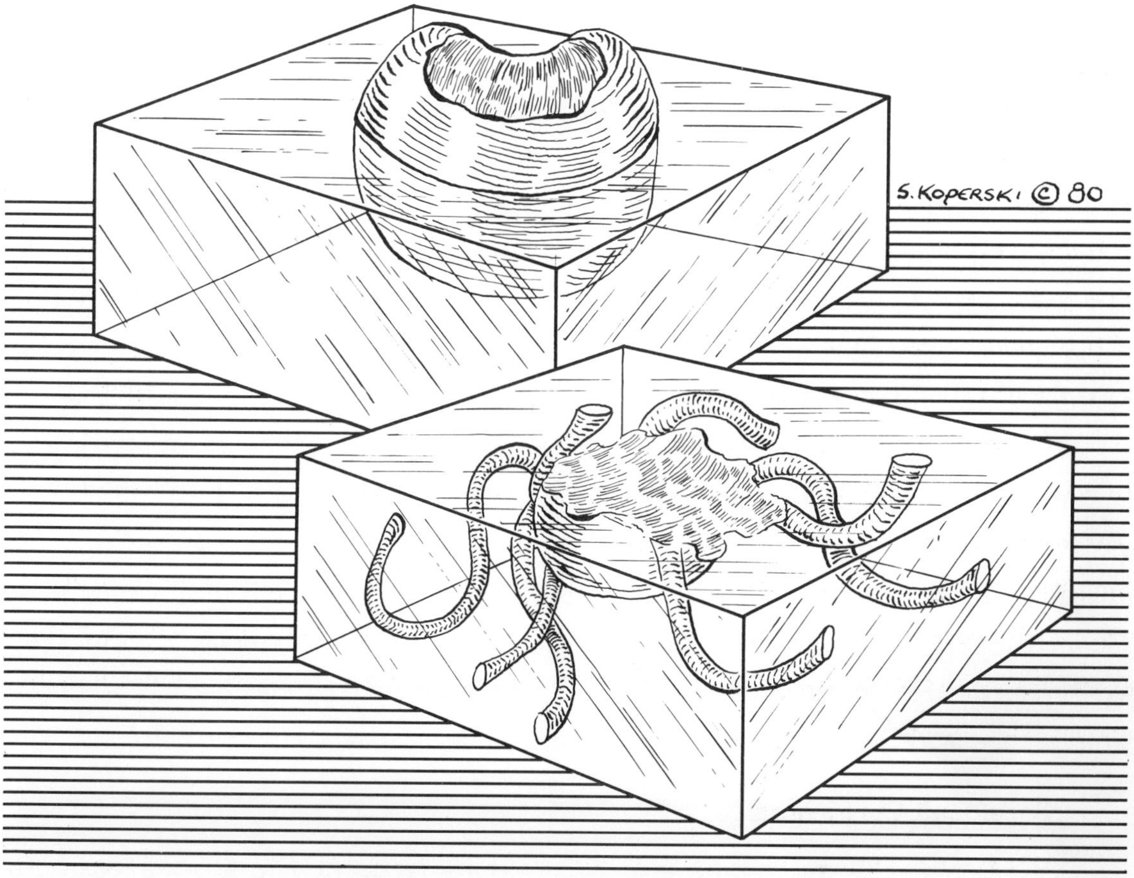

Figure 12-3. **Clinical types of basal cell carcinoma.** Many types of basal cell carcinoma are described. There are, however, only two important differences among them. The single, isolated, nodular basal cell has rolled pearly edges with telangiectasia and sharply defined borders (top). These borders are just as sharp in the subcutaneous plane which is represented by the transparent cube. The central umbilication arises from central necrosis as the tumor outgrows its blood supply resulting in a volcano-like appearance. The second type (bottom) is endophytic, has scaly, vague borders and, most importantly, has subcutaneous extensions (represented here in the cube) much like the roots of a tree. It is these extensions which lead to the higher recurrence rate of this type of carcinoma since one of these foci can easily be missed in excision if a wide border is not taken.

Because inadequately treated basal cell lesions may recur and become more aggressive locally, complete excision is essential. Well-circumscribed lesions should be excised by including a margin of 2 to 3 mm of normal-appearing tissue in the excision. Lesions such as the morpheic and sclerosing basal cell types have ill-defined borders and require a more generous margin, as much as 1 to 1½ cm beyond the visible limits of the lesion. Other acceptable forms of treatment for small discrete lesions include curettage and desiccation. Radiation therapy can be used for palliation or cure in the elderly. Mohs' chemosurgical treatment, which today is really a fresh tissue technique using microscopic mapping, has proven a very accurate method of treatment.

Recurrence of the lesion in the excision scar occurs in 3 to 7 percent of cases and may be insidious and slow to become obvious. When the patient finally seeks therapy, the recurrent lesion is often large and the margins are indistinct. In these cases, specialized treatments may be useful. Mohs' technique of serial excision of the lesion permits the surgeon to excise only as much tissue as necessary to obtain tumor-free margins. In areas of the face where a small excision may result in a large deformity, the advantage of this controlled surgery is obvious. Mohs reports a cure rate of 97 percent.

Reconstruction following excision of basal cell tumors can be accomplished by using split thickness grafts, local flaps or primary closure. Immediate reconstruction is favored if the excision margins are clear of tumor. The method used must take into account the general condition of the patient. Often the simplest method of reconstruction is the best.

Squamous Cell Carcinoma

Squamous cell carcinoma also occurs most frequently in areas exposed to the sun. Seventy-five percent of such lesions occur on the head and neck. The lower lip is the most common site. Several conditions associated with chronic or repeated damage to the skin are known to predispose it to development of squamous cell carcinoma. Areas of irradiation, chronic granulation tissue, chronic osteomyelitis, ulcers of the lower leg and old burn scars have all been sites of squamous cell carcinoma.

Squamous cell carcinoma spreads more rapidly than basal cell carcinoma, more aggressively invading local tissue. More significantly, the squamous lesion has the capacity to spread by way of the blood and regional lymphatics in 5 to 10 percent of cases. Histologically, lesions are classified as well differentiated or anaplastic.

The lesion appears as a raised papular area which soon becomes ulcerated. The ulcerated lesion may become covered with a serous crust or may remain a raw, granular surface. The lesion may become exuberant and exophytic or may remain flat and extend under the skin into the adjacent structures. The best treatment is surgical removal with a margin of 1 to 1½ cm of normal tissue included, followed by immediate reconstruction.

Because of the low incidence of metastatic disease, therapeutic, rather than prophylactic, lymph node dissection is indicated. If the nodes are clinically positive at the time the primary lesion is excised, an in-continuity excision can be performed. Prophylactic node dissection might be recommended in recurrent lesions, in lesions greater than 2 cm in size, and in lesions with highly anaplastic histology. Generally, however, regular examinations are sufficient to follow the lymph node drainage areas.

Malignant Melanoma

Malignant melanoma can arise from any cell capable of producing melanin. It is most common in the skin but can be seen in virtually any organ. It has been reported in the eye, rectum, and on mucosal membranes. The disease is uncommon, having been estimated at 4 to 8 cases per 100,000. Women are more frequently affected than men. Melanomas are rare in Negroes where the incidence is 0.6 per 100,000; when they do occur, they are more likely to be seen on the lower extremity or in nonpigmented areas such as the palms of the hands or soles of the feet.

There are two periods during life when one is at greater risk: at 35 to 54 years of age and at 65 years of age and older. The lesion is very rare in children before puberty, but it has been described as developing from congenital giant hairy nevi.

Genetic factors, exposure to sunlight, and/or repeated trauma have been implicated in the pathogenesis of malignant melanoma. It has been proven, however, that melanoma can arise from preexisting pigmented lesions. While the true incidence is uncertain, it is believed that between 5 and 35 percent of nevi can turn into malignant melanoma. The junctional nevus is the most likely type to undergo malignant transformation.

Hutchinson's melanotic freckle, which is not in itself malignant, is seen in older individuals, chiefly on the face. This lesion is flat, has irregular borders, and is colored with several shades of black and brown pigment. One-third of these cases may become transformed into malignant melanoma. The benign lesion generally spreads superficially, but malignant transformation is indicated by nodularity, a change in pigmentation or irregular borders. Treatment of a melanotic freckle consists of complete excision of the lesion.

Older classifications of malignant melanoma were based upon clinical appearance of the lesion. Superficial spreading malignant melanoma was the commonest type (54 percent) and carried a good survival rate. It was flat and extended slowly in a radial direction. On the other end of the spectrum was the more serious nodular melanoma with a grave prognosis. The lesion is characterized by rapid vertical extension and early metastases.

Newer classifications have linked survival and clinical behavior of the tumor to the depth of microscopic invasion of the skin. Clark described his classification based on the level of the dermis invaded. More recently, Breslow has been able to predict clinical behavior of melanoma based upon the absolute thickness of the lesion in millimeters (Fig. 12-4).

As with other malignancies, clinical staging is important in determining appropriate therapy (Table 12-1). The most significant immediate goal of therapy is to eliminate the local focus of the disease. A radical excision, including excision of normal skin margins 4 to 6 cm beyond the limits of the tumor, is carried out where the anatomical location permits. Recently, authorities have questioned the amount of normal skin excision required to prevent local recurrence. The excision can be asymmetrical so that more of the skin adjacent to the draining lymphatics is removed. Whether the fascia of the underlying muscles should be removed with the specimen or left intact is a subject of controversy.

Table 12-1. Clinical Staging in Melanoma

Stage I. Melanoma presents as a local disease, either intact, recently biopsied, or locally recurrent after inadequate treatment.

Stage II. Melanoma presents as local disease or recently excised for biopsy purposes, with evidence of metastases to the regional lymph node group; this stage also includes melanoma with an unknown primary site.

Stage III. Melanoma which has metastasized to distant organs or to multiple lymph node areas, or melanoma which has spread throughout the skin and subcutaneous tissues at the site of the original disease.

From: McNeer, G., and DasGupta, T.: Prognosis in malignant melanoma. Surgery 56:512, 1964.

When the regional lymph nodes are clinically involved, they should be removed en bloc with the primary specimen if that is practicable. The indications for prophylactic lymph node dissection in the treatment of malignant melanoma are highly controversial. Thin stage I lesions (Clark level I and II, or less than 0.76 mm absolute thickness) very rarely metastasize to the regional lymph nodes and require no lymph node dissection.

In thicker (greater than 0.76 mm) stage I lesions, certain guidelines exist for performing an elective lymph node dissection. Such a dissection should be strongly considered in the case of: (1) Level III to V lesions, (2) tumors with grave clinical signs (e.g., polypoid, ulcerated and rapidly growing lesions), (3) lesions in the immediate vicinity of the regional lymph nodes, and (4) locally recurrent lesions which have been previously adequately treated. Recently some investigators have shown that an elective node dissection improves the survival rate for lesions between 0.76 and 3.55 mm. For lesions thicker than 3.55 mm, the dissection may be useful as a staging procedure, but it has no effect on survival.

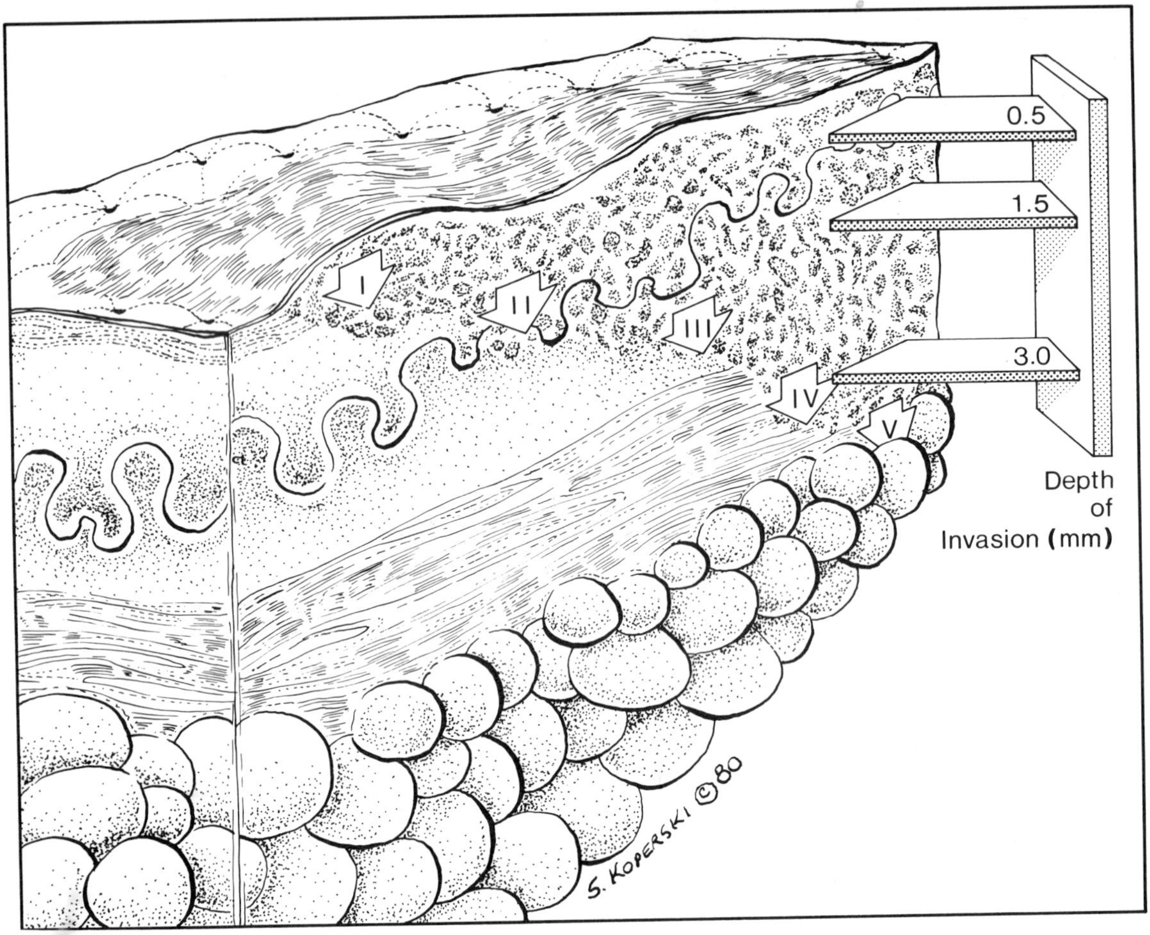

Figure 12-4. **Melanoma classification.** The classification of melanomas is based upon the depth of invasion in the skin. In Clark's classification (indicated by arrows), a Level I lesion is above the basement membrane of the epidermis; Level II penetration goes through the basement membrane to the upper dermis; Level III lesions are confined to the papillary dermis; Level IV lesions are confined to the reticular dermis; and Level V lesions penetrate to the subcutaneous fat, or even deeper. Breslow levels are indicated at the extreme right in a way that permits them to be correlated with Clark's levels. The importance in these classifications lies in their correlation with possible regional lymph node involvement.

For advanced, or stage III, malignant melanoma, no effective therapy exists and palliation is the goal of treatment. Several national studies employing combinations of chemotherapy and immunotherapy are currently in progress to determine the best treatment for advanced disease. Surgical debulking procedures often prove palliative and provide a temporary improvement in the quality of life.

CHAPTER 13

Head and Neck Tumors

The explosion of technology and the proliferation of information regarding head and neck surgery have made it impossible for one physican to remain an expert in all phases of this subspecialty. The patient with a head or neck malignancy should be evaluated and treated by an interdisciplinary team consisting of chemo- and radiotherapists, a surgical oncologist, a reconstructive surgeon and a dental expert. In addition, the research and support services of a major medical center, including speech and occupational therapy, and social services, should be available.

Because of the deforming, often disabling, nature of both the disease and its treatment, the patient and his family should receive ongoing counseling. They should be constantly apprised of the advantages and disadvantages of various treatment alternatives. Ideally, every cancer patient's diagnosis and treatment should be reported to the tumor registry. In that way, studies of the centralized data would contribute to an understanding of the disease and the efficacy of various treatment strategies.

Diagnosis

Head and neck malignancies are frequently diagnosed during physican or dental examination of a patient who complains of a painful mouth ulcer or other lesion that fails to heal. The oral mucosa and alveolus are most frequently involved. Sometimes the lesion is associated with ill-fitting dentures. While this lesion will be the focus of initial attention, other aspects of a careful examination should not be neglected. Alcohol and tobacco are the two most commonly cited carcinogenic agents. Patients who continue to smoke or chew tobacco are particularly prone to multiple intraoral malignancies (Fig. 13-1).

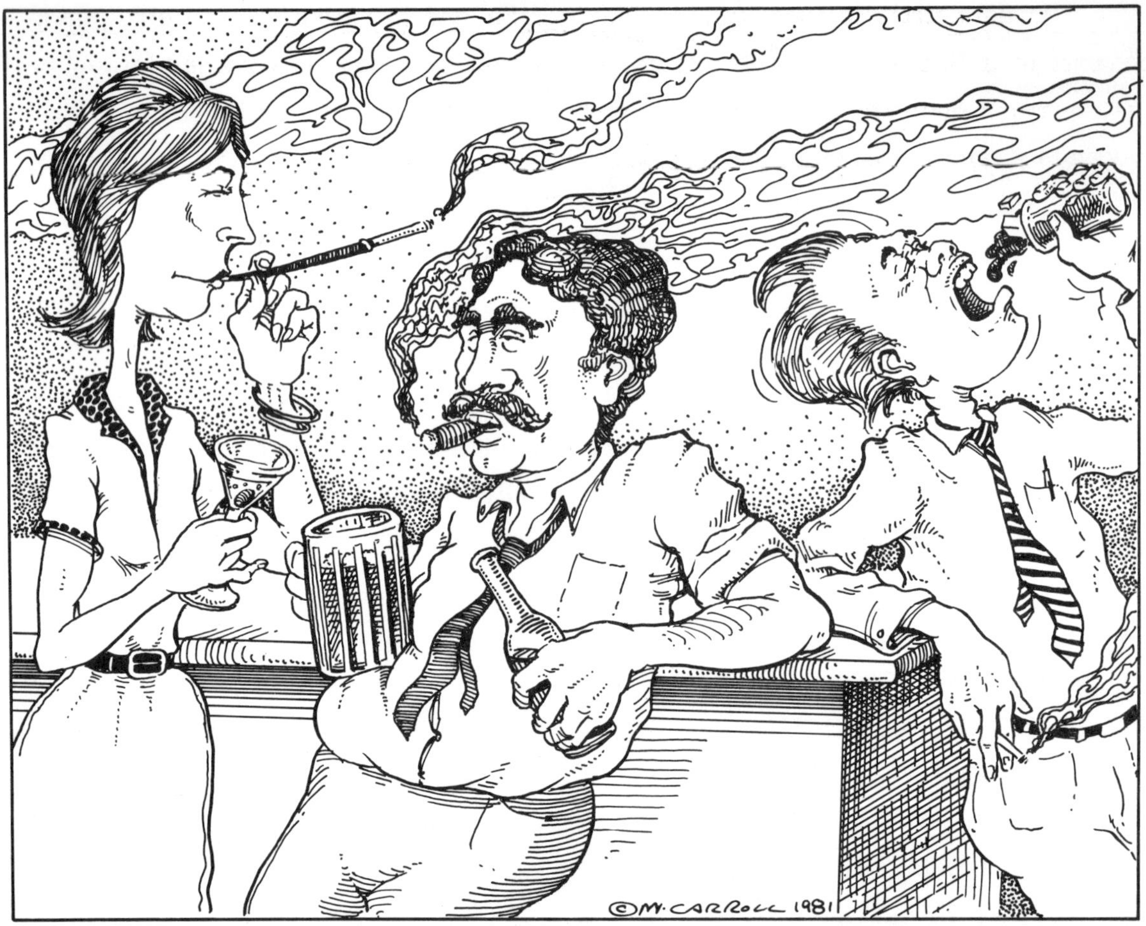

Figure 13-1. **Oral and pharyngeal carcinoma.** Causative factors in oral and pharyngeal carcinoma are tobacco and alcohol. These two agents seem to have a synergistic effect.

The patient should be seated comfortably for the examination in the presence of an adequate light source. Examination gloves, tongue blades and retractors should be at hand. The oral mucosa should be systematically inspected. The lingual and buccal surfaces of the alveolus should be examined, as well as the surfaces of the tongue, cheek mucosa and the mucosa of the hard and soft palates. The lingual and buccal sulcus and alveolus should be explored with bimanual finger palpation. The examiner should palpate for ulcerations, extensions of masses into the adjacent soft tissue, and fixation of lesions to the underlying bone. The examination should include palpation of the cervical lymph nodes and the contents of the submaxillary triangle. Suspicious lesions should be noted and the size and location recorded.

Precancerous lesions include leukoplakia and erythroplasia. Leukoplakia consists of a flat, white patch visible on the oral mucosa. It is caused by higher than normal deposits of keratin as a result of chronic irritation of the oral mucosa by alcohol, tobacco or spices. If an elevated plaque or deep fissures are discovered in an area of leukoplakia, a biopsy is indicated. The region at greatest risk of change in leukoplakia is the floor of the mouth. Erythroplasia is a red, velvety, hyperplastic lesion. It can be seen in areas of leukoplakia and should be considered carcinoma in situ.

The regional lymph nodes should be systematically palpated. Common sites for metastatic lesions are the submandibular triangle and the anterior cervical lymph nodes. Normally, no lymph nodes should be palpable in the submaxillary area or along the anterior edge of the sternocleidomastoid muscle.

Biopsy

Histological diagnosis should always be obtained prior to initiation of definitive treatment. Incisional or excisional biopsies are the most frequently used techniques for tissue diagnosis of intraoral lesions. Incisional biopsies should include an area of normal tissue for the purpose of comparison. All biopsies should be planned so that the scar can be excised in the course of definitive treatment, should that become necessary. Needle aspiration of neck masses frequently fails to provide an adequate tissue specimen and often results in seeding of the tumor. For those reasons, it should be avoided in making the diagnosis.

Staging

As in other forms of cancer, the TNM classification is used to standardize diagnosis and treatment. Following the examination, the patient is classified based on the clinical findings. This classification does not change regardless of the course which the disease subsequently follows (Table 13-1).

Table 13-1. Clinical Staging TNM System

T = Primary tumor
T1 - less than 2 cm
T2 - 2 cm to less than 4 cm
T3 - 4 cm or greater

N = Reginal node metastasis
N0 - none
N1 - hemilateral
N2 - bilateral or contralateral
N3 - fixed

M = Distant metastasis
M0 - none
M1 - present

Stage 1 - T1N0
Stage 2 - T2N0
Stage 3 - T3N0
T1N1
T2N1
T3N1

Stage 4 - T1, T2, or T3, with N2, N3, or M1

American Joint Committee for Cancer Staging and End Results Reporting, and the TNM Committee of the International Union against Cancer (1967).

Treatment

Tongue

Ninety-five percent of the malignancies of the tongue and floor of the mouth involve the squamous mucosa. The epithelial cells of this area are prone to malignant transformation by a variety of common carcinogens. The lesion presents as a nodule with firm, rolled borders, often with an ulcerated center. As the lesion enlarges, the ulcer becomes painful, often prompting the patient to seek medical attention.

Tongue malignancies comprise 20 to 30 percent of intraoral lesions. They are most commonly found in men in the sixth decade of life, usually along the lateral aspect of the middle third of the tongue. Lesions of the anterior two-thirds of the tongue tend to be more differentiated, while those of the posterior one-third do not keratinize and they metastasize early. Metastases to the submental, submandibular neck nodes have occurred in 50 to 60 percent of patients by the time the disease is diagnosed.

Treatment of lesions of the tongue is an area of controversy; there are advocates of both radiation and surgical excision. Small lesions on the tip and dorsum of the tongue are amenable to either modality, but, because of the rapidity and ease of surgical treatment, surgical therapy is generally advised. Surgery is advocated particularly for patients who tolerate radiation poorly. These include the elderly, alcoholics and heavy smokers.

The proper method of treatment of lesions of the middle third of the tongue is particularly controversial. Comparable cure and morbidity rates attend both radiation and surgical excision. When bone or cartilage is invaded, however, irradiation is ineffective and surgical excision is required.

When neck nodes are clinically diagnosed as positive, an en bloc resection of the tongue and ipsilateral neck must be performed and postoperative radiation therapy is indicated if the nodes are histologically positive. T-4 lesions receive combined therapy, with 5,000 to 6,000 rads of radiation given preoperatively followed in six weeks by surgical excision, with en bloc neck dissection.

Prognosis for five-year survival of T1 and T2N0 lesions is 80 to 90 percent. It diminishes steadily with larger tumors or in patients with metastatic disease. Patients with T4N2 lesions have a 20 to 30 percent five-year survival.

Floor of the Mouth

Squamous cell cancer of the floor of the mouth is the most common type of malignant intraoral lesion. Most such cancers occur in the fifth and sixth decades of life and originate from the precancerous lesions of leukoplakia or erythroplasia. These lesions metastasize later than those of the tongue, but they may invade the mandible.

Either surgery or irradiation is effective with T1 and T2N0 lesions, where the mandible is not invaded. Irradiation is commonly preferred in patients who will tolerate it because of the extensive reconstruction which is necessary following surgery to the anterior floor of the mouth. However, in T3 and T4 lesions, where the lymph nodes of the neck are clinically positive, composite resection followed by postoperative radiation is the recommended treatment.

Lesions of the floor of the mouth tend to be less well differentiated than those of the tongue and are often detected later in their course. Because of this, the prognosis is not as good for lesions of the floor of the mouth as it is for lesions of the tongue. A 60 percent survival rate for T1 and T2N0 lesions at the end of five years is reported following irradiation. T3 lesions, with or without nodes, and T2 lesions with nodes have a 25 to 30 percent five-year survival rate following surgical resection.

Lip

Carcinomas of the lip are frequent. The lower lip is the most common site, probably because of its exposure to the sun. Men in the fifth through seventh decades of life are the most commonly affected.

The lesions appear grossly as either large ulcerative or exophytic growths. Lip cancer tends to spread laterally, with metastasis to the submental nodes found in less than 5 percent of patients. Lesions of the upper lip are more aggressive and metastasize with greater frequency.

Small lesions in situ might respond to a stripping of the mucosa, which removes the tumor. Larger lesions must be widely excised. Lymph node dissection might be considered in lesions greater than 2.5 cm. The defect may be closed primarily or with a local flap. The cure rate is 80 to 90 percent in patients with no metastatic disease.

Salivary Glands

Tumors of the salivary glands are relatively rare, comprising 2 percent of all neoplasms. Salivary gland tumors most frequently occur in middle-aged women. Lesions of the parotid gland are more likely to be benign while lesions in the smaller salivary glands are more frequently malignant.

Parotid Gland. Parotid tumors follow the rule of 75 percent: 75 percent of all salivary gland tumors occur in the parotid, 75 percent of these are benign lesions, and 75 percent of the benign tumors are benign mixed tumors (pleomorphic adenoma). These last consist of epithelial cells in nests or strands, intermingled with islands of relatively acellular hyaline stroma.

Benign mixed tumors appear macroscopically as lobulated pink or grey masses. There is a circumscribing pseudocapsule composed of compressed adjacent structures. The lesion rarely involves the branches of the facial nerve which is separated from the tumor by the pseudocapsule. Patients usually present after noticing a painless, slowly enlarging mass anterior to the ear.

There is some evidence that untreated or recurrent benign mixed tumors can undergo malignant transformation.

The next most common parotid gland lesion is Warthin's tumor, or papillary cystadenoma lymphomatosum, which comprises 10 percent of benign parotid tumors. It occurs in the elderly male and has no malignant potential.

Cure can be expected in treatment of 95 percent of the benign tumors with a 5 percent recurrence rate. Recurrences are most frequently associated with surgery in which rupture of the pseudocapsule results in seeding of the tumor. Local recurrences can be very aggressive and may require that branches of the facial nerve be sacrificed during subsequent operations. Additional recurrence may be as frequent as 30 percent.

Malignant tumors comprise 25 percent of parotid lesions. There appear to be two clinical behavioral patterns based on cell type. The first type includes mucoepidermoid and adenoidcystic adenocarcinoma (cylindroma). These represent low-grade malignancies which run a slow course. They are the more common of the two types. These tumors are locally invasive and may involve cartilage, mandible or branches of the facial nerve. Cylindromas, in particular, have a propensity for spreading along the branches of the facial nerve. These lesions can metastasize to the lung and regional nodes, although such metastasis occurs late. Low-grade malignancies have a cure rate of 90 to 95 percent.

The more aggressive malignant parotid lesions comprise the second type. These include squamous cell carcinoma, adenocarcinoma and undifferentiated carcinoma. Patients in this category present with the characteristic clinical picture of a rapidly growing, painful lesion. Paralysis of the facial nerve, as well as regional metastatic disease, may be present at the initial examination. The five-year survival rate for patients with highly malignant lesions is a disappointing 33 percent. The lymph nodes in the superficial parotid lobe may also be the site of metastatic disease, most commonly from lesions in the sinuses, scalp or face.

Before considering treatment of various parotid lesions, it will be worthwhile to review a few facts regarding parotid gland anatomy. The parotid gland lies in close proximity to several important structures. The facial nerve runs between the so-called deep and superficial lobes of the gland after emanating from the stylomastoid foramen. The terminal branching of the nerve into its five trunks occurs within the substance of the gland. The deep lobe of the parotid gland extends medially into the soft tissue of the lateral pharyngeal area. For that reason, lesions of the deep lobe can appear as parapharyngeal masses.

The gland itself lies on top of the masseter muscle; Stensen's duct proceeds anteriorly to penetrate the oral mucosa at the level of the second upper molar. The gland is of variable size, depending on the age of the patient. The great auricular nerve and the auriculotemporal nerve (both sensory nerves) run through the area and are important factors in surgery in this region. The auriculotemporal nerve has been implicated for potential involvement in a condition known as Frey's syndrome.

For most lesions of the parotid gland, treatment consists of superficial lobectomy. A cuff of normal tissue should be removed with the lesion to avoid rupturing the pseudocapsule. The key to success in parotid gland surgery is exposing the facial nerve to avoid damaging it. The nerve can be isolated at the stylomastoid foramen with the aid of a galvanic nerve stimulator and followed distally for lesions located peripherally. Alternatively, the surgeon can isolate the terminal branches of the nerve and follow them proximally in order to locate and excise lesions situated immediately anterior to the ear. Lesions of the deep lobe can be explored by retracting branches of the facial nerve which obstruct the site.

Benign and malignant lesions can be excised similarly, except where the latter obviously invade adjacent structures. In such cases, the surgeon must often remove parts of the mandible, ear cartilage or even branches of the facial nerve along with the tumor. In cases where branches of the facial nerve are sacrificed, they can be repaired primarily with a nerve graft from the great auricular, auriculotemporal or sural nerve.

Recently, postoperative radiation has proved beneficial in treatment of some salivary gland tumors. Radiation is advocated when malignant parotid tissue is known to have been left behind at the time of surgery. Anaplastic tumors should receive postoperative radiation. Radiation may also be useful as a palliative measure.

Paralysis or paresis of the facial nerve is the most common complication of parotid gland surgery. It does not occur in more than 10 to 15 percent of cases. Most frequently, paresis represents a temporary nerve injury which is sustained through aggressive retraction or repeated stimulation with the nerve stimulator. Function is usually restored in two to four months.

Frey's syndrome, or auriculotemporal nerve syndrome, probably affects all but can significantly disturb 15 to 20 percent of parotidectomy patients. Clinically, this syndrome manifests itself as perfuse sweating from the cheek and temple of the affected side during eating. This syndrome is believed to be the result, following surgery, of aberrant connections between the parasympathetic fibers of the seventh cranial nerve and the sweat glands innervated by the sympathetic fibers of the auriculotemporal nerve. These aberrant connections result in sweating of the distribution of the auricular temporal nerve while eating. Relief can often be obtained by a transection of Jacobson's nerve.

Submandibular Gland. Ninety percent of submandibular gland disease is inflammatory in nature. However, when tumors of the gland present, they are more likely to be malignant than in the case of the parotid. Forty percent of submandibular gland lesions are malignant. The lesions are aggressive locally and metastasize early. They are frequently painful. The most common histological type is adenoidcystic or cylindroma. The most common benign tumor is the mixed tumor (60 percent).

Treatment of the benign lesion consists of excision of the gland. Recurrences are extremely rare. Because of the high possibility of malignancy, a frozen section biopsy should be performed at the time of surgery. If the lesion is malignant, radical ablative procedures should be undertaken with inclusion of a neck dissection when appropriate. Postoperative radiation treatment is indicated in the case of high-grade malignant lesions and where tumor is known to have been left behind.

Radical Neck Dissection

As with many types of malignancy, the decision as to whether or not to remove the regional lymph nodes draining the primary site is influenced by many factors. In head and neck cancer, the regional nodes are particularly accessible and can often be removed en bloc with the primary tumor. Because of the intimate association of the lymph node chain with the surrounding structures, it has been taught that the surgeon must excise the anterior portions of the carotid sheath and the jugular vein, as well as the sternocleidomastoid (SCM), omohyoid, sternohyoid and digastric muscles, in order to assure a complete removal of the lymph nodes. The intervening structures, the ansa hypoglossi and the spinal accessory nerves, must also be removed. The contents of the submandibular triangle are often removed as well (Fig. 13-2).

Recently, however, the extent of surgery required to eradicate metastatic disease from the neck has been questioned. In the so-called functional neck dissection, the cervical nodes are removed within a fascial envelope sparing the sternocleidomastoid muscle, jugular vein and spinal accessory nerve. While there has been little experience with this procedure to date, it may prove to be ideal for the patient with a large primary lesion and clinically negative neck in whom a prophylactic neck dissection is contemplated. It may also be of use in patients requiring bilateral neck dissections.

Despite the magnitude of the classical radical neck dissection, the procedure is surprisingly well tolerated by most patients. The patient can ambulate early, has little pain, and, if only a neck dissection has been performed, can take fluids immediately. A tracheostomy is usually not necessary. Preoperative radiation or an en bloc removal of the primary tumor adds considerably to the morbidity of a radical neck dissection.

In the standard surgical procedure, the contents of the neck are exposed through two transverse incisions. This ensures coverage of the carotid artery postoperatively. The skin flaps are elevated, usually in a plane deep to the platysma muscle. The ramus mandibularis of the seventh cranial nerve is identified and protected. The digastric muscle is detached from the mandible, and the contents of the submaxillary triangle are removed, care being taken to preserve the lingual and hypoglossal nerves. Next, the sternocleidomastoid and the external jugular veins are divided and the internal jugular vein exposed.

The posterior margin of the dissection is defined by the border of the trapezius muscle. The spinal accessory nerve is isolated and divided at the border of the trapezius. The specimen is removed in a plane above the prevertebral fascia, thus protecting the brachial plexis and the phrenic nerve. The cutaneous nerves to the neck are transected and removed with the specimen.

The carotid sheath is exposed and the thoracic duct and vagus nerves are identified. At this point, the internal jugular vein is ligated and divided. The dissection proceeds superiorly and the specimen is removed by dividing the jugular vein and the spinal accessory nerve at the base of the skull and transecting the stylohyoid and digastric muscles.

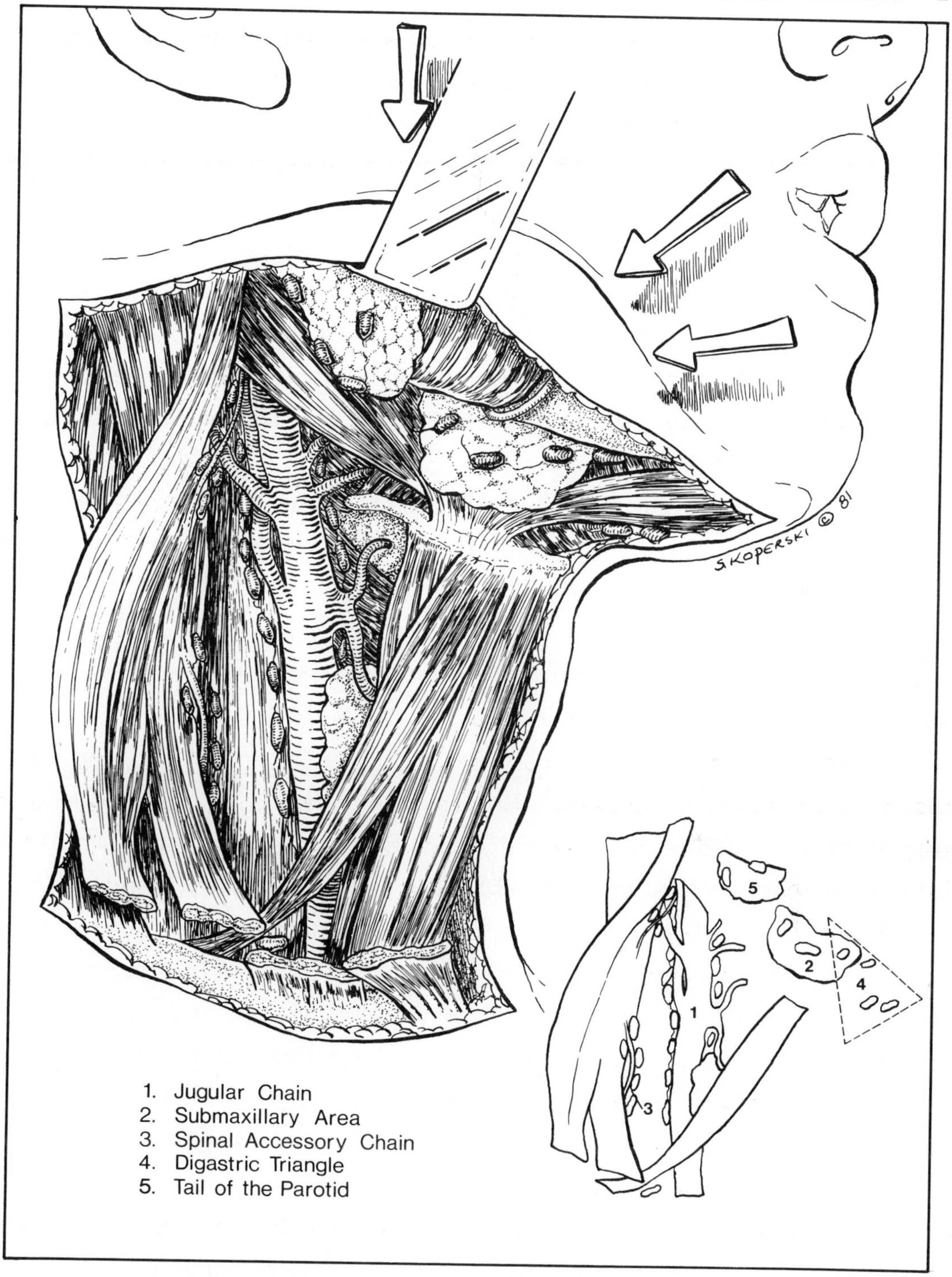

Figure 13-2. **Radical neck dissection.** A radical neck dissection removes the lymph nodes in the jugular chain, submaxillary area, spinal accessory chain, digastric triangle and tail of the parotid gland. In most dissections, therefore, the SCM, omohyoid muscles and jugular vein are removed en bloc. Some authors preserve the SCM muscle, here reflected to show the anatomy of the lymph nodes. The arrows indicate lymph drainage from cheek and lips. Note that most of the drainage from upper and lower lip goes to the submaxillary area.

Next, the wound is irrigated and hemostasis meticulously achieved. Suction drains are placed beneath the skin flaps. The dressing should be minimal. Since the patients are frequently elderly, intensive pulmonary toilet is essential. The patient can ambulate immediately and begin eating early.

CHAPTER 14

Pediatric Plastic Surgery

The plastic surgeon who treats children is confronted with many of the same clinical problems, such as scar revision, skin tumors, facial fractures and hand injuries, seen in adults. There are, however, some problems unique to children; most of these involve the reconstruction of congenital defects.

Cleft Lip and Palate (Primary and Secondary Palate)

One of the most common of such congenital conditions is cleft lip and palate. In any meaningful discussion of cleft lip and palate, it is important to distinguish between the primary and secondary palate since either, or both, can be involved in the deformity. The incisive foramen serves as the demarcation point. The primary palate includes the lip, columella, caudal septum and premaxilla. The secondary palate is posterior to the incisive foramen and consists of the hard and soft palate.

Cleft lip, with or without a cleft palate (secondary palate) occurs in approximately one in every 650 live births. Isolated cleft palate occurs much less frequently. Of all cleft lip and palate defects (CL&P), 25 percent are cleft lip (CL) alone, 50 percent are CL&P, and 25 percent are cleft palate (CP) alone. Males are more frequently affected with CL&P, and the defects tend to be more pronounced. Females have twice the incidence of CP. There is a definite left-sided preponderance in CL&P. There is an incidence of associated anomalies in 29 percent of cleft cases.

Genetic factors are important in the formation of the cleft lip and palate. One-third of all CL&P patients have a positive family history. Families in which CL&P appears have a significantly higher than average chance of producing children with this deformity. CL&P is believed to be multifactorial and of variable expressivity. Children of Oriental parentage are more frequently affected than are Caucasians. CL&P is very rare among Blacks. Genetic counseling should be available to the adult CL&P patient and to the family (Table 14-1).

Table 14-1. Family Incidence

Affected Relatives	Predicted Recurrence (%)	
One sibling	4.4	2.5
One parent	3.2	6.8
One sibling, one parent	15.8	14.9

From Ross, R.B., and Johnston, M.C.: *Cleft Lip and Palate*. The Williams and Wilkins Co., Baltimore, 1972.

In addition to the genetic factors, there are known environmental agents that influence CL&P formation. Certain drugs, including steroids, anticonvulsants, diazepam and aminopterin, have been associated with increased frequency of CL&P. Maternal diseases such as rubella, toxoplasmosis and diabetes increase the incidence of cleft defects.

Embryology

In order to understand the nature of the cleft defect, some appreciation of the normal embryological development of the lip and palate is necessary. As mentioned previously, the primary palate includes the lip, columella, caudal septum and premaxilla. It is formed when the ectoderm of the oral dimple enters the mouth, creating a bilamellar ectodermal membrane. The membrane becomes perforated by the olfactory placodes which create the nasal passages. This thin membrane must be reinforced by an ingrowth of mesodermal tissue or it will rupture prior to birth.

Mesodermal tissue enters the area of the primary palate by migrating medially from both sides and over the top of the head. The mesodermal ingrowth of the maxillary process actually decussates in the midline, and the developing muscle fibers insert into the contralateral philtral ridge. If this mesodermal ingrowth is delayed or incomplete, then the bilamellar ectodermal membrane splits apart leaving a cleft lip (Fig. 14-1).

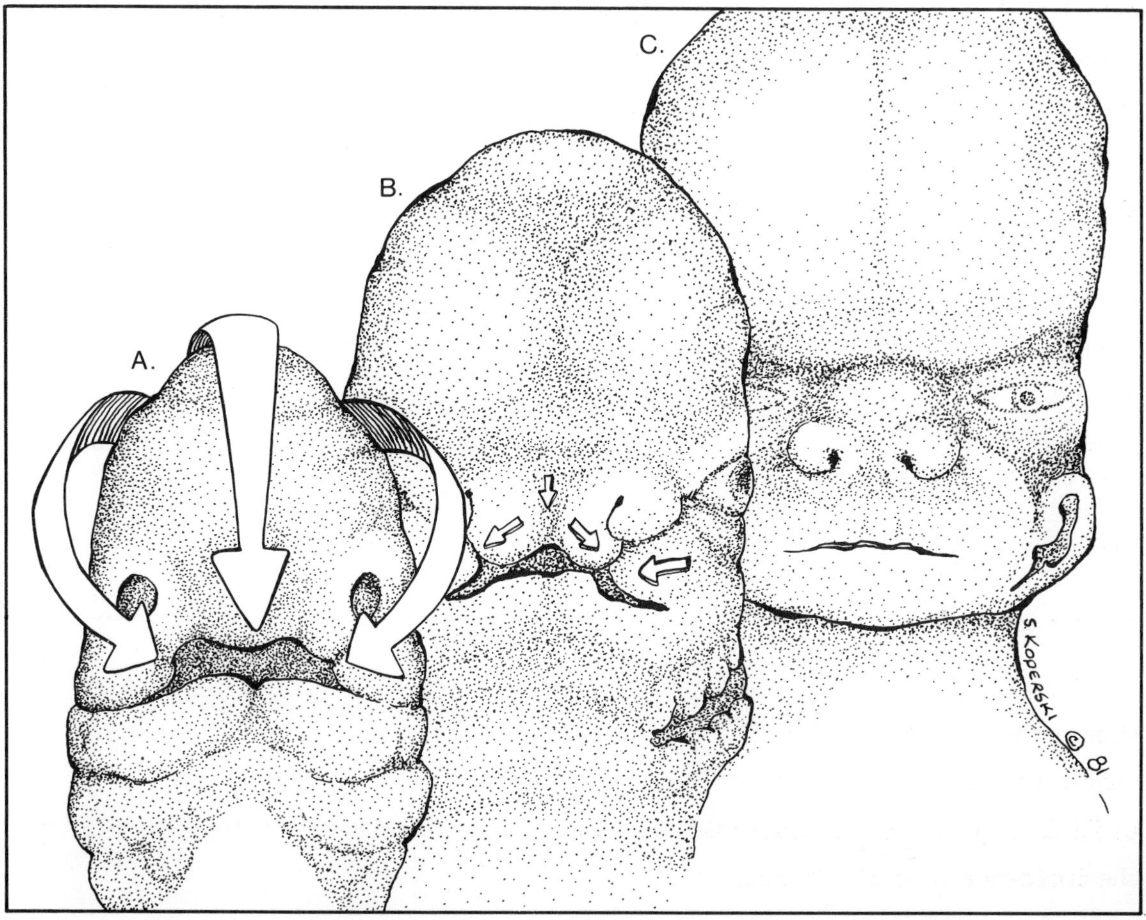

Figure 14-1. **Development of primary palate.** Mesoderm originating as neuro-ectoderm from the paravertebral area migrates over and around the head (A, arrows). Mesoderm ingrowth reinforces the facial processes laterally and in the philtral area (B). With the normal ingrowth of mesoderm, the primary palatal elements fuse completely (C).

In the cleft lip deformity, the muscle fibers run parallel to the margin of the cleft and insert into the alar base rather than crossing the midline. The development of the primary palate takes place in the embryo at from four to seven weeks, and normal mesodermal fusion occurs during this period. The severity of the cleft depends upon when the course of normal embryological development was interrupted.

The secondary palate consists of the hard and soft palate. The embryological development of the secondary palate takes place at from 7 to 12 weeks, and it is during this period that fusion of the palatal processes would normally transpire. By the time the formation of the primary palate is complete, the primordial palatal processes hang vertically on either side of the tongue. At this time, the head, which had been flexed, begins to extend and the tongue drops to a position below the palatal processes. The palatal shelves are manipulated into a horizontal position by the milking action of the tongue. They grow toward one another and fuse in the midline. The adhesive palatal edges are held together while mesodermal elements fuse from anterior to posterior. These processes also fuse with caudal septum, obliterating the intervening ectoderm. This development occurs earlier in males and may explain the higher incidence of CP in females (Fig. 14-2).

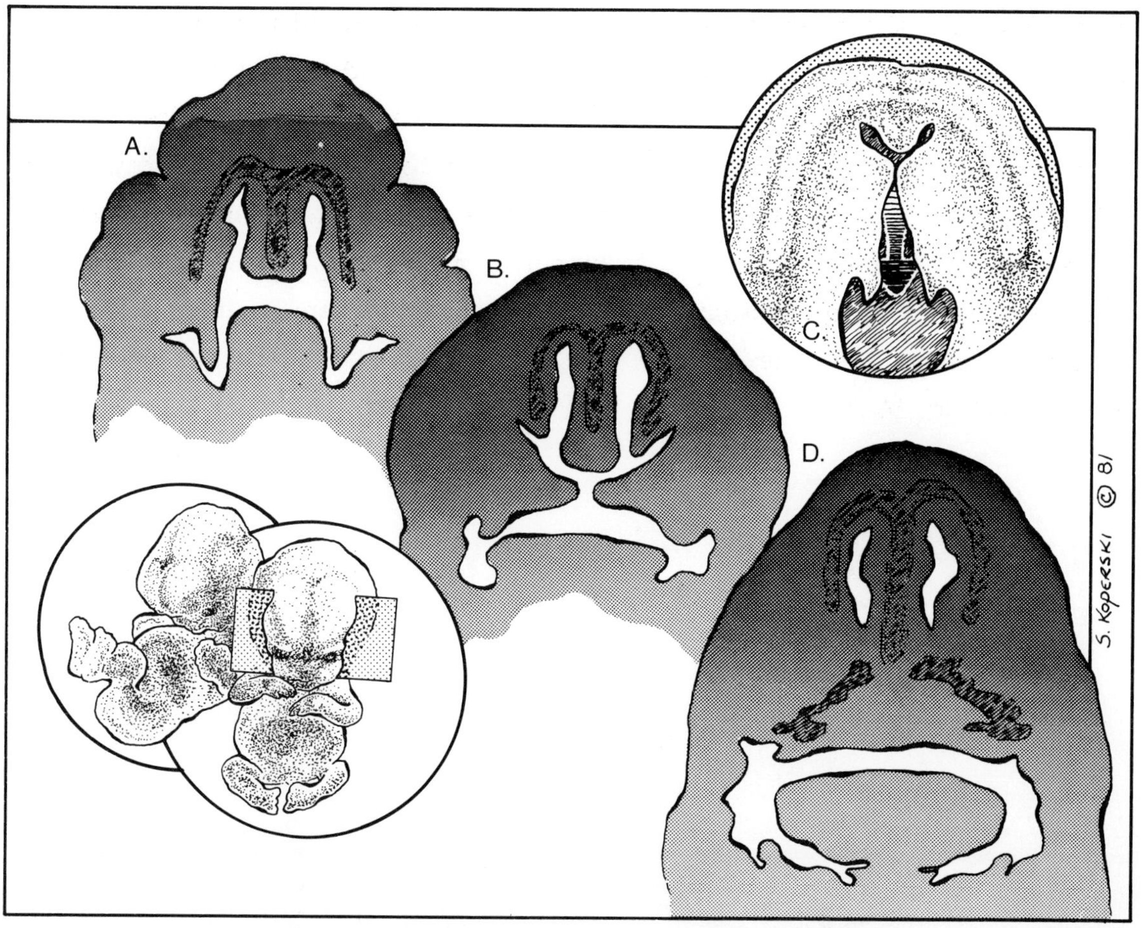

Figure 14-2. **Development of secondary palate from weeks 6 to 9.** Development of the secondary palate is shown in saggital section (inset, bottom left indicates saggital plane). The palatal processes initially hang vertically alongside the tongue (A). As the fetal head begins to extend, the tongue drops below the palatal processes and begins to force them together in a horizontal plane and toward the nasal septum (B). As the palatal processes come into contact, fusion begins and proceeds from an anterior to a posterior direction (C). With the fusion completed, the oral and nasal cavities are more separated (D).

In a submucous cleft of the soft palate, the palatal shelves remain in continuity but there is inadequate mesodermal development. In complete clefts of the secondary palate, the fusion of palatal shelves is disrupted. The abnormal muscle fibers of the levator palati do not cross the midline but run anteriorly and insert into the posterior edge of the hard palate.

Many methods of describing and classifying CL&P deformities have been proposed. The striped Y classification introduced by Kernahan and Stark is the easiest to work with. The classification is based on the embryology of the region. The incisive foramen serves as the reference point in describing the morphology of the cleft. The cleft is visually depicted on the striped Y diagram (Fig. 14-3).

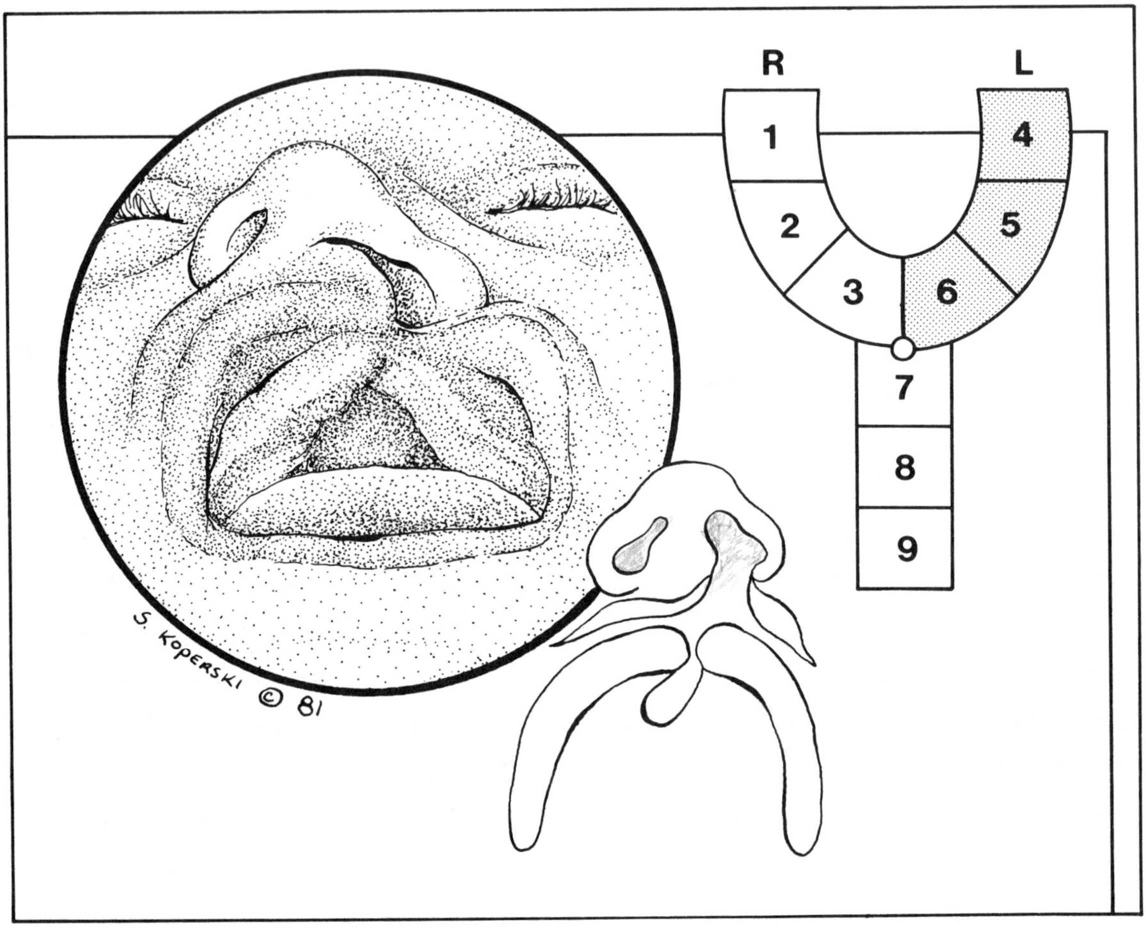

Figure 14-3. **A guide to CL&P deformities.** The striped Y diagram (right) serves as a developmental and anatomical reference for charting CL&P deformities. The incisive foramen, located at the junction of the limbs of the Y, separates the secondary and primary palates. The three portions anterior to the foramen represent the lips, alveolus and anterior hard palate on each side. The posterior segments depict hard palate, soft palate and uvula. A typical defect is shown on the left and is also represented on the striped Y diagram which corresponds to the clinical situation.

The timing and method of treatment of CL&P are matters of controversy. Generally, cleft lip is repaired at an early age. The "rule of ten" has long been the guide for timing cleft lip repair. The infant should be at least 10 weeks of age, weigh at least 10 pounds and have at least 10 grams of hemoglobin prior to surgery. In most cases, cleft lip closure is done between the second and fourth month. If the cleft is particularly wide, a lip adhesion of the skin and mucosa only may be performed initially and a definitive lip repair performed later.

Repair of Cleft Lip

Over the years, many types of cleft lip repair have been developed and many have been replaced by newer methods. The earliest attempts at correction involved simply suturing the paired lip edges together. Because of scar contracture, this resulted in obvious shortening of the lip with a notched, or whistle lip, deformity.

Other techniques were developed by rotating different shaped flaps of local tissue to close the defect. These techniques gave satisfactory results at times but often resulted in lips that were too long or too short. Many of the techniques violated the natural landmarks of the Cupid's bow, producing an artificial-looking lip.

Many centers now employ the technique of Millard. In this procedure, a monobloc of tissue from the lateral portion of the lip is rotated and advanced into the medial segment to lengthen the lip on the repaired side. Kernahan, in contrast, emphasizes that it is of paramount importance to correct the underlying mesodermal (muscle) defect as a separate unit prior to repairing the skin and mucosa. The orbicularis oris muscle fibers must be freed from their abnormal insertion in the alar base and repaired in the midline. Often an extensive dissection and mobilization are required to ensure that the muscle repair is not performed under tension. Kernahan then employs small Z-plasties which lengthen the skin of the lip (Fig. 14-4).

Adequate postoperative care is important to the success of the repair. Lip dressings are not required. The child's arms, however, must be extended with elbow splints to prevent damage to the repair. The patient must be fed with a syringe or medicine dropper, and no sucking is permitted. The child's regular diet is usually well tolerated. The sutures should be removed after five to seven days. This can be done under general anesthesia or with the infant sedated and

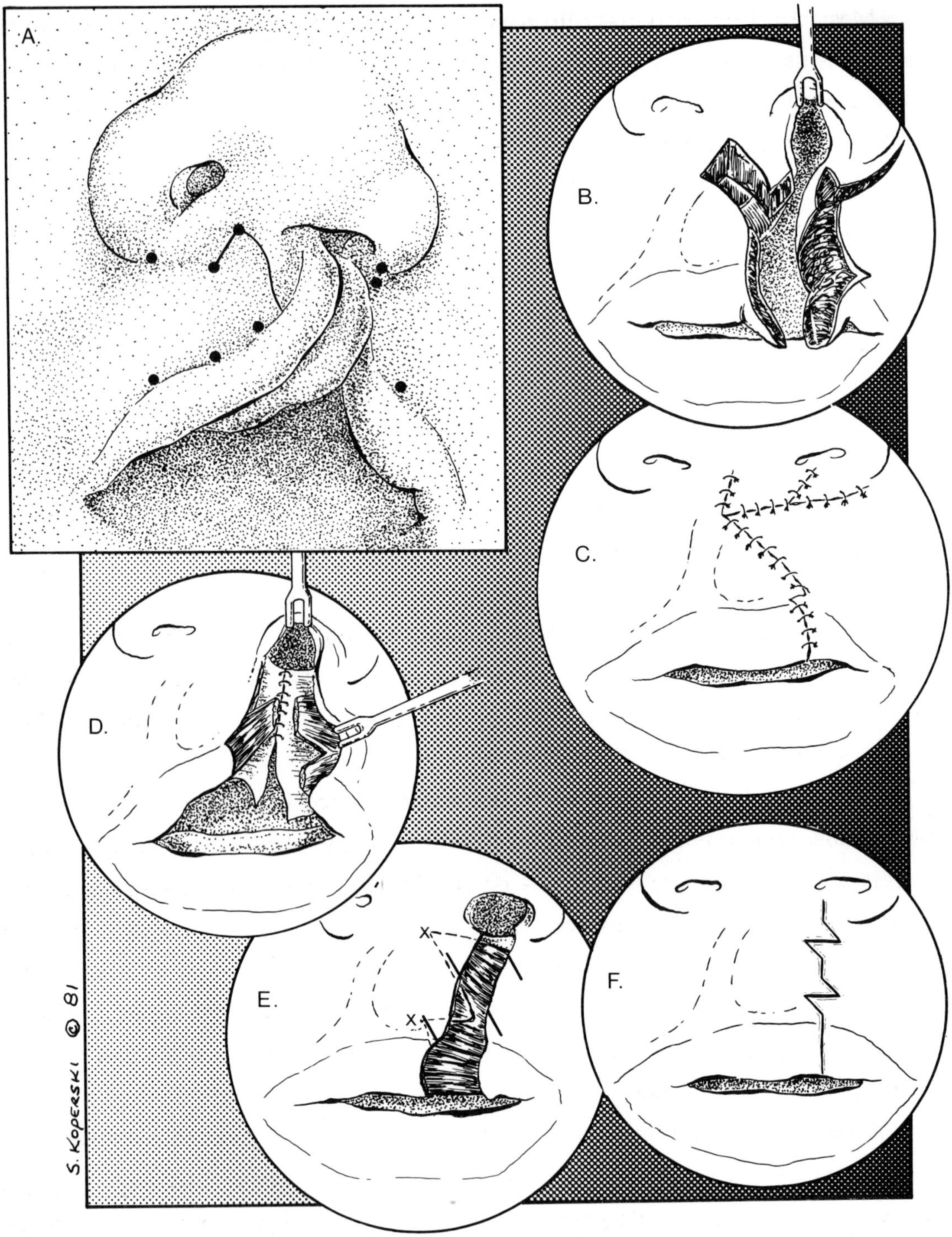

Figure 14-4. **Cleft lip repair.** Basic landmarks of the philtral ridges, the nasal base and the white roll of the lip are marked (A). In the Millard repair, tissue is taken from the lateral side of the cleft and advanced into the medial segment (B). The landmarks of Cupid's bow and the philtrum have been preserved (C). In the Kernahan repair, each of the anatomical layers is dissected and closed separately (D). Great attention is paid to repairing the obicularis muscle as a separate unit (E). The skin length is established with small Z-plasties (F).

Most children with cleft lip have an associated nasal deformity. While the extent of this deformity varies, the usual features include a deformed alar cartilage on the cleft side with a nostril fold, external nostril groove and nostril overhang. The alar domes are at different heights, and the alar base is recessed on the cleft side. The nasal septum is usually deviated to the normal side.

Some surgeons advocate nasal revision at the time of cleft lip repair. Others believe that it is impossible to achieve a satisfactory result on the delicate cartilage of the newborn infant and argue that corrective rhinoplasty should await full growth of the nose and face.

Treatment of Cleft Palate

Isolated cleft lip presents few problems beyond the aesthetic deformity. This is not at all the case with a cleft palate. A host of long- and short-term functional difficulties ranging from poor feeding to hearing and speech disorders can result from a cleft palate. Because of this, a multidisciplinary team, consisting of plastic surgeon, orthodontist, audiologist, otolaryngologist, speech therapists and social workers, is necessary to follow the progress of the cleft palate patient. These support services are generally available only in a large medical center.

The immediate problem confronting the parents of a child with a cleft palate is how to effectively feed the infant. A baby with a cleft cannot create adequate sucking pressure. Because of this, attempted breastfeeding or bottle-feeding using standard nipples results in the rapid fatigue of the child and the frustration of the parents. The parents must be instructed to cut a larger hole in the standard nipple and hold the baby at about 45° upright so that suction is not required to deliver the baby's formula. Children usually gain weight rapidly once this procedure is established.

A majority of patients with cleft palate will develop repeated episodes of serous otitis media. This is due to improper function of the tensor palati muscles, resulting in inadequate aeration of the middle ear. Appropriate treatment consists of myringotomy and evacuation of the transudate in the middle ear. Continuous ventilation is provided with a transtympanic plastic tube. Frequent follow-up examinations must be made in order to avoid permanent hearing loss. These examinations in the infant can be coordinated with the same anesthetic used in the surgical procedures.

The most serious challenge confronting the cleft palate patient is the development of normal speech. An airtight closure of the palate against the posterior pharyngeal wall is essential for normal speech. Defects in the normal sphincteric velopharyngeal closure mechanism allow air to escape into the nasal pharynx, obscuring the normal sound pattern. This is called velopharyngeal incompetence.

The goal of cleft palate repair is to create a normal velopharyngeal valve by reconstituting the muscular sphincter action of the levator palati sling. The parents of the patient should be made to realize that years of intensive speech therapy may be necessary before the child can achieve adequate communication skills. In some cases, a secondary surgical procedure may be necessary.

Generally, cleft palate repair can be performed from age 8 to 18 months. Early closure of the cleft palate has the advantage of reducing the incidence of middle ear disease and may facilitate normal speech development. Closure of the palate should not be delayed beyond 18 months because such delay will interfere with normal speech development.

In some centers, dental prostheses are applied shortly after birth. These aid in the infant's feeding and prevent excessive collapse of the bony structures. These devices are usually well tolerated by the infant. They are removed at the time of palate closure.

In some centers, primary bone grafting is undertaken to correct defects of the alveolar bone and to stabilize the maxillary dental arch. Adult dentition will often erupt through these bone grafts, and they can be used by the orthodontist later in life to manipulate teeth. In other centers, however, bone grafting is reserved for correcting alveolar deficiencies in older children.

Repair of Cleft Palate

Surgical correction of clefts of the hard and soft palate is performed under general anesthesia. A small amount of local anesthetic with epinephrine is injected to minimize blood loss. In the case of older children, blood for transfusion should be available.

Various techniques are used for closing the palatal defect. While the technical details differ, a multilayered closure is the underlying principle common to all repairs. Great care must be taken in dissecting the delicate structures. Oral and nasal mucosal flaps are elevated along the midline. The flap from the undersurface of the bony palate must be elevated carefully to protect the palatal vessels. These flaps are moved to the midline, and the layers are approximated individually in repairing the cleft. The raw donor site areas left laterally close in rapidly and present no problem (Fig. 14-5).

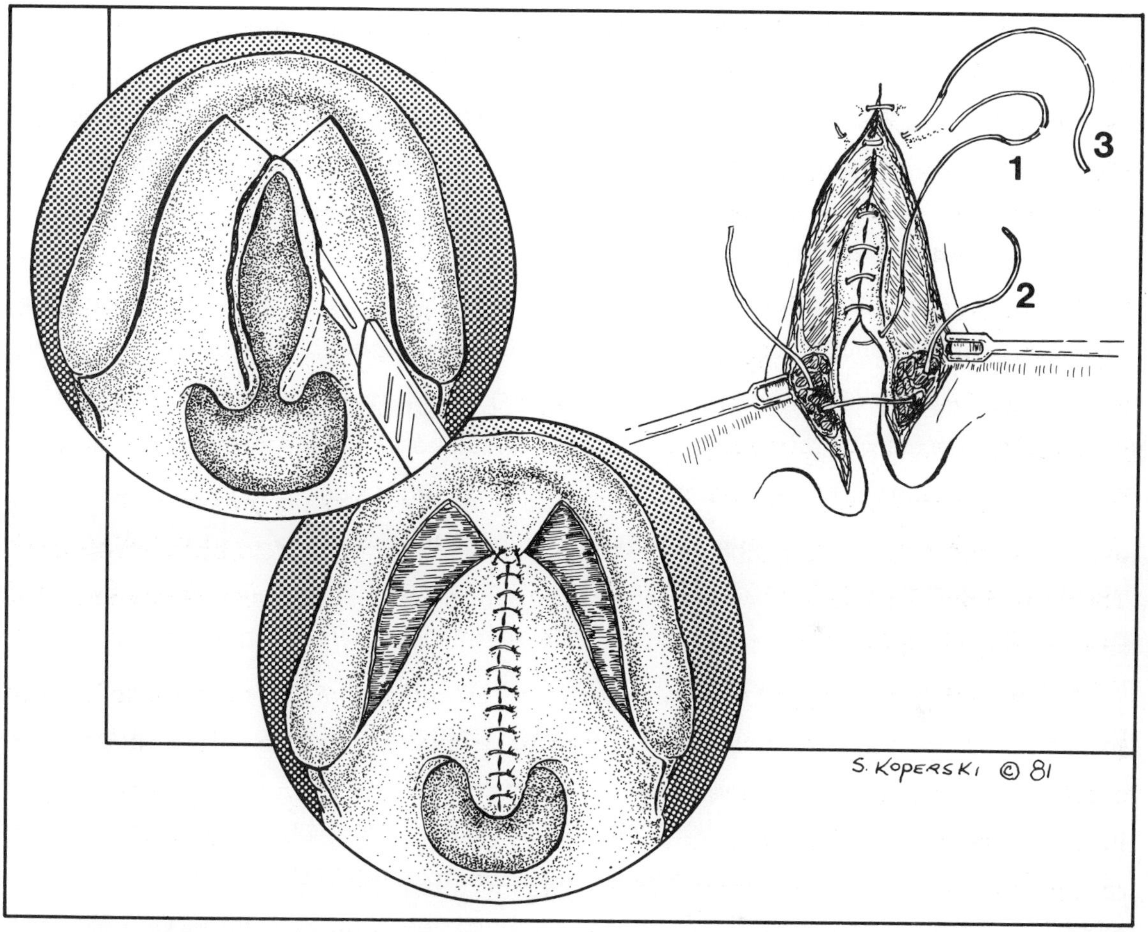

Figure 14-5. **Cleft palate repair.** The surgeon makes an incision and elevates mucoperiosteal flaps from the hard palate. The abnormal insertion of the levator palati on the posterior portion of the hard palate must be separated (top left). Three layers are closed separately (right). The nasal mucosa is repaired first (1); then the levator palati muscle is closed in the midline reconstituting the levator sling (2); finally the oral mucosa is closed (3). The M-incision allows lengthening of the palate (lower inset).

As with cleft lip, repair of the underlying mesodermal defect in a cleft palate is essential. The levator palati muscles have an abnormal insertion into the posterior edge of the hard palate. The muscles must be isolated and reapproximated in the midline to construct the velopharyngeal sphincter.

Postoperative care is similar to that following cleft lip repair. The patient's elbows must be splinted for 10 days to avoid disrupting the repair, and the child is fed through a syringe or a medicine dropper. Because of the extent of the intraoral surgery, prophylactic antibiotics are recommended in many centers.

As the child grows older, additional procedures may be necessary. Orthodontic manipulations, once the permanent dentition begins to erupt, are the most common of these. Also as previously mentioned, bone grafting may be performed at a later date.

Velopharyngeal Incompetence

It may become apparent that the child with a cleft palate is developing difficulty with speech. In some cases, intensive speech therapy may prove sufficient to improve communication. In others, speech therapy is ineffective and further surgery is necessary. Lateral static and cinefluorographic studies are used to evaluate the condition of the velopharyngeal opening (Fig. 14-6).

In patients with obvious velopharyngeal incompetence and in patients with marginal closure who have failed a trial of speech therapy, a pharyngeal flap may help. The procedure consists of raising a superiorly based flap from the posterior wall of the pharynx to narrow the velopharyngeal opening. The free inferior edge of the flap is inserted into the posterior edge of the repaired soft palate.

This mass of tissue in the posterior pharynx keeps the main stream of air from escaping into the nasopharynx during speech, yet small streams of air can enter the nasopharynx around the lateral ports of the flap. These portals prevent oral breathing. Immediately following the pharyngeal flap procedure, however, the airway should be checked carefully. A suture may have to be placed in the tongue so that it can be retracted to secure the airway until recovery from anesthesia is complete.

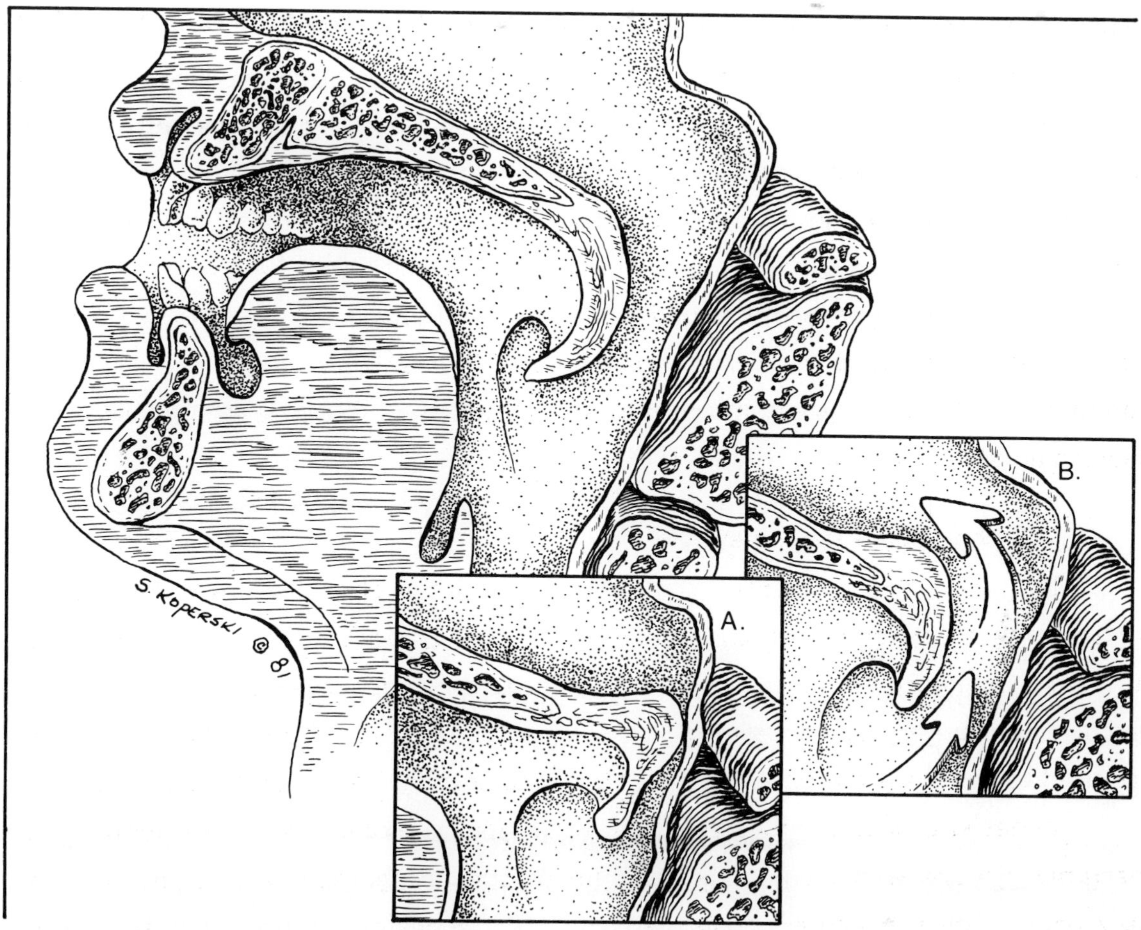

Figure 14-6. **Velopharyngeal closure.** Normal pharyngeal closure is accomplished when the levator palati muscle elevates the soft palate against the posterior pharyngeal wall to close off the nasopharynx (A). In patients with CP, the muscle action may be inadequate or the soft palate itelf may be too short, resulting in an escape of the vocal stream into the nose, (B, arrow).

Primary soft palate repair permits normal speech to develop in 60 to 70 percent of patients. Following pharyngeal flap or other secondary procedures, another 70 to 80 percent of these patients will no longer have nasal air escape. However, intensive speech therapy will be necessary to help the patient unlearn the compensatory articulation errors previously developed. Patients who have secondary procedures performed in adulthood do not fare as well in speech improvement as do children. As an alternative or as an adjunct to the pharyngeal flap, some centers advocate building up the posterior pharynx with silicone or Teflon so that Passavant's ridge is closer to the palate.

Craniofacial Anomalies

Recent developments in the field of pediatric reconstructive surgery have made it possible to offer some degree of correction to children with severe deformities of the skull and facial bones. The severe deformities in this group of patients present one of the most significant challenges to the reconstructive surgeon. It is no longer necessary for these people to live their lives as social outcasts. While there are a number of clinical entities, only the most common will be dealt with here.

The masses of dense mesenchyme that later develop into the bones of the cranium and face, have made their appearance in the form of a primitive cartilage by the end of the embryo's sixth week. By the end of the seventh week, ossification centers are present in the maxilla, mandible and malar bones. It is not until the eighth week that ossification centers appear in the cranial bones. It is because of this relatively late development of cranial ossification that severe cranial deformities can exist without concomitant facial bone deformities.

The cause of these severe craniofacial deformities is not known. Drugs such as thalidomide have been implicated in some cases. For some reason, however, the normal, orderly intrauterine processes are interrupted. In some cases, the sutures at the base of the skull fuse prematurely producing craniostenosis. In other cases, such as Treacher Collins syndrome, hypertelorism and facial clefts, the deformities may be caused by mesodermal fusion defects similar to those in CL&P.

Orbital Hypertelorism

Orbital hypertelorism is abnormally increased distance between the eyes. The reference point for measurement of the intraorbital distance is the medial orbital wall at the level of the lacrimal groove. The measurement is taken from radiographs or directly at the time of surgery. Normal adult intraorbital distance is 25 to 28 mm.

Orbital hypertelorism is associated with many clinical conditions. It is present in Apert's syndrome, in midfacial clefts, and as an isolated finding. Several conditions resemble true orbital hypertelorism. Telocanthus, or lateral displacement of the medial canthal ligaments, can occur following trauma or associated with various syndromes.

The anatomical basis of orbital hypertelorism is an increase in the mass of the ethmoidal air cells. The increase in width is limited to the anterior portion of the ethmoidal cells, causing a divergence of the axis of the orbits from the midsaggital plane. Fortunately, however, the apices of the orbits are not displaced laterally and the optic foramina are in their normal anatomical position. This fact makes the correction of hypertelorism possible.

Exposure of the orbits is attained by reflecting a scalp flap anteriorly. The neurosurgical team exposes the floor of the anterior cranial fossa. Osteotomes are used to separate the orbits from their attachments to the skull. A bar of frontal bone is left to serve as a rigid framework for securing the repositioned orbits.

Next, an appropriate segment of the anterior ethmoidal air cells is moved, and the orbital boxes are displaced medially. When the air cells are removed from the parasaggital location, the cribiform plate can be left undisturbed in the midline. Interosseous wires and bone grafts maintain the new position of the orbits. The medial canthal ligaments are reattached to their insertions with wires. The skull flap is replaced and the soft tissue is closed. Postoperative care follows standard craniofacial routine (Fig. 14-7).

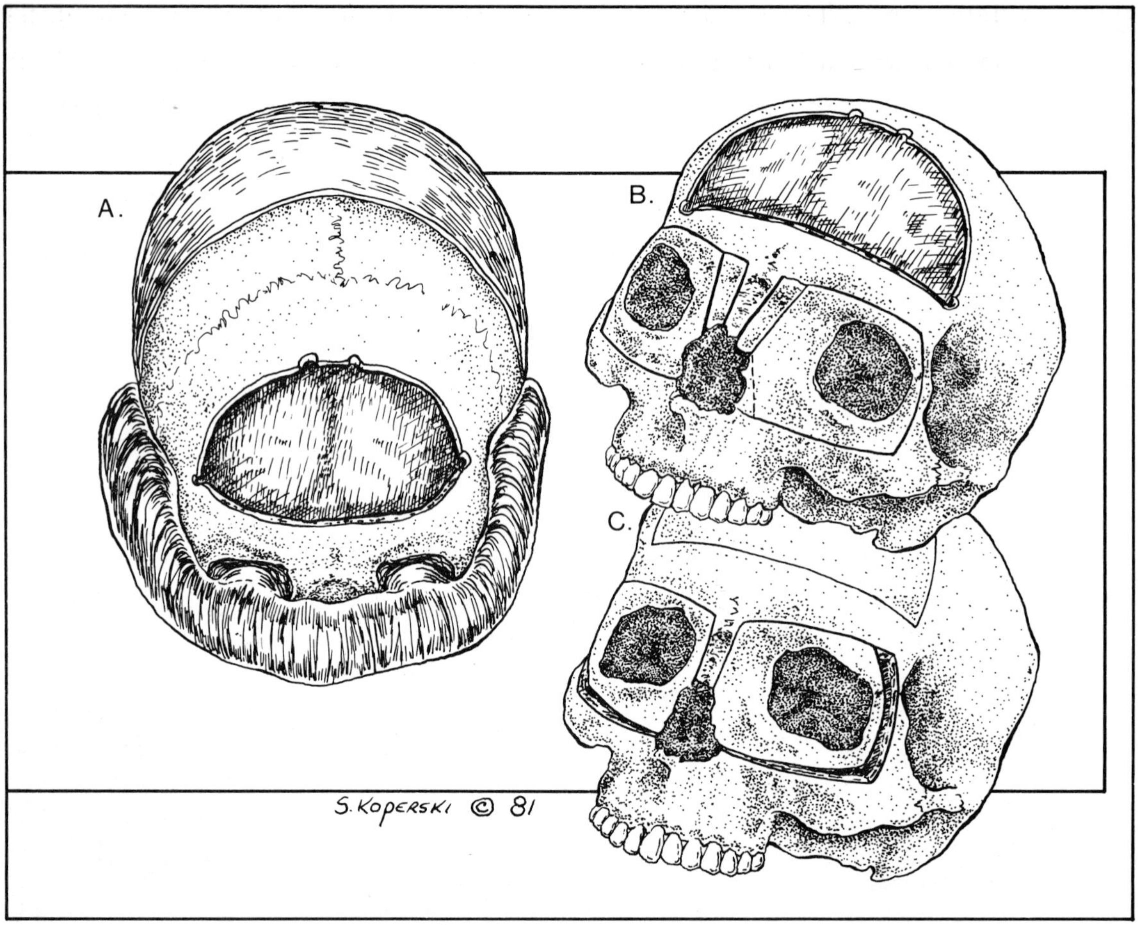

Figure 14-7. **Orbital hypertelorism surgery.** The skull and orbits are explored by reflecting the soft tissues of the scalp and face. The neurosurgical team exposes the floor of the anterior cranial fossa (A). Osteotomies are performed to mobilize the bony orbit and its contents (B). Bone is resected from the paramedian area and anterior cranial fossa on either side of the cribiform plate. Interosseous wires and bone grafts are used to stabilize the fragments (C).

Crouzon's Disease, Apert's Syndrome

One of the more severe types of craniofacial anomalies, craniofacial stenosis, is illustrated by Crouzon's disease and Apert's syndrome. In patients with these conditions, the cranial sutures synostose, or fuse, prematurely. Because of this early fusion, there is compensatory growth of the other cranial bones and an abnormal skull and facial contour result. Any combination of cranial sutures may fuse.

The deformities of the skull in Crouzon's disease and Apert's syndrome are variable. Generally, there is a tall skull with a broad, often bulging forehead. Fusion of sutures at the base of the skull results in abnormal orbital growth, and these patients are often exophthalmic and hyperteloric. Maxillary hypoplasia with a relative prognathism is present. The patients have what is called a "dish face" in which the center portion of the face is recessed relative to the forehead and the chin. In addition, in the case of Apert's syndrome there are anomalies of the hands and feet, usually in the form of syndactyly. Mental retardation may be present; it is usually mild with Crouzon's disease but is more severe with Apert's syndrome (Fig. 14-8).

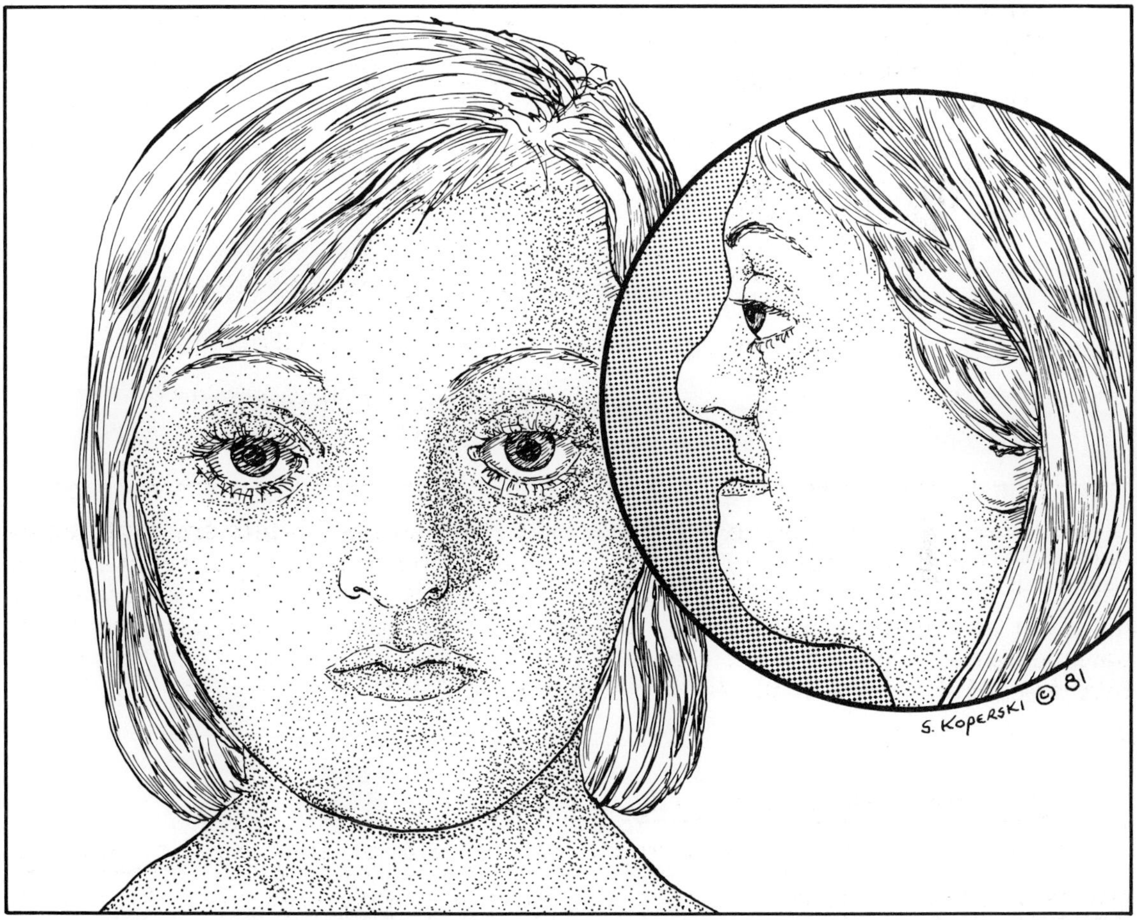

Figure 14-8. **Crouzon's disease.** Crouzon's disease patients often have a "frog-like" appearance. The midface bones are retruded, resulting in exophthalmos and exotropia. There is relative prognathism (inset).

Many of these patients have increased intracranial pressure caused by the premature synostosis of the cranial sutures. Neurosurgical decompression should be undertaken as soon as increased intracranial pressure is detected. Decompression consists of a cranioplasty in which the fused sutures are excised and the cranial contents allowed to expand.

The reconstructive surgical procedure is similar in both Crouzon's disease and Apert's syndrome. The procedure is designed to relieve the exophthalmos and to correct the midface hypoplasia and relative prognathism. There is a tendency at present to perform the reconstructive surgery at an early age because of the progressive nature of the midface hypoplasia. However, the surgery is technically easier when the child is a bit older. The long-term effects of this type of surgery on facial growth and development are currently under investigation.

Like many other aspects of reconstructive surgery, the correction of craniofacial defects requires a team approach. Neurosurgeons, anesthesiologists, geneticists, orthodontists and oral surgeons are necessary for comprehensive patient care. Preoperative evaluation consists of undertaking cephalometric studies of the skull. A computerized axial tomographic study provides useful information about the size and shape of the orbital cavities. Preoperative dental models are useful. Often tracheostomy must precede the reconstructive procedure.

The operative procedure requires both plastic and neurosurgical specialists. The bones of the skull and face are exposed through a bifrontal scalp incision. The soft tissues of the scalp and face are reflected anteriorly in the subperiostial plane. The orbital contents are freed circumferentially from their bony attachments to the orbits. Care must be taken to protect the optic structures at the apex of the orbit. The neurosurgical team exposes the anterior cranial fossa and the roof of the orbits.

The plastic surgeon then uses a saw and osteotomes to perform the appropriate osteotomies. The osteotomy lines resemble those of a Le Fort III facial fracture and permit the orbits and midface to be moved forward. The surgeon employs bone grafts and intermaxillary fixation to stabilize the fragment once it is placed in position. The hypertelorism can be corrected at the same time by resecting the abnormal tissue from the midline and wiring the orbits together.

The postoperative neurological status of the patient must be monitored closely. Any change in visual acuity usually calls for surgical exploration. Prophylactic antibiotics are used routinely because of the exposure of the cranial contents to nasal and oral secretions. Other routine measures include elevation of the head and protection of the cornea. If tracheostomy has not been performed, close observation of the airway must be maintained because of the high degree of postoperative edema. Secondary procedures are frequently required.

Anomalies of the Branchial Arch

Cleft lip and palate are the most common congenital problems seen by plastic surgeons. Anomalies of the branchial clefts and pouches are also common, although they are rarely of the functional significance of CL&P.

Anomalies of the first and second branchial arches are among the most frequently encountered. Clinically, they appear as underdevelopment or malformation of the facial structures arising from the first and second arches, pharyngeal pouch and first branchial cleft. Complete hemifacial microsomia may be present in the syndrome. Hemifacial microsomia consists of hypoplasia of the external and middle ear, mandible, zygoma, maxilla and associated facial muscles, muscles of mastication and parotid gland. Often macrostomia and first branchial cleft sinus are associated findings.

There appears to be no consistent mode of inheritance found with these anomalies. The syndrome has been associated with the malformation caused by thalidomide ingestion during pregnancy. Bilateral involvement is seen in 10 percent of patients.

Treatment consists of reconstruction or augmentation of the specific structures involved. (Reconstruction of the external ear will be covered later in this chapter.) Onlay bone grafts are an effective means of correcting mandibular, maxillary and zygomatic hypoplasia. The ribs are the best source for autogenous grafts, although Silastic and irradiated cartilage allografts have been used. The associated soft tissue deficiencies rarely require reconstruction.

Branchial Cleft Cysts

Occasionally the remnants of the second and third branchial cleft or pouch fail to disappear. When this occurs, the epithelium-lined passage can fill with fluid secretions resulting in a branchial cleft cyst. The cyst may have an external sinus along the anterior border of the SCM muscle, usually below the level of the thyroid cartilage. The opening of the internal sinus is located along the posterior tonsillar pillar. Fistulas occur when there are openings on the skin and in the pharynx. Branchial cleft cysts may become infected and drain serous or purulent fluid.

These branchial cleft cysts are the most common anomaly of the branchial arch. They lie beneath the anterior edge of the SCM muscle on the surface of the carotid sheath. They are lined with squamous epithelium, but lymphoid tissue is always present in the cyst wall.

Treatment consists of complete excision of the embryological remnant. Infection of the cyst must be controlled prior to surgery. The sinus or fistula must be followed from the anterior SCM border, superiorly through the carotid bifurcation to the opening at the posterior tonsillar pillar (if there is one). Exposure is effected through a series of transverse "stepladder" incisions. Total excision is required because any residual cyst can trigger a recurrence of the infection.

Ear Reconstruction

The external ear is formed from the mandibular and hyoid arches. The mandibular arch forms the tragus, crus, helix and conchal floor and the hyoid arch forms the rest. Total absence of the auricle, or a significant deformity therein, can have severe psychological consequences. Hypoplasia of the ear can occur in isolation or in association with other head and neck syndromes. Other anomalies, particularly of the genitourinary tract, may be associated with congenital defects of the ear.

The ear must be reconstructed before the child becomes psychologically traumatized. Ninety percent of the growth of the ear has occurred by age five. It is practical to begin reconstruction at this age, before the child has entered school and before the attention of the patient and his peers has become focused on the deformity. Many surgeons begin reconstruction during the summer preceding the child's sixth birthday.

Reconstruction of the ear is commonly performed in three stages. In the first stage, the cartilage foundation of the new ear is established. A graft is obtained from the cartilaginous portions of the contralateral sixth, seventh and eighth ribs. The surgeon carves a rigid framework representing normal anatomical landmarks. The cartilage segments can be stacked upon one another to obtain a maximal projection from the side of the head.

Then the surgeon creates a thin subcutaneous pocket through a small incision placed anterior to the auricular vestige. The deformed cartilage vestige is removed and the cartilage graft inserted into the subcutaneous pocket. The skin is drawn into the interstices of the cartilage framework by means of a suction catheter. Suction is maintained postoperatively for several days.

The second procedure is performed six weeks later when the surgeon transposes the soft tissues of the microtic vestige to create an ear lobule. This can usually be done on an outpatient basis, using a Z-plasty type of transposition.

In the third procedure, the surgeon adds refinements to the reconstructed ear. A tragus is constructed, using a cartilage and skin composite graft. This graft can be taken from the opposite ear and can be combined with a contralateral otoplasty if necessary. In most cases, adequate lateral projection of the ear has been obtained with the cartilage graft. A release of the reconstructed ear from the skull with a skin graft is generally not necessary.

Syndactyly

Anomalies of the upper limbs are about as common as cleft lip and palate. The incidence is 1 to 625 live births. In the past many severe anomalies of the upper limb were caused by thalidomide. Most anomalies of the hand are spontaneous, although 5 percent have a hereditary basis.

One of the most commonly encountered anomalies consists of syndactyly or fusion of several fingers. The syndactyly may consist simply of skin webbing between the fingers. In more complex cases, there is associated fusion of the bones, and fingernail bed.

The presence of a skin web rarely represents a functional disability of the infant's hand. Surgery can be performed between the ages of three and four when the structures are large enough to work on. When syndactyly involves fingers of different lengths, the longer finger may become deviated toward the shorter digit. The two fingers should be separated as soon as such distortion becomes apparent in order to prevent permanent deformity.

The principles of incision placement discussed in Chapter 7 must be observed in syndactyly repair. The incisions are made in a zigzag pattern to avoid a linear scar which might result in a scar contracture. Flaps are cut so that the web space and one finger are covered as much as possible by the flaps. It is particularly important that flap skin cover the sides of the finger used for apposition to the thumb.

Usually a full thickness skin graft is required to cover the remaining finger. The groin is a suitable donor site for this graft. A stent is applied to hold the graft in place, and the hand is immobilized with a bulky dressing. The dressing is removed at the end of a week.

CHAPTER 15

Hand Surgery

Injuries to the soft tissue of the hand are extremely common, particularly among industrial workers. Punch presses, knives, lawn mowers and snow blowers are common causes of hand injuries. While the care of hand injuries crosses several disciplines, the skills of the plastic surgeon are of vital importance in reconstruction.

Diagnosis and treatment of hand injuries should always be approached with a keen appreciation of the close relationship between anatomy and function. The examination of the hand is an exercise in applied anatomy, and evaluation of the functional and sensory capabilities of an injured hand must be undertaken with the anatomy of the involved structures in mind.

Data describing the mechanism and the site of injury, plus all sensory and functional impairment, should be kept in an orderly and standardized form. Especially useful are diagrams showing the injury, the range of motion and the sensation of the digits. The diagrams can be used to evaluate progress following reconstruction and as a basis for the final disability evaluation.

Examination

Inspection will reveal a great deal regarding any functional impairment. Abnormalities of the bony skeleton will be immediately apparent. Tendon lacerations can be diagnosed by noting any abnormal positioning of the digits. Presence or absence of sweating can indicate the neurological condition of the hand.

It is best to perform a sensory evaluation at the outset of the examination, before the patient becomes apprehensive or uncooperative. Objective evaluation of the sensory status of the peripheral nerves should be conducted with a sharp pin and a dull instrument. It is best that the patient's view of his hand be obstructed during sensory testing. The location of the injury and the pattern of sensory loss indicate the site and nature of any peripheral nerve damage (Fig. 15-1).

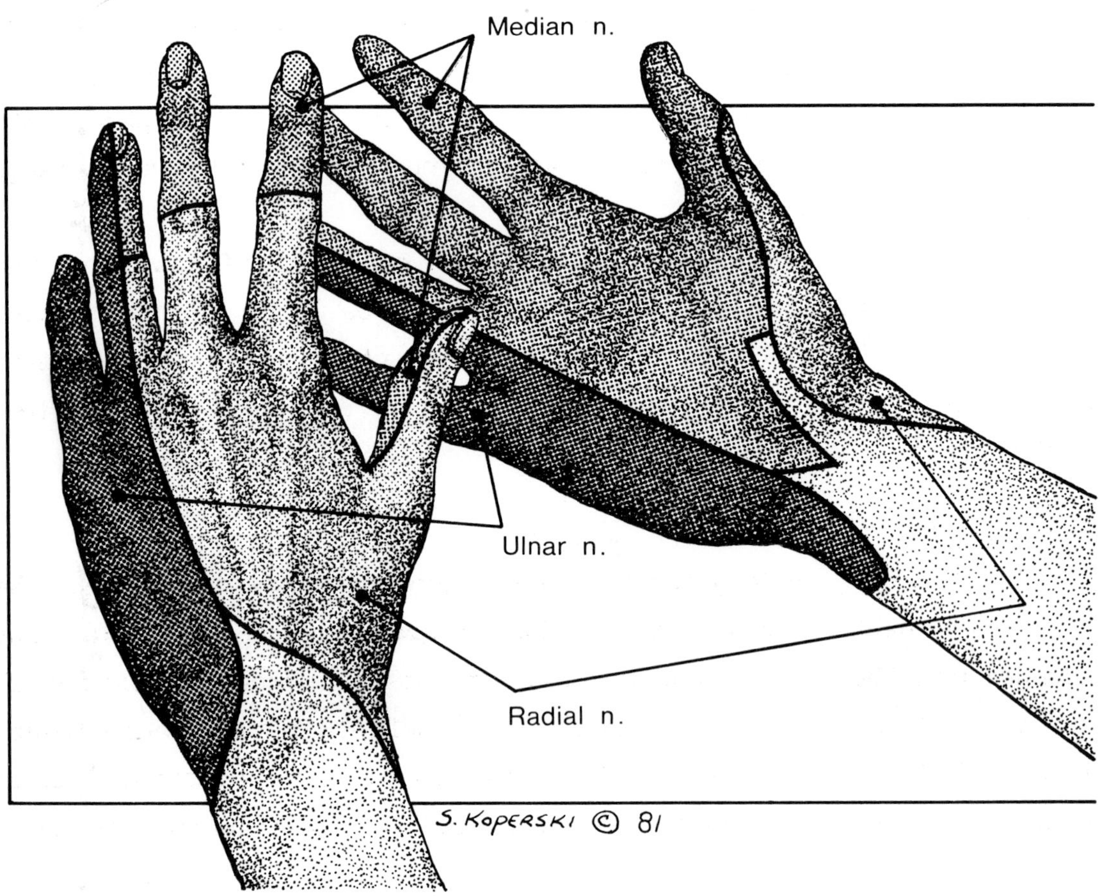

Figure 15-1. **Sensory nerves of hands.** Sensation for the hand is provided by the median, ulnar and radial nerves. The ulnar nerve provides sensation from the front and back of both the little finger and the ulnar aspect of the ring finger. The median nerve provides sensation from the palmar aspect of the thumb, index and middle fingers, and the radial half of the ring finger (stippled). The median also provides sensation from the distal dorsal aspect of these fingers. The radial provides sensation only from the dorsum of the radial aspect of the hand and thumb (cross-hatched areas).

The motor ability of the hand is evaluated next. The patient is asked to make a fist and to extend his fingers. Any impairment in the range of motion of any joint is recorded. The examiner then manipulates the affected part to determine passive range of motion and degree of joint flexibility. Each joint must be examined individually to determine its active and passive range of motion.

This information is recorded as the observed active motion versus the potential range of motion. A normal proximal interphalangeal (PIP) joint has a range of motion of from 0° at full extension to 120° at full flexion. An abnormal finger that straightens to 20° and flexes to 80° is recorded as ROM = 20/80. The passive range of motion, if different, is recorded in a similar manner. An uninjured distal interphalangeal (DIP) joint in which the flexor tendon to the finger is lacerated will have an active range of motion of 0/0 but a passive range of motion of 0/90.

X-rays of the hand should be a part of any examination following trauma. In most cases any foreign bodies, including glass, will be visible. A marker taped to the skin helps determine the location of a foreign body. The pattern of many common hand injuries can be delineated from a general evaluation such as that described above.

Bones and Joints

Fractures of the long bones of the fingers are easily diagnosed by the accompanying pain, deformity and swelling. Fractures of the metacarpals and phalanges must be reduced and immobilized. It is important to correct all angulation and rotational deformities at the time of reduction. Fractures which fail to retain their anatomical reduction, or which are innately unstable, such as middle phalanx fractures, must be immobilized with percutaneous Kirschner wires.

In open fractures, or fractures refractory to Kirschner wire stabilization, direct interosseous wiring may be done. In this method, two sets of small holes are drilled through the bones on each edge of the fracture site. Two 28 gauge wires are passed through the holes and tightened to impact the fragments together. It is known that fractures heal best when the fragments are impacted together. Interosseous wire fixation is so stable that mobilization of the hand is begun earlier than when fractures are fixed with Kirschner wires (Fig. 15-2).

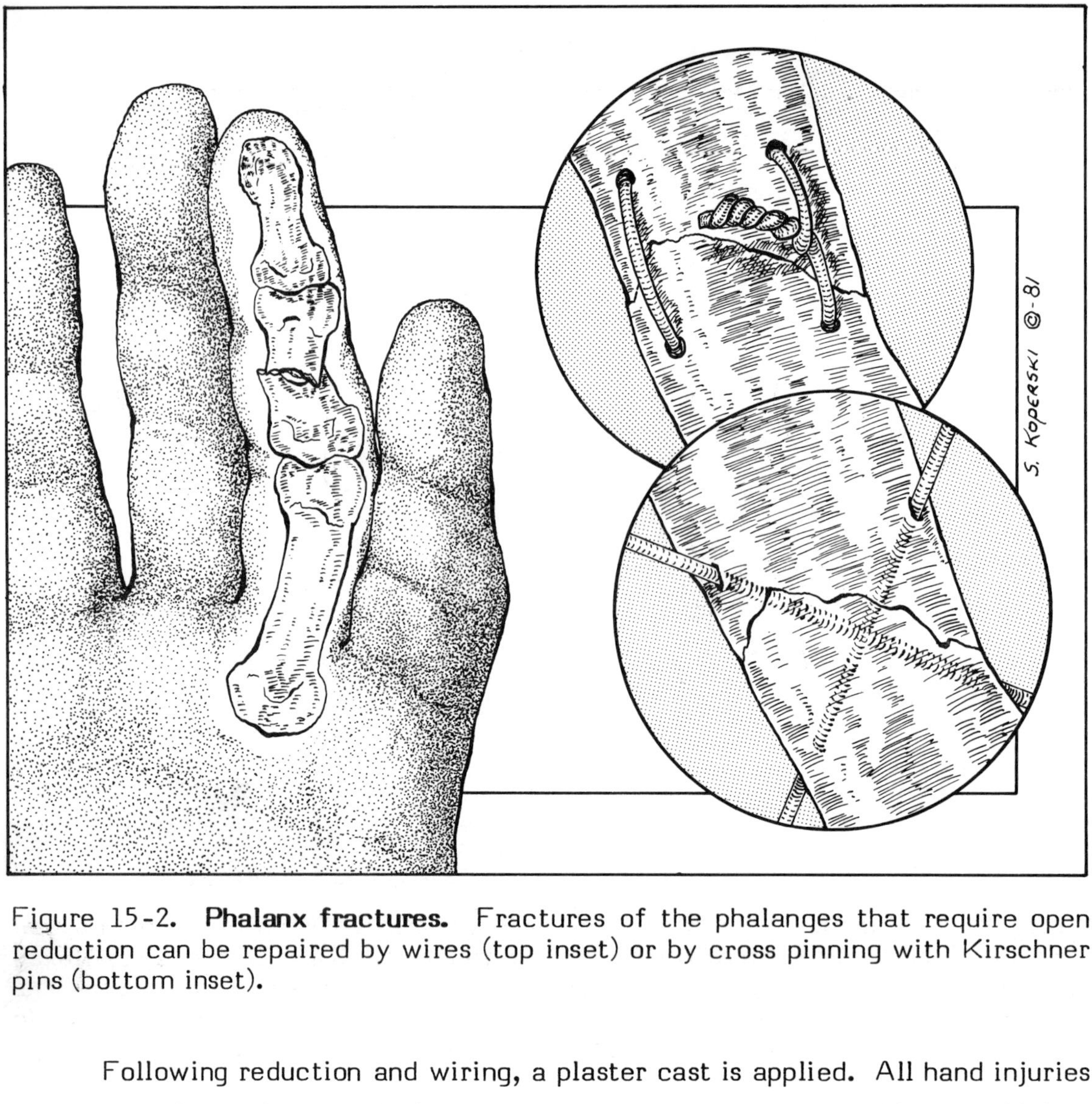

Figure 15-2. **Phalanx fractures.** Fractures of the phalanges that require open reduction can be repaired by wires (top inset) or by cross pinning with Kirschner pins (bottom inset).

Following reduction and wiring, a plaster cast is applied. All hand injuries should be elevated to minimize edema and postoperative stiffness. Unless contraindicated by the specific injury, the hand should always be immobilized in the "position of function." The position of function is designed to minimize the ill effects of prolonged splinting of the hand and consists of the extension of the interphalangeal (IP) joints, the palmar abduction of the thumb, and the flexion of the metacarpophalangeal (MCP) joints. The IP joints must be extended to eliminate the rapid and irreversible contraction of the volar plate that ensues when the fingers are flexed for prolonged periods of time. The thumb should be abducted in the palmar plane to avoid contracture of the first web space. If the MCP joints are not kept flexed, the collateral ligaments will contract and prevent flexion when the splint is removed (Fig. 15-3).

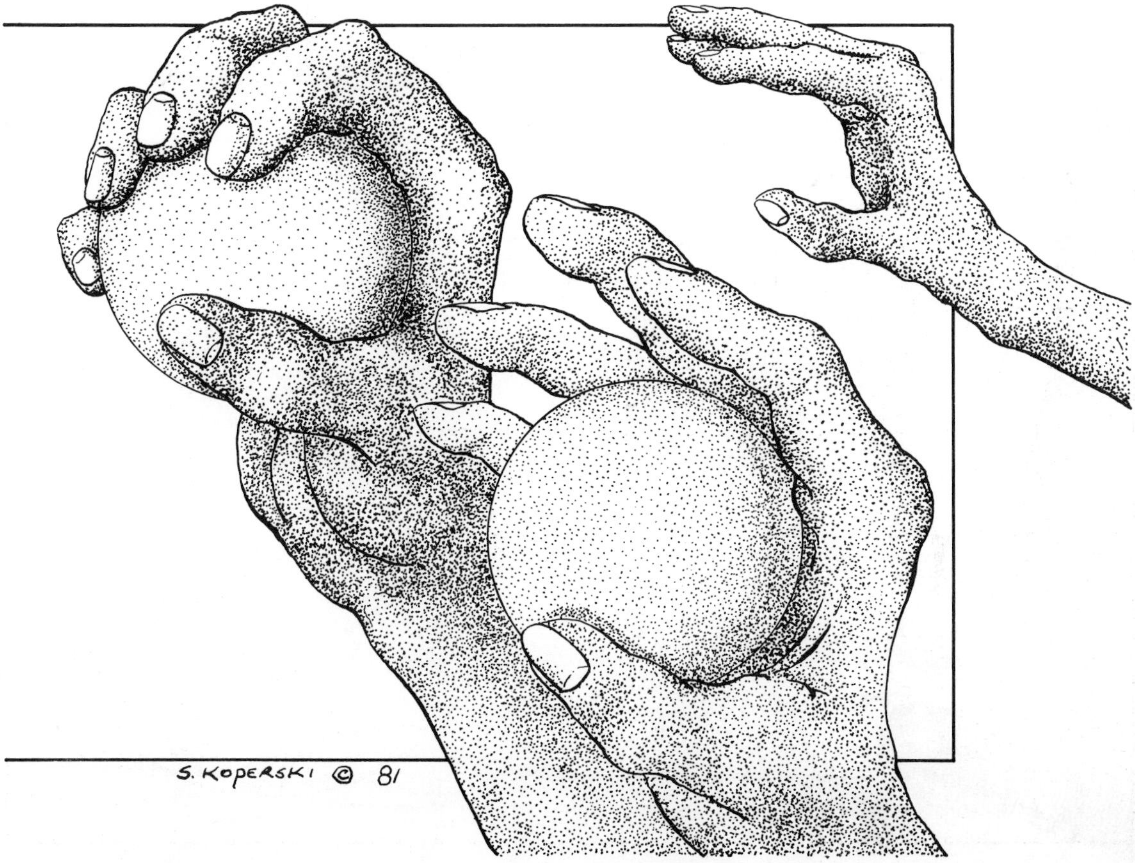

Figure 15-3. **Position of function.** The hand position assumed in grasping a ball is an excellent description of the position of function. The MCP joints are flexed and the thumb is in opposition (left). Some hand surgeons prefer that the phalanges be in extension, to keep the collateral ligaments taut (center). In either case, it is important to keep the wrist in extension (right).

Fracture avulsions and ligament injuries of the fingers are more subtle than are long bone fractures. The mallet finger, a commonly encountered injury, is caused by forceful striking of the tip of the finger, often with a ball. The force of impact causes a separation of the extensor mechanism of the DIP joint. It may include avulsion of the dorsal base of the distal phalanx where the tendon inserts. In such a case, the patient is unable to fully extend the digit at the DIP joint.

Mallet finger injuries should be splinted in full extension continuously for six weeks. An episode of flexion at the DIP will tear the healing tendon. The avulsed fragment can be directly wired if the initial fracture is open or if the fragment represents more than 25 percent of the affected joint surface (Fig. 15-4).

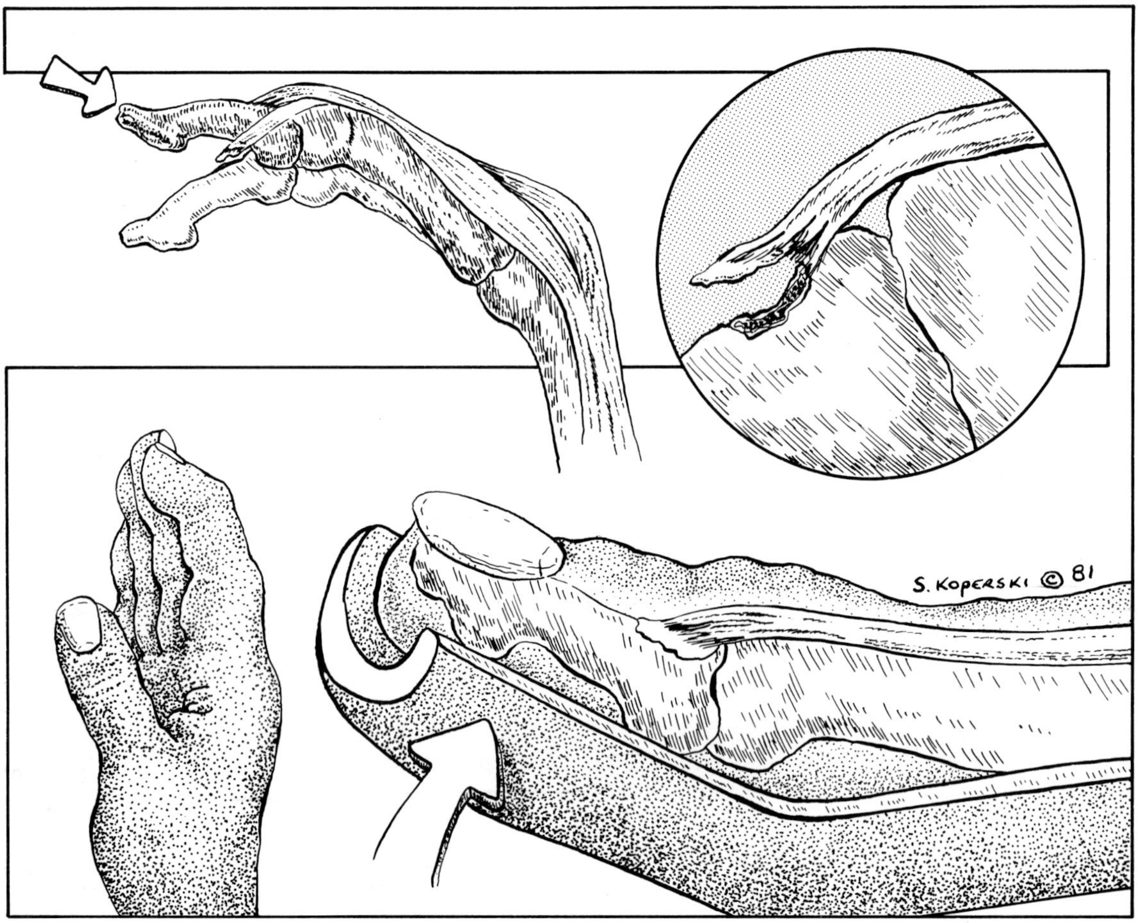

Figure 15-4. **Hyperflexion injuries to the phalanges (mallet finger).** Avulsion of the insertion of the long extensor tendon results from a direct blow on the fingertip, caused most commonly by miscatching a ball (inset). The injury results in inability to extend the distal phalanx (bottom). Treatment includes hypertension of the DIP joint by splinting. Open reduction may be necessary if the bone avulsed enters the joint space.

Another serious injury is caused by forceful hyperextension of the proximal interphalangeal joint. The resultant stress on the volar plate of the joint causes an avulsion of the distal part of the joint. If less than 40 percent of the joint surface is involved and the fragment is in good alignment, the injury can be splinted at 30° flexion for two weeks. Where more of the joint surface is avulsed, or if the fragment is widely separated, repair of the volar plate with wiring of the fragment must be undertaken. After three weeks of immobilization, the joint is permitted some motion, but only with a splint in position to block the extension of the finger beyond 30° (Fig. 15-5).

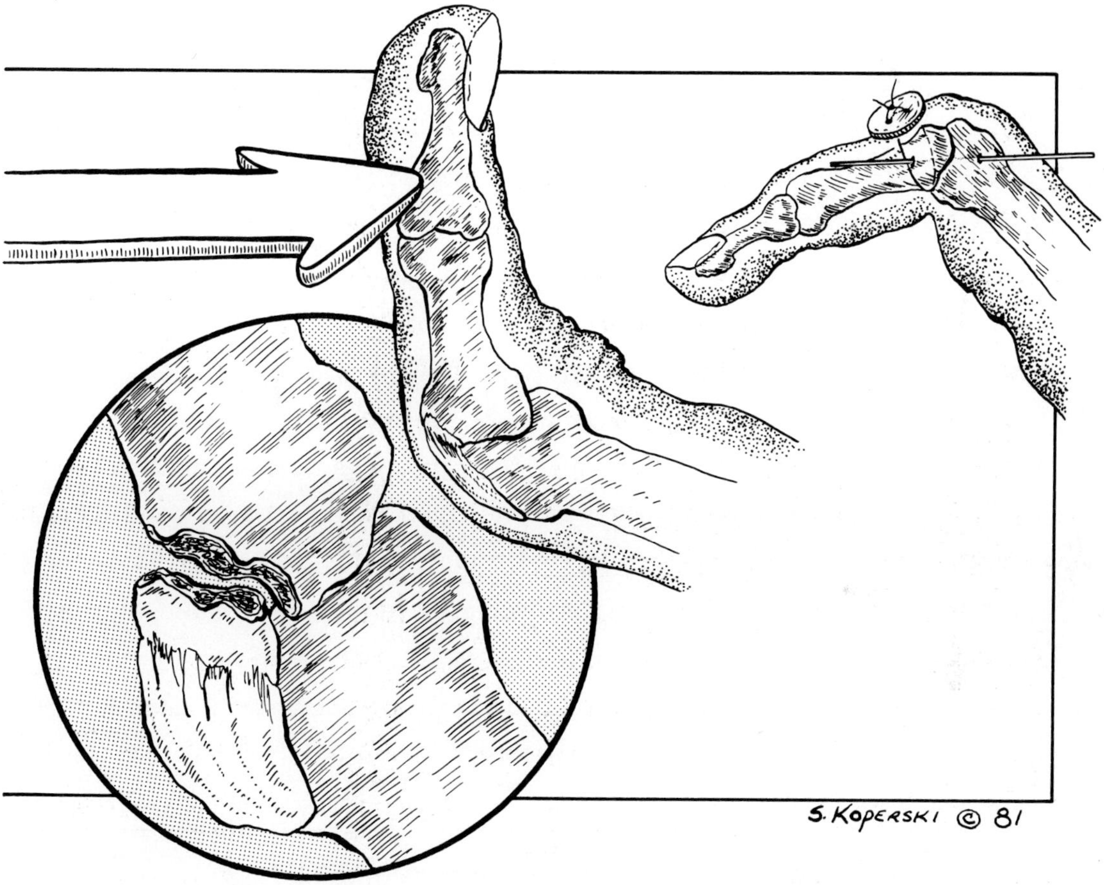

Figure 15-5. **Hyperextension injuries to the phalanges.** In these injuries, hyperextension of the volar plate (arrow) tears off a piece of bone, which usually enters part of the joint (circular insert). Open reduction by pin and/or wire is usually required (right).

Muscles and Tendons

Evaluation of the motion of the joints must take into account the action of both the intrinsic muscles of the hand and the extrinsic muscles that act on the hand from a distance.

The intrinsic musculature is innervated by a combination of the median and ulnar nerves. Generally, the thenar muscles are innervated by the median nerve and the lumbricals and interosseous muscles by the ulnar nerve. There is an interconnecting network that allows some cross innervation of these structures. The cross innervation is of variable extent.

The extrinsic muscles act on the finger joints from a distance through the tendons. Extrinsic extensor tendon function is evaluated by the ability of the patient to extend the IP and MCP joints. With the MCP joints slightly flexed, the phalanges can be extended by either the extrinsic or the intrinsic system acting on the common extensor hood.

The intrinsic muscles flex the MCP joints to 90°. The extrinsic muscles are responsible for the remaining flexor motion of the MCP and for flexion at the phalanges. The flexor profundus tendon passes through an opening in the flexor superficialis tendon and inserts at the base of the distal phalanx. An intact profundus tendon provides flexion at the DIP joint.

The superficialis tendon inserts on the base of the middle phalanx and provides flexion at the PIP joint. Because the profundus tendon can also flex this joint, its action must be blocked when testing the superficialis tendon by holding the adjacent fingers in hyperextension. If the finger to be tested flexes at the PIP joint, the superficialis tendon is intact. With the finger flexed at the PIP, the DIP should be flaccid and relaxed, indicating that the profundus tendon is not participating in flexion of the PIP joint. Because of the independent action of the flexor profundus to the index finger, the superficialis tendon test does not give good results on that digit.

Tendon Lacerations

Because of the intimate relationship between the flexor superficialis and profundus tendons, scar formation following tendon laceration and repair can cause significant functional impairment. This is especially true following repair when both tendons have been lacerated at the same level. As scar tissue forms, it can cement the tendons to one another and to the surrounding soft tissue, making active flexion impossible.

Scar tissue adhesions are most disabling in the "critical zone" or "no man's land" extending from the distal palmar crease to the level of insertion of the superficialis tendon at the base of the middle phalanx. It is here, where the profundus tendon passes through the narrow fibro-osseous tunnel and the insertion of the superficialis tendon, that the tendons are in their most intimate contact (Fig. 15-6).

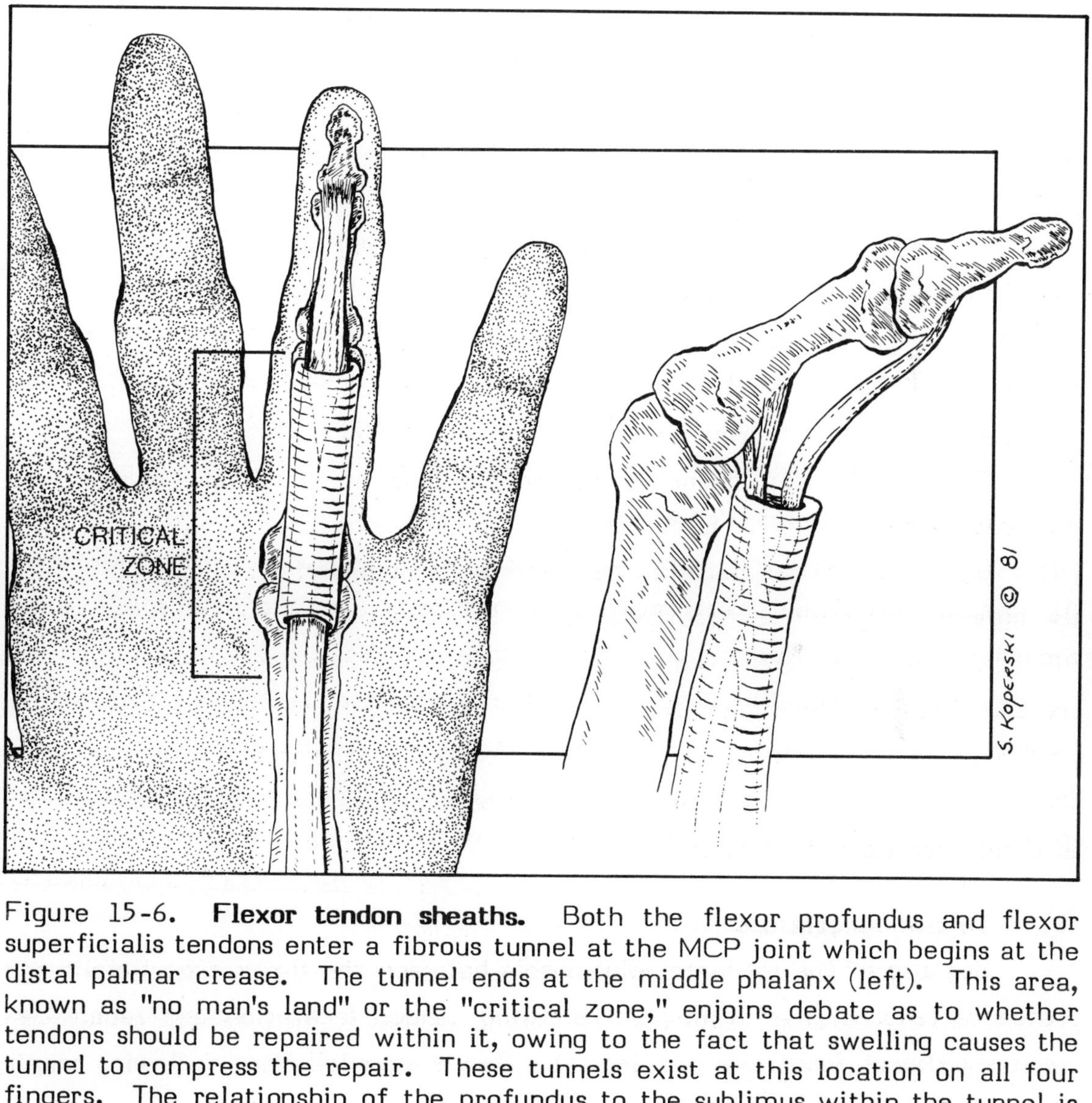

Figure 15-6. **Flexor tendon sheaths.** Both the flexor profundus and flexor superficialis tendons enter a fibrous tunnel at the MCP joint which begins at the distal palmar crease. The tunnel ends at the middle phalanx (left). This area, known as "no man's land" or the "critical zone," enjoins debate as to whether tendons should be repaired within it, owing to the fact that swelling causes the tunnel to compress the repair. These tunnels exist at this location on all four fingers. The relationship of the profundus to the sublimus within the tunnel is shown (right).

Because of the frequency of poor function following tendon repairs in this region, there is a controversy regarding their management. Some practitioners do not perform a primary tendon repair of lacerations in the critical zone. They advocate closing the skin and later, when the wound has healed, performing a primary tendon graft employing the palmaris longus or plantaris tendon. The joints must be passively exercised and kept mobile during this waiting period.

Recently, primary suture of tendon lacerations in the critical zone has returned to favor. The tendons are repaired, as with other tendon lacerations of the hand, with fine atraumatic suture. The tendon sheath in the vicinity of the repair may be excised or, in some cases, transposed between the tendons to diminish the likelihood of adhesions between the repair sites.

The timing of primary tendon repairs is also controversial. In many centers, the tendons are repaired as soon as possible following laceration. Equally good results can be obtained, however, when the skin is closed and delayed primary tendon repair is undertaken within 10 days following surgery. Because of the devastating effect of an infection on tendon repairs, any potentially contaminated wound should be closed and a delayed primary tendon repair undertaken at the appropriate time.

In the past, primary tendon repairs were splinted in the position of function for three weeks while the tendon healed. The longer a tendon is immobilized, however, the more likely is the development of firm adhesions to the adjacent soft tissue. Early mobilization of the finger is believed to minimize the risk of such adhesions and is advocated today in most centers.

The finger should be passively manipulated so that no tension is placed on the tendon repair. This is accomplished by means of an extension block splint. A dorsal splint is applied to prevent full extension of the finger and tension on the anastomosis. A small hook is attached to the fingernail and connected to the wrist with an elastic band. The elastic band passively flexes the finger, and the intact extensor tendon straightens it against the splint (Fig. 15-7).

The finger can be mobilized in this protected manner within the first several days following repair. The splint is maintained for three weeks. Following this guarded period, active range of motion exercises can begin. By the end of the fifth week, the hand is unrestrained and active use should be encouraged.

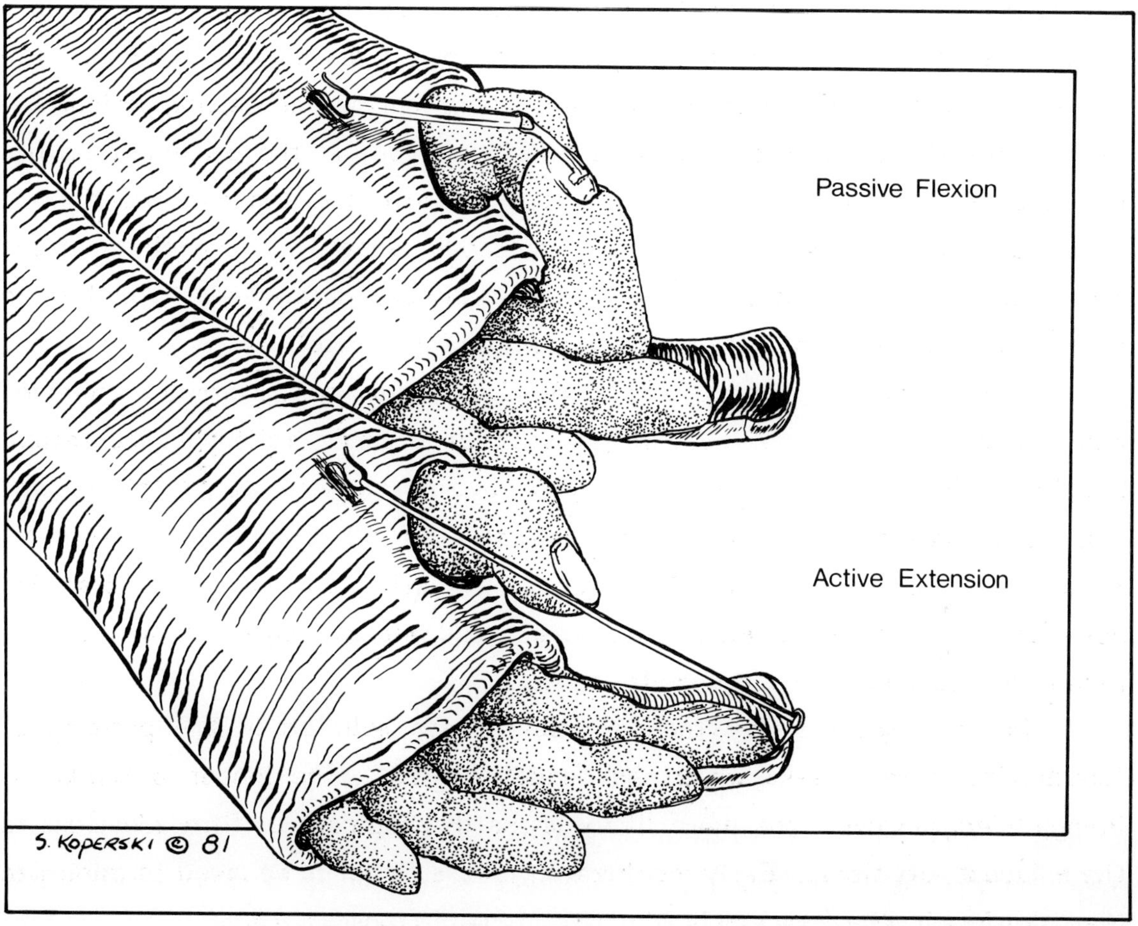

Figure 15-7. **Flexor tendon repair.** A cast which allows passive flexion of the tendon, and hence no muscle pull on the repair, may decrease adhesions surrounding the repair (top). A rubber band is glued from the cast to the finger nail so that no active flexion is required by the flexor tendon (in this case, the wrist is flexed to relax the tendons). Active extension counteracts the rubber band (bottom).

Because of the loose connective tissue on the dorsum of the hand, extensor tendon adhesions are not a significant problem. Extensor tendon injuries on the dorsum of the hand can be repaired immediately, or a delayed primary repair can be performed. Because the extensor tendons are thinner and the sutures have less holding power, these repairs must be protected from active motion longer than flexor tendons. Protective splints must remain in place for five weeks for injuries distal to the MCP joint and for four weeks for injuries proximal to this joint.

Nerves of the Hand

The median and ulnar nerves are frequently damaged in hand injuries. They are both mixed nerves, with the ulnar nerve having a greater proportion of motor fibers and the median more sensory fibers. The sensory innervation to the hand is well established, and this knowledge can serve as a guide to diagnosis of nerve damage.

The ulnar nerve innervates the flexor carpi ulnaris and the ulnar half of the flexor profundus in the forearm. It also supplies the intrinsic musculature of the hand except for those areas innervated by the median nerve (flexor pollicis brevis, abductor pollicis brevis, and opponens). Evaluation of the intrinsic musculature serves to test the motor function of the ulnar nerve. The interossei are evaluated by asking the patient to place the hand on a table and spread and adduct the fingers. The first dorsal interosseous muscle can be palpated on the radial side of the index metacarpal when the patient presses against the thumb.

Failure to perform these two tests indicates a lesion of the motor branches of the ulnar nerve.

Froment's, or the adductor pollicis, sign is pathigmanic of ulnar nerve lesions. The patient is asked to grasp a piece of paper between thumb and index finger and to resist the examiner's attempts to remove it from his grasp. The thumb with a paralyzed adductor pollicis muscle will involuntarily flex at the IP joint because of the compensatory action of the flexor pollicis longus (FPL) which is innervated by the median nerve (Fig. 15-8).

The median nerve innervates the palmaris longus, flexi carpi radialis, the flexor superficialis group, the FPL, and the radial half of the flexor profundus. In the hand the median nerve supplies the muscles of the thenar eminence and the two radial lumbricals. The motor branch of the median nerve is tested by having the patient approximate the thumb to the tips of the digits in the form of an O. This indicates that the opponens muscle is intact.

The abductor pollicis brevis is innervated exclusively by the median nerve. Its function can be tested by having the patient rest the supinated hand on the table. The patient is asked to touch an object above the thumb, causing the thumb to be raised in a plane 90° to the table. Failure to perform this test indicates paralysis of the motor branch of the median nerve to the abductor pollicis brevis.

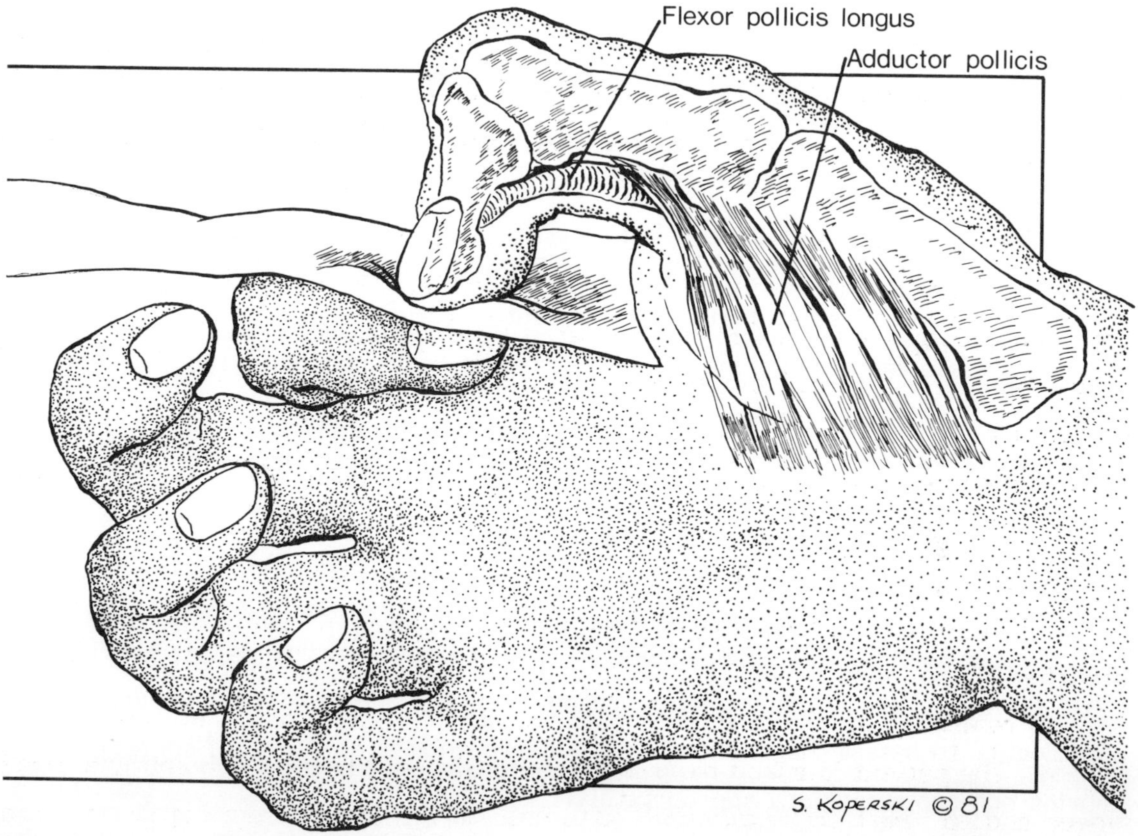

Figure 15-8. **Froment's sign.** Froment's sign is exaggerated flexion of the distal phalanx of the thumb. This results from overcompensation of the FPL in an attempt to overcome the paralysis of the adductor pollicis due to ulnar nerve injury.

The radial nerve supplies the wrist and digital extensors as well as those to the thumb. In the hand it is a purely sensory nerve. Sensory loss over the dorsum of the first web space and the dorsum of the thumb, index and long fingers indicates radial nerve lesions.

Peripheral nerve injury can range from neurapraxia following contusion or prolonged pressure to avulsion injuries with loss of large segments of nerve. Following the transection of a nerve, a neuroma develops at the cut end. Percussion over the neuroma produces a tingling sensation called Tinel's sign. Following a successful nerve repair, the Tinel sign progresses distally as the nerve regenerates. The regenerating axons grow at a rate of 1 mm per day distal to the wrist. Because of this slow growth, it usually takes a year for complete functional recovery following a nerve repair at the wrist.

Nerve Repair

Several factors affect the outcome of the repair of peripheral nerves. The age of the patient is significant. Young children always exhibit good functional recovery following successful repair. However, after the age of six, there is a definite decrease in the quality of functional recovery. This presumably results from the inability of older patients to completely "relearn" the new pattern of sensation following nerve regeneration. Nerves that are cleanly divided by a sharp object do better than those subjected to crushing, tearing or stretching forces.

The timing and type of repair of peripheral nerves have been subjects of controversy. It is now believed that nerves that are cleanly divided are best repaired immediately or delayed to 10 days following injury. If a delayed primary repair is performed, the epineurium and perineurium are edematous and hold sutures well. It is best to wait two to three weeks to repair nerves that have sustained blunt trauma and crushing injury. This gives the surgeon an opportunity to assess the viability of the nerve ends at the time of surgery and to debride nonviable sections appropriately.

There has been considerable debate regarding the benefits of different types of nerve repair. Traditional epineural repairs have been accomplished with the naked eye or using mild magnification. Blood vessels in the epineurium and the mesoneurium can be used for achieving correct rotational alignment. A disadvantage of the epineural repair is that the individual fascicular groups are free to rotate within the epineural sheath (Fig. 15-9).

With the advent of the operating microscope, it has become possible to isolate individual fasciculi and suture the perineurium. While this type of repair provides a precise alignment, the presence of many sutures within the nerve results in a proliferation of scar tissue. Extensive dissection is required to isolate the individual fasciculi, a process which predisposes to edema and scar tissue.

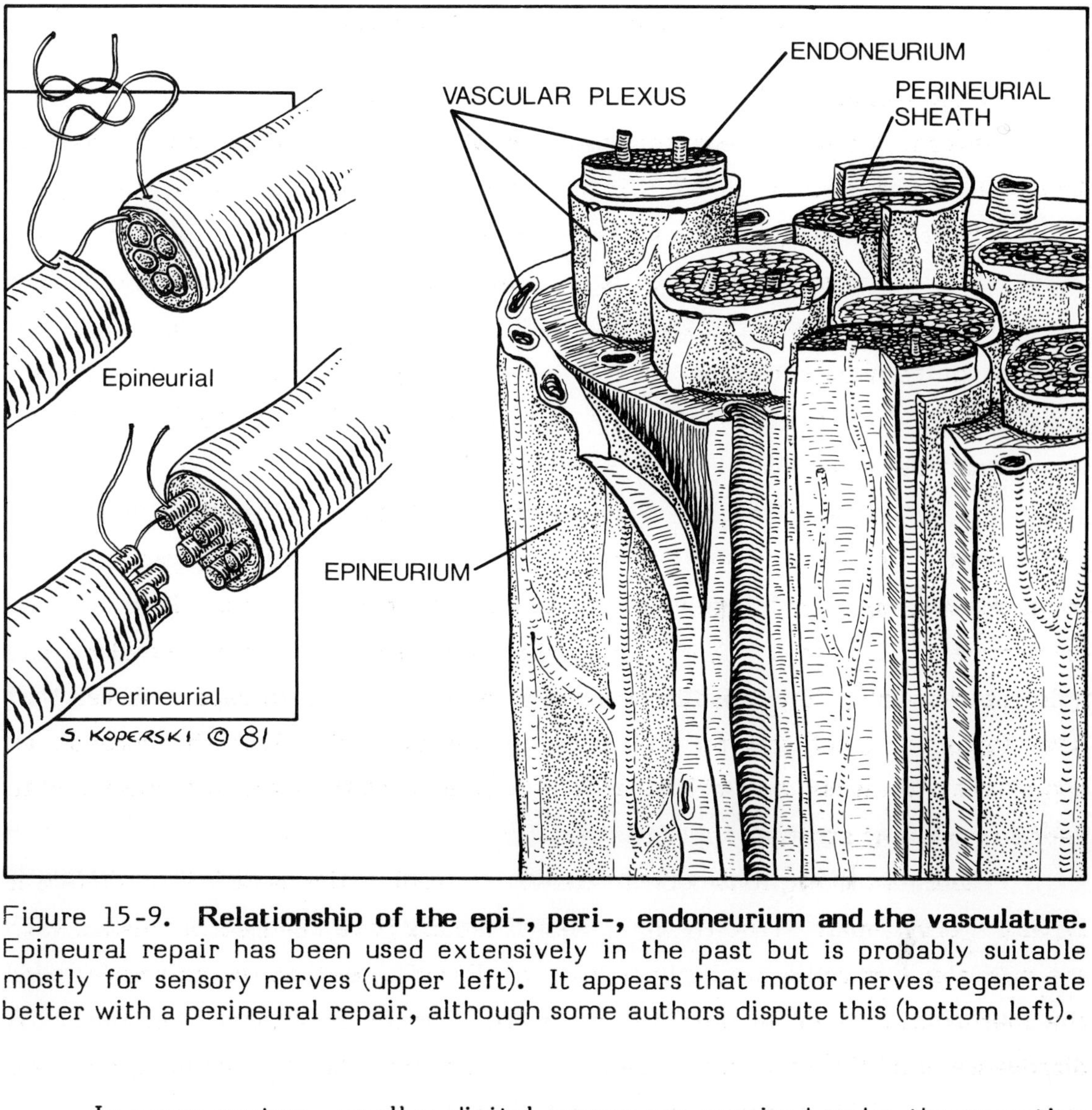

Figure 15-9. **Relationship of the epi-, peri-, endoneurium and the vasculature.** Epineural repair has been used extensively in the past but is probably suitable mostly for sensory nerves (upper left). It appears that motor nerves regenerate better with a perineural repair, although some authors dispute this (bottom left).

In many centers, smaller digital nerves are repaired under the operating microscope by means of an epineural technique and 10-0 or 11-0 suture. Larger nerves, such as the median nerve at the wrist, are repaired under magnification using a group fascicular repair. The epineurial cuff is resected, several fascicular bundles are dissected, and the perineurium is approximated with several sutures. The group fascicular repair provides precise approximation while introducing less suture material and dissection to the nerve repair.

Tension on the nerve anastomosis can ruin an otherwise excellent repair. It has been shown that even a mild degree of tension on nerve repairs stimulates connective tissue proliferation which prevents regenerating axons from crossing the nerve repair site. To avoid this problem, a nerve graft should be used when segments of a nerve have been avulsed or require extensive debridement. It has been shown that regenerating axons will cross the two anastomoses required for nerve graft more readily than they will cross one repair site under great tension.

Fingertip Injuries

Trauma to the tip of the finger is a common problem. Most of these injuries can be treated in the emergency room. The goal of treatment is to close the wound, obtain rapid healing, and return the patient to productive activity as rapidly as possible. The simplest and most direct method of tissue replacement is the best.

For wounds that cannot be closed primarily, a split thickness skin graft offers the most expedient form of wound closure. This is best used when some soft tissue remains to cover the distal phalanx, but the graft can be applied to bone or tendon, or even to the nail bed to obtain rapid wound closure (Fig. 15-10).

Split thickness skin grafts can be cut (freehand) from the hypothenar eminence or the thigh. Often the graft can be made to overlap the wound edges and be secured quite nicely with tapes. This obviates the necessity of sutures, which is especially helpful in the case of young children. The edges do not survive and peel off. This maneuver does not work well in full thickness grafts as the bridging effect causes survival of the graft distal to the wound edge, resulting in a raised area. Full thickness skin grafts may be taken from the palmar crease, cubital fossa or the thigh. (Grafts taken from the forearm consistently result in unsightly scarring.) The graft is tacked into place in an edge-to-edge fashion and secured with a compression or stent dressing. The patient is instructed to keep the hand elevated. The dressing is changed after five days. The patient can return to work when the wound is closed.

If the wound is superficial and small, i.e., less than a square cm, it will epithelize rapidly with good results in some patients and a graft may not be necessary. Of course, in any of these injuries if the severed skin is available and reasonably clean, it may be completely defatted and utilized as a free graft.

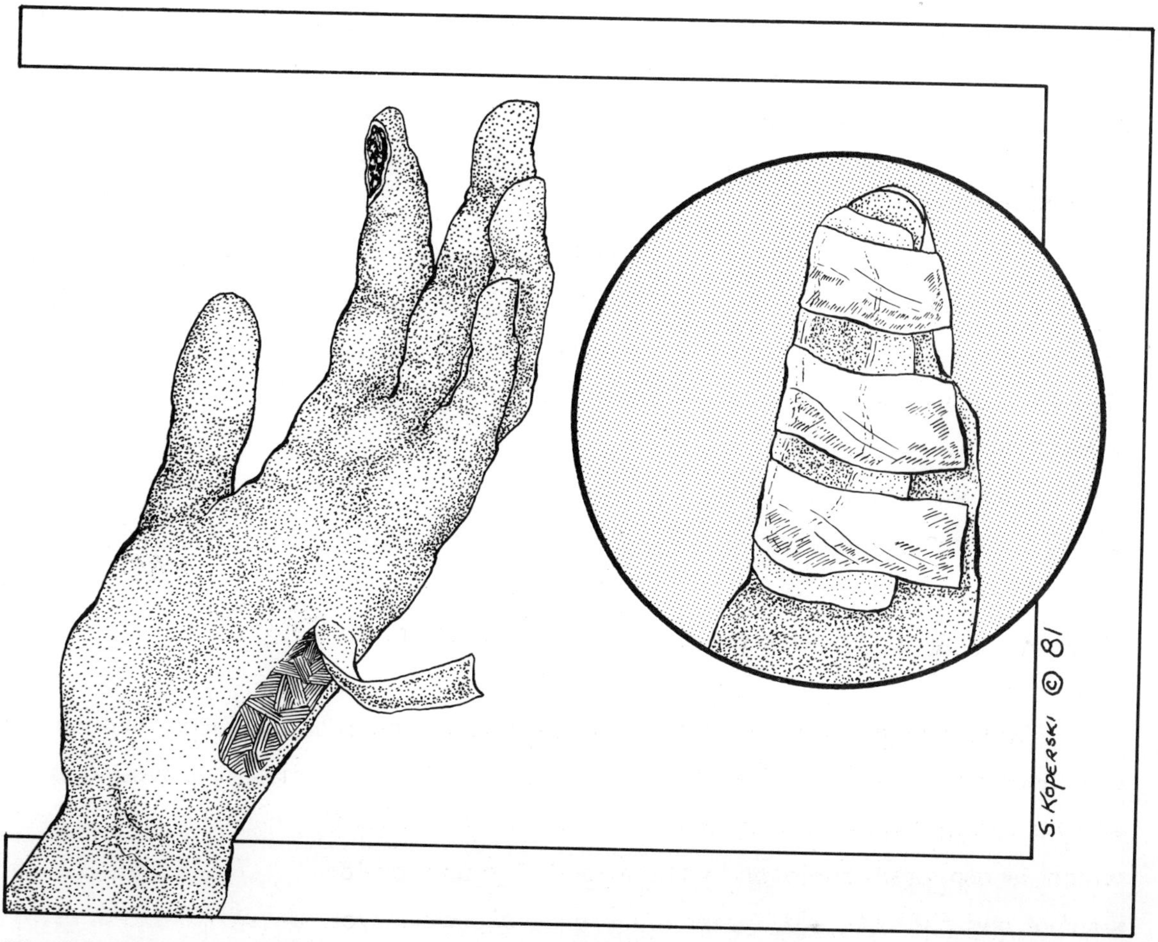

Figure 15-10. **Fingertip repair by skin graft.** A split thickness skin graft from the hypothenar region offers excellent coverage for finger wounds that have soft tissue loss. The graft is cut larger than the wound and can be taped to the recipient area (inset).

Injuries in which considerable bone is exposed are not suitable for skin grafting and require flap coverage for closure. In injuries to the tips of the three ulnar fingers, where length is not essential, the bone can be shortened to facilitate a primary closure. Maintenance of length is more important in the thumb and index finger to preserve the proper pinch relationship. These fingers should not be shortened unless absolutely necessary.

Many types of flaps have been advocated for closure of fingertip injuries. Most of these employ donor tissue from the palm or adjacent fingers. To utilize these sources, the hand must be immobilized, often in an unfavorable position, for two weeks. Because of the stiffness resulting from such immobilization, this method is unsuitable for elderly patients. Once the pedicle has been divided, intensive physical therapy is often required to regain useful function. Flaps from adjacent fingers must rely upon the recipient bed nerve supply for reinnervation. These fingers never again have normal sensation.

The best fingertip closure is obtained from local tissue moved into the defect with an intact neurovascular pedicle. The tissue of the volar aspect of the finger can be advanced on a subcutaneous pedicle by dividing the skin and the vertical fibrous septa attaching the flap to the periosteum. The proximal defect is closed in a V-Y manner. This flap provides good cover and normal tip sensation (Fig. 15-11).

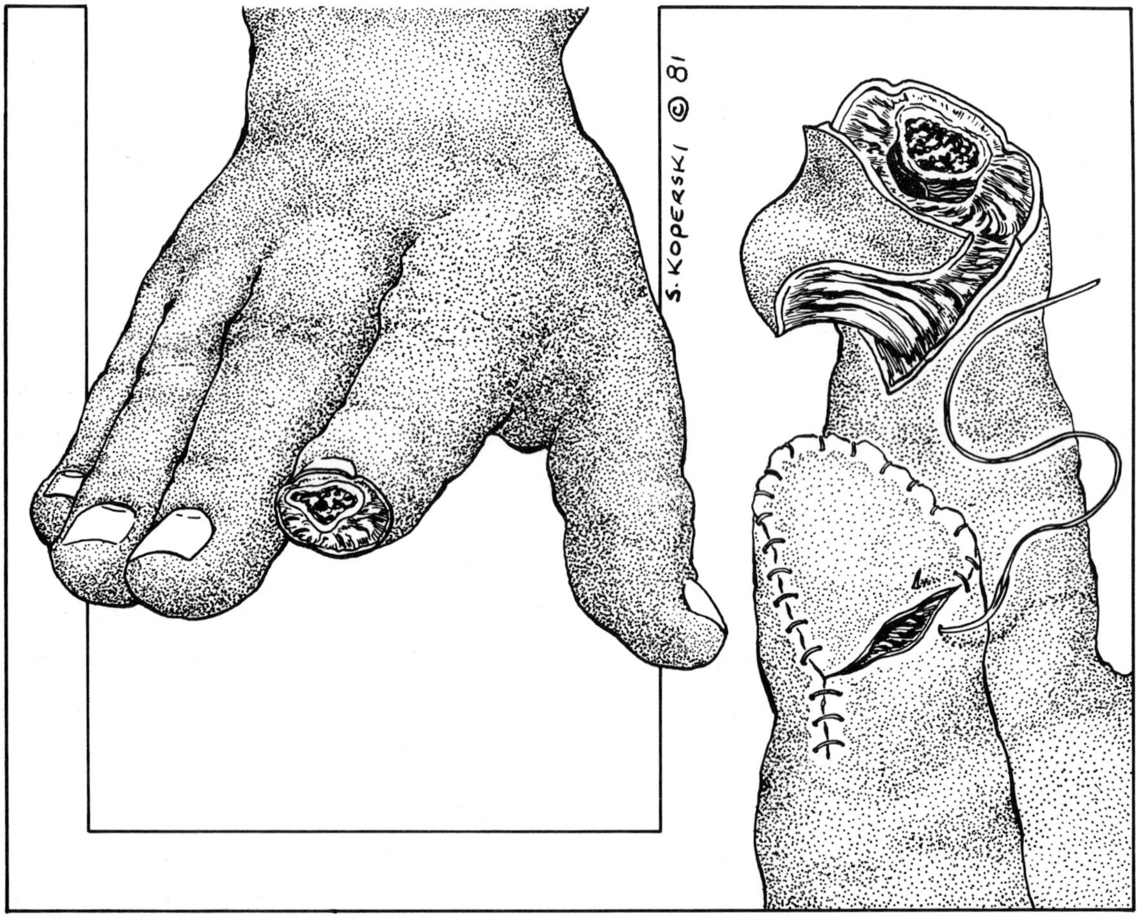

Figure 15-11. **Fingertip repair by skin flap.** When bone is exposed, a flap must be used for coverage (left). For small areas, a subcutaneous V-Y pedicle from the volar aspect of the finger provides the necessary padding (right).

Where large amounts of soft tissue have been lost following crush, avulsion or degloving injuries, distant flaps must be employed for closure. While flaps from the abdomen, chest wall and opposite arm have been used, the most convenient flap is the groin flap. This flap is based on the superficial circumflex iliac artery. The flap is hairless and thin. The donor site is inconspicuous and can be closed primarily. The flap is divided and inset three weeks following its elevation. Secondary procedures are necessary to reinnervate the groin tissue with a neurovascular island flap from an adjacent digit.

As microsurgical techniques have become more sophisticated, a one-stage reconstruction of the thumb and index finger has become possible. A completely amputated thumb can be reconstructed using a toe as a free flap. Degloving injuries or large avulsion injuries can be repaired using a free flap from the first web space of the foot. The deep peroneal nerve which innervates the first web space of the foot can be anastomozed to a digital nerve and sensory capacity restored at the same time the soft tissue deficit is reconstructed. Replantation surgery is described in detail in Chapter 16.

Chronic Hand Ailments

The reconstructive surgeon is often sought for advice regarding chronic ailments of the hand. The elderly are particularly prone to such chronic problems as Dupuytren's contracture, median nerve compression (carpal tunnel syndrome), and tenosynovitis (the trigger finger syndrome).

Median Nerve Compression (Carpal Tunnel Syndrome)

The median nerve is the most vulnerable structure confined within the carpal canal by the transverse carpal ligament. The precise cause of compression of the median nerve in the carpal tunnel is unknown. Suggested mechanisms include congenital anatomical variations, post-traumatic scarring, the degenerative changes of aging, and space occupying lesions.

The typical patient is a postmenopausal female complaining of parasthesias and numbness over the distribution of the median nerve. Typically, the symptoms awaken the patient from a sound sleep. The symptoms are relieved by elevating the extremity and by exercising the hand. The presumed cause of these nocturnal symptoms is related to a local accumulation of edema fluid which is relieved by elevation and exercise.

Objective findings may be difficult to elicit early in the course of the disease. The symptoms may be simulated by pressure or tapping over the carpal tunnel. In the Phalen test, the wrist is acutely flexed for one minute, compressing the median nerve. The symptoms may be intensified by this activity. Relief is produced by returning the wrist to a neutral position.

In more advanced, long-standing cases, obvious clumsiness may be apparent in tasks requiring dexterity of the thumb and index finger. Compression of the motor branch of the median nerve can result in atrophy of the thenar musculature. In equivocal cases, measurement of nerve conduction velocity is required to confirm the diagnosis. Motor latency of greater than 5 milliseconds is considered abnormal.

In mild cases where there is no thenar muscle atrophy, a trial of nonoperative therapy may be warranted. An extension splint sometimes successfully relieves the nocturnal symptoms. Steroids and local anesthetic injected into the carpal tunnel may resolve the symptoms. Triamcinolone, in 10 mg doses, is injected every two weeks for a maximum of three times. Great care must be taken not to inject any of the steroids into the nerve itself. There is often a transient reaction of increased pain following the injection. Ultimately, 20 to 40 percent of patients will show significant improvement and will not require surgery.

When splinting and steroid injections are not successful, or when there are objective signs of nerve compression, surgical release of the median nerve is indicated. The median nerve is explored through an incision in the palm that extends to the proximal wrist crease. Great care must be taken not to damage the motor branch during this exploration. The motor branch originates most commonly from the radial side of the nerve at the distal limits of the carpal tunnel. In long-standing cases, the main trunk of the median nerve may have an hourglass shape at the site of compression. In such cases, it may be necessary to perform an internal neurolysis. In this procedure the scar tissue compressing the nerve is released under the operating microscope.

Dupuytren's Contracture

In 1832, Dupuytren, the surgeon who first classified the depth of thermal burns, published a description and method of cure of the disease which now bears his name. The exact cause of Dupuytren's fasciitis is not known. It is believed that an inflammatory process in the subcutaneous space of the palm induces a secondary contracture of the palmar aponeurosis. Aberrations in myoblast function are undoubtedly important in the etiology of the deformity.

The disease primarily affects Caucasians, particularly of Anglo-Saxon lineage, in the later decades of life. Dupuytren's disease is more common in epileptics and has been associated with alcoholism and tuberculosis. While a specific injury may cause or aggravate the fasciitis, there is little proof that prolonged manual labor causes the disease.

Heredity is probably the most significant factor in the etiology of the disease. The age of onset is younger and the severity of the disease is greater in the presence of a strong family history. There may be involvement of areas beside the hand in Dupuytren's disease. The most common sites are in the plantar aponeurosis of the foot and over the Achilles tendon.

The only effective treatment for Dupuytren's disease is a surgical fasciectomy. When the fingers are deformed to the degree that the patient can no longer touch his palm on a flat surface, surgery must be considered. If undertaken, the procedure should be performed under tourniquet control. Magnification is advisable because of the proximity of the fascial bands to the neurovascular structures. The principles of elective incisions should be observed in order to prevent scar contractures. To prevent such contractures, Z-plasties are often required. Skin grafting may occasionally be necessary in very severe cases.

Following surgery, the hand is placed in a bulky dressing for 10 to 14 days. The dressing should permit the patient to exercise his fingers. Because of the tenuous blood supply to the skin flaps, the sutures should remain in place a minimum of 14 days.

Tenosynovitis

Stenosing digital tenosynovitis, or the trigger finger syndrome, is most commonly seen in middle-aged women. The syndrome presents as a painful blocking of flexion and extension of the involved digit. The symptoms are usually produced by active flexion and the finger may become stuck in a flexed position. The pain may be referred to the PIP joint. The most commonly involved site, however, is the tendon sheath over the MCP.

De Quervain's stenosing tenosynovitis involves the tendon sheaths of the abductor pollicis longus and extensor pollicis brevis tendons in the first dorsal wrist compartment. The triggering phenomenon is generally not present in De Quervain's Disease. There is local tenderness over the radial styloid where the inflamed tendon sheath may be palpated. Finkelstein's test produces the symptoms by a passive tensing of the tendons. This is accomplished by adducting the thumb in the palm and deviating the wrist ulnarward.

A trial of intrathecal steroid injections may sufficiently control the inflammatory process. A treatment of up to four injections of triamcinolone at weekly intervals may alleviate the symptoms. When this is ineffective, or if the digit is repeatedly locked in flexion or extension, surgical release of the tendon sheath is required.

This is performed under local anesthesia with a brachial tourniquet. A longitudinal or transverse incision is made in the distal palm over the metacarpal heads of the affected fingers (or over the radial styloid for De Quervain's disease). Care must be taken to avoid damage to neurovascular structures. Also the affected pulley must be divided in such a way as not to damage the underlying tendon. The release is tested by having the patient flex and extend the fingers.

A bulky dressing is applied and left in place for three to seven days. The fingers should be actively flexed and extended during this time. Normal use of the hand may begin after 10 to 14 days. The most serious complication of the procedure is damage to a sensory nerve. Painful neuromas of the sensory branch of the radial nerve following surgery for De Quervain's disease can be particularly disabling.

CHAPTER 16

Microsurgery

Microsurgery is one of the most rapidly expanding fields in plastic and reconstructive surgery. The term refers to the use of magnification during operative procedures. The operating microscope is the instrument for this magnification and has facilitated reconstructions that would be impossible employing traditional techniques. While microsurgery is applicable to every surgical subspeciality, it has been most fully exploited in plastic surgery.

The field of microsurgery emerged when consistently high grade optical instruments became available. In 1953, Carl Zeiss, Inc. began mass production of the operating microscope. The new instrument permitted ophthalmologists to improve their surgical procedures and to devise new ways to reconstruct the anterior segments of the eye. For the first time, otolaryngologists could perform precise middle ear surgery. Neurosurgeons began using magnification to aid in their dissections and in revascularization of the cerebral cortex. Plastic surgeons began to use the microscope for improved nerve repair and digital replantation.

Today, most surgical subspecialties employ the operating microscope routinely. Orthopedic surgeons use it for free bone transfers; urologists use it for vas deferens reconstruction; and obstetrical specialists use the microscope to reconstruct fallopian tubes. Microsurgery has become an integral part of every surgical subspecialty.

The Microscope

The essential components of the operating microscope are the objective lens, the binocular assembly, and the magnification changer (Fig. 16-1).

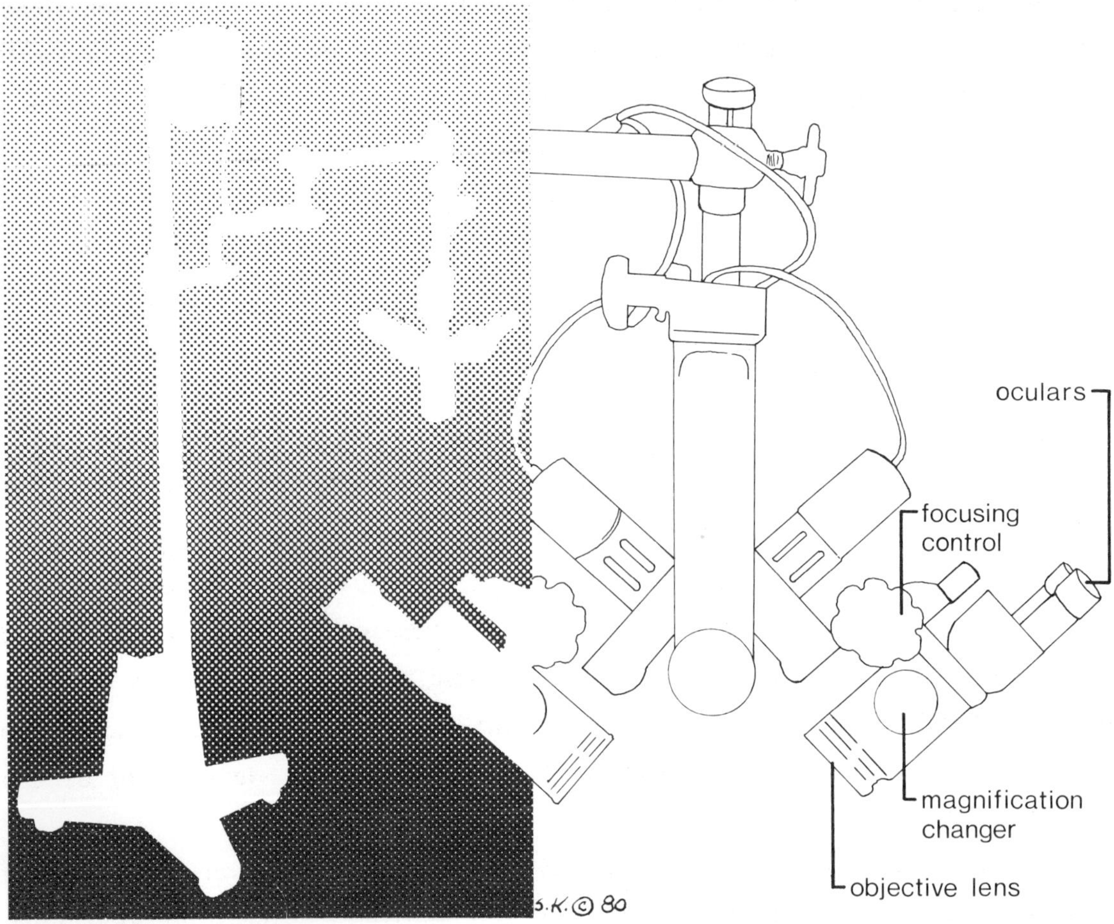

Figure 16-1. **Operating microscope.** The operating microscope, shown as a floor model (left) and in close-up (right), has allowed accurate approximation of blood vessels and nerves. This work, pioneered by Buncke, has revolutionized tissue transfer techniques.

The objective lens forms an image of the object which is subsequently magnified by the binocular assembly. The objective lens is the component that determines the surgeon's working distance from the operative field. Interchangeable objective lenses are used as the situation requires. A 150-200 mm objective provides a working distance which is appropriate for hand surgery. This distance allows for easy clearance of the surgeon's hands and the instruments underneath the operating scope. When the surgical field is located deeper in the body, additional working distance can be provided by a 300 mm objective lens.

The binocular assembly provides the base of magnification. The oculars consist of a series of lenses which provide a specific degree of magnification.

The oculars can be changed to increase or decrease the fixed base of magnification. The eyepieces most commonly used in microvascular surgery magnify 12.5X. The two eyepieces are arranged with parallel, rather than convergent, optics to permit accurate judgment of the depth of the operative field.

Most modern operating microscopes are equipped with a foot pedal-activated zoom magnification changer. This motorized unit changes the distance between two lenses, rendering a continuously variable range of magnification from 4.0X to 31X, depending on the particular microscope.

The power of magnification describes the dimensions of the area visualized, not the dimensions of a specific object within the visual field. There is not a linear relationship between the power of magnification and the increased size of the object. For instance, a 10X magnification renders a threefold enlargement, while a 40X magnification increases the size of the object about 14 times.

There is an inverse relationship between the power of magnification and the size of the visual field. With greater magnification, the size and depth of the operative field are diminished. The zoom mechanism allows the surgeon to adjust the power of magnification and the size of the visual field as the operative situation dictates.

Most modern operating microscopes are equipped with accessories that permit the surgeon to work without taking his eyes from the field. In addition to the foot-activated zoom mechanism, there is a foot-activated automatic focus switch and a switch that makes the microscope move in the vertical or horizontal axis. This permits the surgeon to change his field of vision without touching the microscope.

Most operating microscopes can be equipped with 35 mm still and video cameras. These permit the surgeon to make teaching records and allow other personnel in the surgical suite to follow the progress of the operation. Modern microsurgery is a team effort, and most operating microscopes are equipped with binocular stereoscopic assemblies for use by the assistant.

An effective assistant can significantly facilitate a microsurgical operation. The assistant can irrigate the field, greatly improving the surgeon's view of the anastomotic site. The assistant can hold the vessels together, expose the vessel lumen and even tie sutures, thus permitting the primary surgeon a moment of relaxation before placing the next stitch.

Instruments

Most microsurgical forceps are derived from jeweler's forceps. These delicate instruments have fine atraumatic tips to minimize tissue damage. Their shoulders are narrow to avoid obstruction of the operative field. The forceps can be lengthened so that they rest comfortably in the first web space between the surgeon's fingers. They are used for manipulating tissue and tying sutures.

The design of microsurgical needle holders is taken from the spring-loaded ophthalmic needle holder designed by Castroviejo. Most surgeons prefer a slightly curved tip on the needle holder to permit a better angle of approach to the tissues. Spring-loaded scissors of various sizes are essential for microdissection and for cutting sutures. Scissors with a serrated blade are particularly useful for cleanly transecting small nerves prior to anastomosis.

Hemostasis is critical to successful microsurgery. The standard unipolar electrocautery used for macrosurgery dissipates the electrical impulse through the surrounding tissues en route to a ground plate on the patient's skin. Unipolar coagulation of small branch vessels during a dissection could lead to electrical damage to the parent vessel that would compromise the success of a vascular anastomosis.

To circumvent this problem, the bipolar cautery is used in microsurgery. Electrodes are attached to the two mutually insulated arms of a jeweler's forceps. The electrical current passes from the active tip through the tissue to be coagulated and out the ground tip. Far less electrical damage is produced with the bipolar coagulator, and more precise coagulation is possible.

Hemostatic clamps and clamp approximators are commonly used in microsurgical procedures. Microclamps must be strong enough to occlude the vessel lumen during an anastomosis but must not cause damage to the vessel. It has been determined that closing pressures greater than 30 g per square mm cause endothelial damage that can result in subsequent thrombosis at the point of occlusion.

Most of the clamps used in neurosurgical procedures have excessive closing pressures. Ackland has developed flat, smooth-bladed clamps of various widths with closing pressures less than 30 g per square mm for use in microvascular procedures. The clamps can be mounted on a metal rod with an adjustable interclamp distance to create a clamp approximator. The vessel or nerve to be sutured is grasped in the clamps which are then moved together so the anastomosis can be performed without tension.

Irrigation solutions are indispensable in keeping the vascular lumen and operative field free of debris. A heparin-saline solution is used to irrigate the vascular lumen, to clean the tips of the micro instruments, and to irrigate the field. This solution decreases the "stickiness" of the operative field and prevents the sutures from adhering to the local tissue.

Vasodilators are used topically to prevent vasospasm of the vessels being anastomosed. A dilated vessel has better flow when the clamps are removed and is less likely to thrombose than a vessel in spasm with sluggish flow. Lidocaine or bupivacaine solutions are most frequently used to promote vasodilatation in microvascular surgery.

Suture

For many years, the absence of commercially available microsutures was the obstacle limiting the progress of microsurgery. In 1966, 10-0 (122μ) nylon suture swaged to a 139μ needle was made available. This permitted the successful anastomosis of vessels less than 1 mm in diameter.

The size of the needle in relation to the suture remained a problem; the passage of the needle left a large hole which could not be filled by the attached suture material. Further progress resulted in sharper, smaller diameter needles which leave less of a hole in the blood vessel wall. Currently 50 to 70μ curved needles and 10-0 suture are used for anastomosing vessels in the range of 1 mm. The body of the needle is round to avoid tearing the vessel wall.

Microvascular Technique

Successful end-to-end anastomosis of blood vessels in the 0.75-1.5 mm range is a mainstay of microvascular reconstructive surgery. Proficiency with this technique facilitates the digital replantations, free flap transfers and vasectomy reversals that are common today in major reconstructive centers.

The principles of a successful vascular anastomosis were described by Carrel in 1902. They are as follows:

- Clamps are applied to control bleeding.
- A segment of adventitia is resected.
- Three guide sutures are placed approximately 120° apart.
- The vessel is converted into an equilateral triangle by traction on two of the guide sutures, and coaptation sutures are placed.

Carrel received the Nobel Prize in 1915 for his work. Most of the steps he described are practiced today on a microscopic level.

The placement of three guide sutures 120° apart, called concentric triangulation, permits the surgeon to separately anastomose the three limbs of an equilateral triangle. The guide sutures serve as reference points for the anastomosis. Traction on them lifts the portion of the vessel being anastomosed away from the opposing blood vessel lumen. This prevents the potential catastrophe of catching the posterior wall in a suture and thus inadvertently suturing the lumen closed.

Usually 8-10 sutures are required to anastomose vessels in the 1-1.5 mm range. Meticulous attention to detail is essential because the first attempt at an anastomosis is usually the best. The vessel wall and lumen should be manipulated minimally to avoid damage.

The lumen is cannulated with the tips of a jeweler's forceps. The needle is passed full thickness through the vessel wall until it can be observed between the tip of the forceps. With this technique, the opposite wall is not caught in the suture. It is prudent not to attempt to catch both vessel ends in one pass.

The suture is pulled through slowly and care is taken not to cut through either lumen. The first knot is tied so that there is coaptation of the intima. Excess tension must be avoided. Square knots are used to complete the time and the suture is cut by the assistant.

Some surgeons wrap the arterial anastomosis with a vein cuff or piece of plastic. This supports the anastomosis when the clamps are removed and prevents blood leakage which might cause a reflex spasm in the vessels.

Following completion of the anastomosis, first the distal, then the proximal hemostatic clamp is removed. Back bleeding should easily cross the anastomosis when the distal clamp is released, demonstrating patency of the anastomosis. Patency can also be tested by performing the "strip test" on a segment of vessel distal to the anastomosis. Two jeweler's forceps are used in this procedure. One is applied upstream, occluding the vessel; the other is placed adjacent to it and is used to strip a 3 mm segment of vessel clear of blood. The proximal clamp is released. If the stripped segment fills with blood, the anastomosis is patent.

Replantation Surgery

The development of microsurgical technique has made possible the replantation of severed hands and digits. In replantation surgery, all the concepts of bone, nerve, tendon and vascular reconstruction come into play; however, one should not lose sight of the fact that retention of function remains the paramount goal. A stiff, successfully replanted digit without protective sensation is useless to the patient. It has been said that good function is not the most important thing in hand surgery: it is the only thing.

Successful replantation surgery can be accomplished most readily in a major clinical center where the patient has access not only to the microsurgical team but to appropriate rehabilitative services as well. The input of multiple specialty services is essential to a successful outcome.

Digital replantation is indicated in cases of amputation of multiple digits or the thumb. Replantation of single digit amputation is extremely controversial. However, it should be considered in the case of children, in certain occupations, or for aesthetic reasons. The isolated index finger should generally not be replaced because the hand can usually function better in its absence, utilizing a normal third finger.

Sharp guillotine amputations have the most favorable prognosis. Injuries with a moderate degree of crushing component also carry a good prognosis. Avulsion injuries sustained from blunt objects, such as lawn mowers and snow blowers, cannot as readily be replanted successfully because of the extensive tissue damage. Multiple level injury is a direct contraindication to replantation. Replantation should only be attempted on a patient in stable general condition after other serious injuries have been attended to.

All amputated parts should be recovered from the site of injury and sent with the patient to the replantation center. While an amputated part may not be suitable for replantation, sections of it can often be used for reconstruction of other damaged digits. The amputated parts should be cleaned of debris, wrapped in a saline-soaked gauze, and placed in a clean plastic bag. The bag should be sent to the replantation center in an ice bath in order to cool, but not freeze, the part. Partial amputations should also be cooled in an ice bath for transportation. Fingers have been successfully replanted up to 20 hours following amputation when properly cooled (Fig. 16-2).

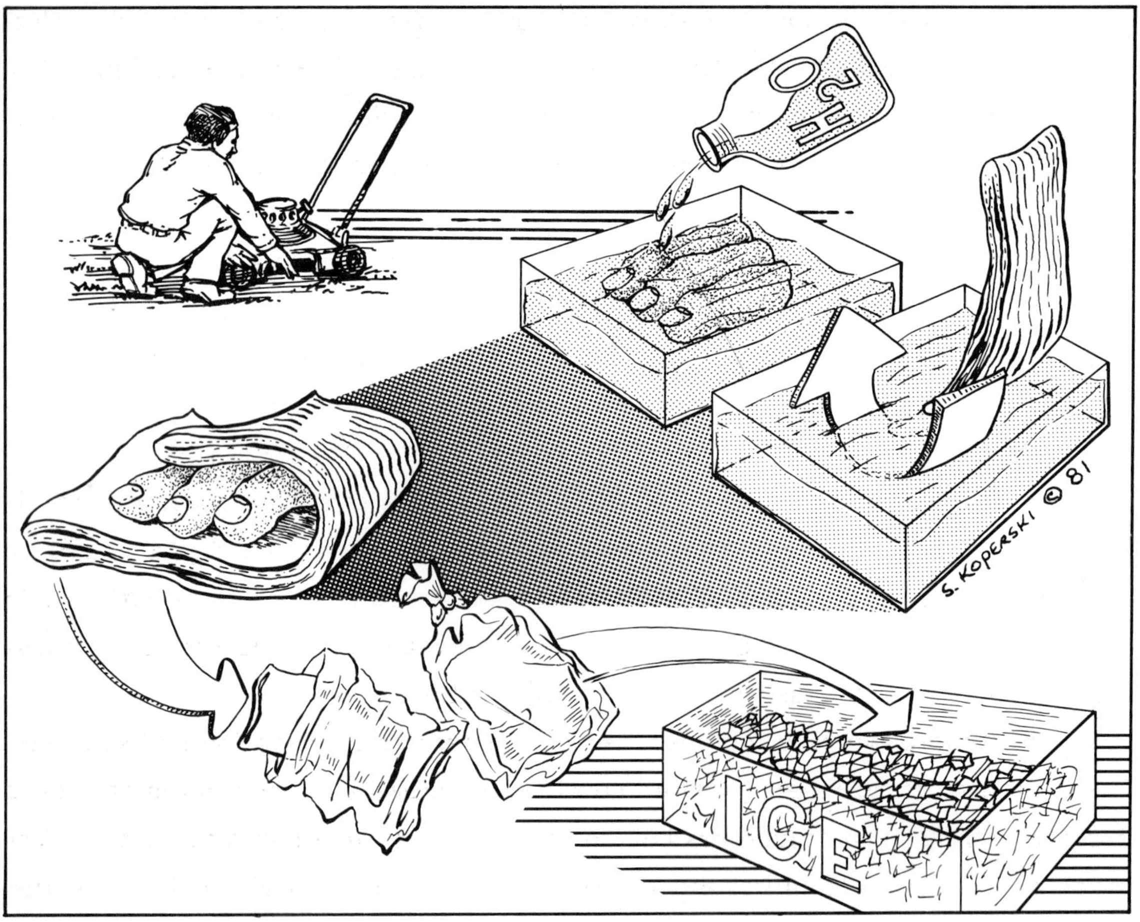

Figure 16-2. **Transport of amputated appendages.** When possible, amputated parts should be saved for possible replantation. They should be (clockwise from top right) washed in water or, preferably, sterile saline (if available), wrapped in a clean or sterile cloth, placed in a plastic bag and stored in ice, being delivered with the patient.

The stump is cleaned and placed in a sterile dressing. Bleeding should be controlled with pressure, and instrumentation of the stump should be avoided. The patient's general condition should be stabilized prior to transportation to a replantation center. Major amputations are a source of considerable blood loss, and this fluid must be replaced during transport.

At the replantation center, appropriate studies, including x-rays of the amputated part, should be obtained. The amputated part can be examined under the operating microscope and the structures labeled while the patient is being prepared for surgery. A second team can label the appropriate structures at the stump once the patient is asleep.

The order of repair of structures of the finger is controversial. Most authors agree that bone stabilization is the first step. This can be accomplished with K-wires or, better yet, with an intraosseous wiring technique. Following bony fixation, most surgeons repair the extensor and flexor tendons prior to anastomosis of the vascular structures.

The anastomosis should only be performed on healthy-appearing vessels. The proximal stump should bleed readily when the clamp or tourniquet is removed. Vein grafts should be used so that the anastomosis is performed under no tension. When possible, both digital arteries and one dorsal vein should be repaired.

Following revascularization, the digital nerves should be anastomosed. It is of paramount importance that a good primary repair of the digital nerve be effected whenever possible. Repair of digital nerves is much more difficult in subsequent operations because of scar tissue formation. A successful replantation without protective sensation is of no use to the patient.

Postoperative care includes the usual measures of elevation and splinting. Great care must be taken to avoid constrictive dressings. Heparin is employed postoperatively in some centers but can result in considerable blood loss. Most centers use low molecular weight dextran, aspirin and dipyridamole to reduce platelet adhesiveness and fibrinogen activity.

After 7 to 10 days, the revascularization of the finger should be secure. If intraosseous wiring has been used, mobilization of the finger can begin at that time. While it is rare that the full range of motion is recovered following replantation, a subsequent tenolysis can significantly improve the situation.

Microvascular surgery has vastly broadened the scope of reconstructive surgery. Patients who have sustained amputation of digits, extremities, genitalia or scalp now have a reasonable hope of successful replantation. With conventional methods, they could harbor no such expectation.

Microvascular surgery has permitted the detachment and transfer of island flaps as free flaps to reconstruct a variety of defects. Most commonly the groin flap or latissimus dorsi flap is used to reconstruct soft tissue defects. Free flaps are most useful in the distal third of the leg. In this area, conventional techniques are difficult to apply and are generally not reliable.

Successful microvascular surgery has raised the possibility of transferring all varieties of tissue. Already ribs and fibular bone grafts have been transferred with microvascular techniques to reconstruct the mandible and extremities. The omentum has been transferred to provide a bed for skin grafting. The great toe, complete with its neural and motor attachments, has been used successfully to replace an amputated thumb. Jejunum has been employed to reconstruct the esophagus. Future microsurgeons will undoubtedly discover new applications and improved reconstructive techniques in this continually expanding subspecialty.

Index

Reading List

Converse, J.M. (ed.): *Reconstructive Plastic Surgery*, W.B. Saunders Co., Philadelphia, 1977.

Daniel, R.K., and Terzis, J.K.: *Reconstructive Microsurgery.* Little, Brown & Co., Boston, 1977.

Gillies, H., and Millard, D.R.: *The Principles and Art of Plastic Surgery.* Little, Brown & Co., Boston, 1957.

Goldwyn, R.M.: *The Unfavorable Result in Plastic Surgery.* Little, Brown & Co., Boston, 1972.

Goldwyn, R.M.: *Long Term Results in Plastic and Reconstructive Surgery.* Little, Brown & Co., Boston, 1980.

Grabb, W.E., and Smith, J.W. (eds.): *Plastic Surgery*, ed. 3. Little, Brown & Co., Boston, 1978.

Grabb, W.E., Rosenstein, S.W., and Bzoch, K.R.: *Cleft Lip and Palate.* Little, Brown & Co., Boston, 1972.

Mathies, S.J., and Nahai, F.: *Clinical Atlas of Muscle and Musculocutaneous Flaps.* C.V. Mosby Co., St. Louis, 1979.

McDowell, F.: *The Source Book of Plastic Surgery.* The Williams & Wilkins Co., Baltimore, 1977.

McDowell, F.: *Series of Plastic Surgery Indexes*, vols. I-V. The Williams & Wilkins Co., Baltimore, 1977.

Rees, T.: *Aesthetic Plastic Surgery.* W.B. Saunders Co., Philadelphia, 1980.